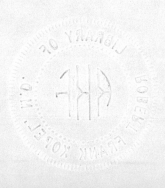

Critical Care
State of the Art

Edited By

T. JAMES GALLAGHER, MD

Professor of Anesthesiology and Surgery
Chief, Division of Critical Care Medicine
University of Florida College of Medicine
Gainesville, Florida

WILLIAM C. SHOEMAKER, MD

Professor of Surgery
University of California, Los Angeles
Los Angeles, California

THE SOCIETY OF CRITICAL CARE MEDICINE
VOLUME 9   1988

Printed in the United States of America.

The Society of Critical Care Medicine
251 East Imperial Highway, Suite 480
Fullerton, California 92635

First Printing, March, 1988

Library of Congress Catalogue Number:
LOCC #80-644205

International Standard Book Number:
ISBN #0-936145-11-0

Standard Address Number:
SAN #275-5505;3

Contributing Authors

NANCY L. ASCHER, MD, PhD
Associate Professor of Surgery, University of Minnesota, Minneapolis, Minnesota

ERIC S. BERENS, MD
Surgical Fellow, Department of Surgery, Washington University School of Medicine, St. Louis, Missouri

ROBERT S. BONSER, MB, BCh, MRCP(UK), FRCS(Eng)
Medical Fellow, Department of Surgery, University of Minnesota, Minneapolis, Minnesota; Senior Registrar, National Heart and Chest Hospital, London, United Kingdom

MICHAEL CALDWELL, MD
Associate Professor of Surgery, Department of Surgery, Rhode Island Hospital, Providence, Rhode Island

FRANK B. CERRA, MD
Professor of Surgery, Department of Surgery, University of Minnesota Medical School, Minneapolis, Minnesota

NICOLAS V. CHRISTOU, MD, PhD, FRCS(C), FACS
Associate Professor of Surgery, Departments of Surgery, Microbiology, and Immunology, McGill University, Montreal, Quebec, Canada

JOSEPH M. CIVETTA, MD
Professor of Surgery, Division of Surgical Intensive Care, Department of Surgery, University of Miami School of Medicine, Miami, Florida

MARILYN R. CLEAVINGER, MSBME
Artificial Heart Program, University Medical Center, Tucson, Arizona

JACK G. COPELAND, III, MD
Professor and Chief, Department of Cardiovascular and Thoracic Surgery, Arizona Health Sciences Center, Tucson, Arizona

RONALD FERGUSON, MD
Director, Division of Transplantation, Ohio State University, Columbus, Ohio

LAZAR J. GREENFIELD, MD
Professor and Chairman, Department of Surgery, University of Michigan Medical Center, Ann Arbor, Michigan

BARTLEY GRIFFITH, MD
Associate Professor of Surgery, Department of Surgery, University of Pittsburgh School of Medicine, Pittsburgh, Pennsylvania

DOUGLAS W. HANTO, MD, PhD
Assistant Professor of Surgery, Department of Surgery, Washington University School of Medicine, St. Louis, Missouri

JAMES R. JACOBS, PhD
Assistant Medical Research Professor, Department of Anesthesiology, Duke University Medical Center, Durham, North Carolina

STUART W. JAMIESON, MB, BS, FRCS(Eng)
Professor of Cardiovascular and Thoracic Surgery, Minnesota Heart and Lung Institute, Minneapolis, Minnesota

PHILIP D. LUMB, MB, BS
Associate Professor of Anesthesiology and Surgery, Department of Anesthesiology, Duke University Medical Center, Durham, North Carolina

JOHN S. NAJARIAN, MD
Jay Phillips' Professor and Chairman of the Department of Surgery, University of Minnesota, Minneapolis, Minnesota

GUIDO O. PEREZ, MD
Professor of Medicine, University of Miami School of Medicine; Director, Dialysis Unit, Veterans Administration Medical Center, Miami, Florida

ROBERT H. POSTERARO, MD
Associate Professor, Department of Radiology, Texas Tech University School of Medicine, Lubbock, Texas; Fellow in Magnetic Resonance Imaging, Duke University Medical Center, Durham, North Carolina

CARL E. RAVIN, MD
Professor and Chairman, Department of Radiology, Duke University Medical Center, Durham, North Carolina

MARC I. ROWE, MD
Professor of Surgery, University of Pittsburgh School of Medicine; Chief of Surgical Services, Children's Hospital of Pittsburgh, Pittsburgh, Pennsylvania

EUGENE R. SCHIFF, MD
Professor of Medicine, Chief, Division of Hepatology, University of Miami School of Medicine; Chief, Hepatology Section, Veteran's Administration Medical Center, Miami, Florida

MARK W. SHELTON, MD
Surgical Fellow, Department of Surgery, Washington University School of Medicine, St. Louis, Missouri

RICHARD G. SMITH, MSEE, CCE
Artificial Heart Program, University Medical Center, Tucson, Arizona

SAMUEL D. SMITH, MD
Critical Care Fellow in Pediatric Surgery, Children's Hospital of Pittsburgh, University of Pittsburgh School of Medicine, Pittsburgh, Pennsylvania

PETER G. STOCK, MD
Medical Fellow, Department of Surgery, University of Minnesota, Minneapolis, Minnesota

RIYAD Y. TARAZI, MD
Medical Fellow, Deparment of Surgery, University of Minnesota, Minneapolis, Minnesota.

THOMAS R. J. TODD, MD, FRCS(C)
Acting Head, Division of Surgery, Associate Professor, Division of Thoracic Surgery, Toronto General Hospital, University of Toronto, Toronto, Ontario, Canada

ALAN S. TONNESEN, MD
Associate Professor, Department of Anesthesiology, University of Texas Health Science Center, Houston, Texas

W. DAVID WATKINS, MD, PhD
Professor and Chairman, Department of Anesthesiology, Professor of Pharmacology, Duke University Medical Center, Durham, North Carolina

THOMAS L. WHITSETT, MD, FACP
Professor of Medicine and Pharmacology, Cardiovascular Division, University of Oklahoma Health Sciences Center, Oklahoma City, Oklahoma

Preface

This book is the ninth volume to be published as a supplement for the registrants of the Society of Critical Care Medicine's Annual Educational and Scientific Symposium, and contains the invited plenary lectures in extended form for the 1988 meeting. The chapters review the three main subject areas of this year's symposium — a) Multiple Organ Failure, b) Transplantation, and c) Critical Care Technology. The contributors to this volume of *Critical Care: State of the Art* are experts in their disciplines; we hope that you, the reader, will appreciate the timely and thorough discussions about these subject areas.

These volumes have evolved from soft-cover syllabi into free-standing hard-cover publications of potential interest to the vast majority of critical care practitioners. A unique feature of *Critical Care: State of the Art* is the limited lag time between the dates of manuscript submission and publication, thus providing the reader with the most current information.

As in previous editions, this year's volume was organized, assembled, and produced by Betty Stevenson and René Arché with the support of the SCCM crew. It is timely and fitting that the Society continues to sponsor and publish the latest information, methods, and concepts which will enlarge our understanding of the rapidly expanding field of critical care medicine.

T. James Gallagher, MD
William C. Shoemaker, MD

Table of Contents

Volume Nine

Chapter 1

The Evolution of Solid Organ Transplantation

Ronald M. Ferguson, MD, PhD

Outline

Educational Objectives

In this chapter the reader will learn:

1. to appreciate the historical development of solid organ transplantation.

2. to understand the role of government regulation and reimbursement in kidney, heart, and liver transplantation.

3. that the future problems in transplantation relate to the availability of donor organs and how government regulates their distribution.

> Man does not burst like a bubble — he falls apart piece by piece. Clinical transplantation must replace exhausted parts as they fall (1).

The current state of the art in solid organ transplantation represents the realization of ancient dreams and myths and is the result of the scientific evolution of thought concerning somatic cellular genetics, immunobiology, and clinical surgery. Over the past 75 years, the marriage of these disparate disciplines has been necessitated by the importance each has upon the other in realizing the goals of successful transplantation of human organs. Other chapters in this text address the specific medical and technical advances that have been made, many very recently, in the field for each transplantable organ. This chapter provides an overview of the field of solid organ transplantation that gives an historical perspective to this new and rapidly emerging field of surgery, and defines problematic areas for the future as transplantation grows and extends. The historical perspective deals with scientific discovery and the application of these discoveries to clinical transplantation. The discussion of future considerations is focused primarily on the role of transplantation in society, with particular emphasis on governmental regulation.

1

An Historical Perspective

The Mythical Period

The expression of human yearnings for longevity and immortality are fantasies that have been preserved in the writings and art of both early Eastern and Western cultures. The most famous is the Greek Chimera, a fabulous monster having a lion's head, a goat's body, and a serpent's tail. This mythical monster has come to represent a successful transplant of foreign tissue. Indeed, the colophon of the American Society of Transplant Surgeons has as its central focus the mythical chimeric monster. The oldest records of the idea of transplanting organs stems from the ancient Chinese medical literature. In the second century BC, Pien Ch'iao is reported to have been able to painlessly operate and successfully exchanged the hearts of two patients. Hua T'o, whose writings were known around AD 190, was also said to have "Transplanted many tissues and organs including the heart" (2). In the West there is the classical legend of the saints Cosmos and Damian. They are the patron saints of medicine who lived in the third century BC and flourished under Diocletian. Legend has it that when approached by a patient who had undergone amputation, but still had a great desire to walk, Cosmos and Damian successfully transplanted the leg of a Moor who had recently died. This famous legend became a favorite subject of subsequent medieval artists and was frequently painted (3). Despite the questionable accuracy of these stories, the fact remains that the transplantation of organs was a dream and a fantasy of even the ancients.

Experimental Transplantation

The modern era of experimental transplantation began with John Hunter (1728-1793). Hunter was interested in the development, growth, and natural history of teeth. As an application of this interest he had "successfully" replaced a premolar of a man who had, only hours before, had this tooth knocked out. This led to a series of experiments on transplanting teeth into the highly vascularized comb of a cock. These experiments had a significant influence on Brown-Sequard (1817-1894), who extended Hunter's observation by successfully transplanting the tails of rodents and cats into a cock's comb. The theoretical basis for such transplantations derived from the Huntarian concept that successful transplantation is "founded on the disposition of all living substances to unite when brought into contact with one another" (4). In extending his experience in experimental transplantation, Brown-Sequard brought upon the field its first public and professional scandal. In an attempt to rejuvenate old male dogs, testes from young guinea pigs were transplanted into these unbemused recipients. Brown-Sequard was so encouraged by these early results that similar experiments were performed in humans. As has been its history, the drama and fantastic expectation of transplantation were out of proportion to the practical reality or scientific understanding of the time. Others "commercialized" the concept and an unfortunately large number of human "sex gland transplants" were performed by a rather large number of individuals whose spirit and intent was far more a business venture than a medical curiosity. The reality of failure led to ridicule and widespread charges of false claims by the medical profession (5).

By the turn of the century, the concepts which Hunter had formulated about transplantation were clearly present at a time of scientific revolution in experimental and clinical medicine. The approximation of vascular beds of two organs had been performed with the Huntarian approach of opposing the transplanted organ into the highly vascularized bed of a cock's comb or by parabiosis, a technique developed by Bert (who was heavily influenced by Brown-Sequard's work) (6).

Alexis Carrel began to pursue the technical problem of a vascular anastomosis at the University of Lyon in France at the turn of the century. In 1905 he came to Chicago to work with the physiologist, Charles Claude Guthrie. In a series of publications between 1905 and 1910 (7, 8), the technical details of a "uniformly successful vascular anastomosis" were published. These included an extraordinary series on transplantations of the heart, kidney, ovaries, thyroid, and parathyroid glands. These two exceptional investigators parted ways, and in 1912 Charles Guthrie's scholarly book, *Blood Vessel Surgery*, was published (9). In that same year, Alexis Carrel was awarded the Nobel prize "in recognition of this work on vascular suture and the transplantation of blood vessels and organs."

The early transplantation experiments were successful only in the short term, i.e., hours to days of survival. The concept of histocompatibility and genetically determined biologic individuality within a species at that time was only beginning to be appreciated. The work in 1900 of Landsteiner and Miller (10) laid the basis for blood group testing in vitro by recognizing isoagglutination and relating this to transfusion practice. In the 1920s it became commonplace to ascribe failure of immediately vascularized experimental allografts to blood group differences, and the concept of blood groups as determinants of individual constitution within a species was promulgated (11). Of course, this was far too simple a view, and in the 1930s the stimulus and application of genetic theory led to the understanding that tissue differences within a species played a more significant role in the expression of inherited biologic individualism than blood group specificities.

A critical intermediary in this evolution of thought of transplantation biology and somatic genetics was provided in the 1930s by Peter Gorer. In 1937 Gorer identified the first histocompatibility antigen and related this to the rejection of tumor allografts (12). Subsequent work led Gorer in 1938 to unequivocally say that genetically determined factors "present in the grafted tissue and absent in the host are capable of eliciting a response which results in the destruction of the graft" (13). Although Carrel, as early as 1908, had recognized that influences other than technical factors were responsible for his first graft failures (14), it was not until the work of Gorer that a rational biologic basis of understanding was put forth. This provided the first link in the necessary marriage of the disciplines of surgery and somatic cellular genetics that would ultimately develop and evolve into clinical transplantation. It also laid the scientific foundation for the subsequent studies of Sir Peter Medawar (15).

History has shown us that the necessities of war can mold the direction of medical thought. Such was the case in 1943 when the War Wounds Committee of the British Research Council approached Peter Medawar with a proposition of applying current thoughts on transplantation biology to skin allografting therapy of burn victims resulting from the bombings of Britain. In an elegantly simple series of experiments in rabbits, Medawar clearly demonstrated that skin allografting displayed the three fundamental characteristics of an immune response: a) the recognition of nonself, b) antigenic specificity, and c) specific memory. The histologic picture of progressive cellular infiltration, the destruction of the graft, and the adoptive transfer of specific immunity by cells from grafted recipients, but not serum, all provided the necessary systematization of a conceptual paradigm whereby tissue-specific antigens that define genetically determined biologic individuality are recognized as nonself, and antigen-specific cellular-mediated immune responses are elicited that have the capability to destroy any tissue bearing the sensitizing antigen. The groundwork had been laid and scientific understanding was sufficient for clinical application in humans.

A Clinical Introduction — The Early Days

Between 1906 and 1930, several attempts at human transplantation were made. In 1906 Jaboulay (16) placed the kidneys of a goat and a sheep into the extremities of two patients. Unger, during this same time period, attempted the transplantation of a monkey kidney into a young girl with acute renal failure (17). In 1933, the first human-to-human kidney transplant was performed by the Russian surgeon, Voronoy (18). An accident victim had suffered a severe head injury and served as the donor. Voronoy performed six human-to-human kidney transplants between 1933 and 1949; none were successful. In 1946, Hume and Huffnagle became the first to succeed by providing a human kidney placed in the upper extremity vessels of a patient with acute renal failure. The kidney functioned long enough to allow recovery of the patient's native renal function after acute renal failure (19); she eventually fully recovered. In the few years that followed, the Boston and Paris groups each performed a series of allografted kidneys in humans without any immunosuppression (20, 21). One patient maintained life-sustaining renal function for several months prior to rejecting the graft. All others failed.

Additionally, the feasibility of the concept of organ replacement therapy in humans had been clearly established by the Boston group in 1954. In a daring experiment, a team headed by John Merrill and Joseph Murray transplanted a kidney from an identical twin to his brother, who was suffering from chronic renal failure. The kidney functioned normally and rejection was not observed. The problem of solid organ transplantation was clearly defined. The lesson was simple — overcome the immunogenetic barrier and transplantation would be successful. As the work of Medawar and Gorer had predicted earlier, recognition of the graft and its immunologic destruction proved to be a formidable obstacle to successful nonidentical twin transplantation.

The first attempts to abort the host immune response again emanated from Boston and Paris (22). Beginning in 1958, a series of patients was treated with whole-body x-irradiation prior to transplantation. There was some modest success, but the immunosuppressive therapy was harsh and associated with severe toxicity leading to excessive morbidity and mortality. This coupled with the lack of long-standing immunosuppression caused these investigators to question its long-term utility. By 1959, despite the lack of success of x-irradiation, anticipation was high and the expectation of realizing the ancient dream of clinical organ replacement therapy in man must have been intense. The laboratory experience had defined the immunologic nature of the problem, and the clinical success of the identical-twin transplant had demonstrated the technical feasibility. The time was ripe for new discovery.

Dr. Robert Schwartz, working in Boston, provided the next conceptual breakthrough that laid the foundation for pharmacologic immunosuppression. In

1959, Schwartz and Dameshek (23) reported that the antimetabolite 6-mercaptopurine (6-MP) could block the formation of antibody to xenogeneic protein. The importance of this observation was immediately apparent to Mr. Roy Calne, then a young surgical investigator in London. Calne and Zukowski began a new era of clinical transplantation by demonstrating the effectiveness of 6-MP and later the derivative "BW-322" or azathioprine. In the canine renal transplant model, long-term survivors were achieved with functioning grafts and little or no cellular infiltrate on biopsy. Within 18 months, the experimental success in dogs was translated into man, and in 1962, the first successful patients were transplanted in Boston, Denver, and Paris utilizing only azathioprine as immunosuppression (24). Shortly thereafter, the effect of corticosteroids on the reversal of acute rejection episodes in man was described by Goodwin et al. (25), and the now-classical approach of prophylactic azathioprine and corticosteroids to prevent, rather than treat, rejection was provided by Starzl et al (26).

It is difficult to overemphasize the importance of the work done in the early 1960s. The demonstration that pharmacologic immunosuppression could prevent and treat the immunologic attack on an allograft and lead to a successful transplantation provided the necessary link to realize the expectations of this therapy. The remainder of the 1960s provides an excellent example of progress realized by the close working relationship between two very different disciplines, surgery and immunology. The surgeons needed a greater understanding of the pathophysiology of rejection in order to prescribe more effective therapies. The immunogeneticist saw real clinical application of his basic research efforts. The discipline of transplantation took on new breadth and depth. The discovery by Dusset in Paris of the HLA locus in man (27) and the technical developments by Paul Terasaki (28) in applying microlymphocytotoxicity testing to HLA typing and cross matching for transplantation are two very important examples of this time period. Kidney transplantation had become feasible for treating patients with end-stage renal disease. At this same time, hemodialysis was emerging as an alternate to transplantation in treating patients with end-stage renal failure. The two therapies were viewed as complementary, dialysis being performed until transplantation could be undertaken.

The Veteran's Administration (VA) was the first governmental institution to see the need for an organized delivery system for end-stage renal disease services. In 1963, the VA embarked on a program that by the end of the decade had established over 40 dialysis centers and over a dozen kidney transplant centers serving approximately 1,000 VA beneficiaries, and performing between 150 and 200 kidney transplants yearly. During the first half of the 1960s, most of this country's transplantation activity was centered within the VA system (29). The VA was uniquely qualified because of its nationally networked system of health care to veterans and provision of a regionalized program for the treatment of end-stage renal failure. Thus, in the 1960s, the VA system became the prime mover in the care of the end-stage renal disease patient for two simple reasons: first, it had the network to organize a system of service delivery, and second, it financed the organization, thereby making dialysis and transplantation reimbursable. This was to dramatically change in 1972.

There were other notable firsts in the 1960s. Starzl et al. (30) performed the first orthotopic liver transplantation and established the only successful liver transplant program in the United States. In addition, and based on the pioneering work of Shumway, Barnard (31) performed the first cardiac allograft in man in South Africa in 1967. This was followed by a flurry of activity. Over 100 cardiac transplants were performed in 1968 and nearly twice that number in 1969. The number of centers performing cardiac transplants grew precipitously during that 18-month period. Unfortunately, the clinical expertise in diagnosing and treating rejection and the use of immunosuppressive drugs was not sufficiently developed to allow long-term success. By the end of 1969, the average 3-month survival following heart transplantation was a dismal 17%. Shumway's group at Stanford was the only center persisting; systematically going from the dog lab to the clinic, Shumway described rejection as an electrocardiographic and histologic diagnosis confirmed by heart biopsy and pioneered new immunosuppressive protocols for cardiac transplantation. Gradually, by the late 1970s the Stanford group had nearly single-handedly led cardiac transplantation into the realm of a respectable therapy with credible long-term survival (32).

Clinical Acceptance — Transplantation and Medicare

The 1970s were replete with significant clinical contributions and gradual growth of transplantation. Kidney transplants remained the focus of this time frame with cardiac, hepatic, and pancreatic transplantation remaining limited to only a few centers and with results that lagged considerably behind those obtainable with the kidney. The focus on renal transplantation was multifactorial. The pool of potential recipients was concentrated within a pool of dialysis patients. The surgical techniques for transplanting the kidney were less technically demanding than those for the liver. Techniques allowed for up to 72 h of preservation for kidneys, but only very short-term preservation of a few hours for hearts and livers. In addition, there was a larger cadaveric donor pool for kidneys than for either the heart or the liver.

While all these factors are certainly true and contributed to the focus on kidney transplantation, perhaps the most significant factor that focused attention on renal transplant was the simple fact that they were not considered experimental. They were, therefore, reimbursable under Medicare's new End-Stage Renal Disease Program (ESRD). The origins of the ESRD derived from the developments during the 1960s in renal transplantation and dialysis, the government's response to these life-giving therapies, and the ethical and social issues accompanying the emergence of such technology. In 1964, Congress, through the NIH, established a program of transplantation immunology within the National Institute of Allergy and Immunology in response to the recent advances in immunosuppressive therapy and the expectations for clinical application in transplantation. The intent was to stimulate and support research in understanding and application of renal transplantation. The VA program for renal failure had begun a year earlier and was a leading force in delivering renal transplant services in the mid-1960s. In 1966, the Bureau of the Budget established a committee of experts to analyze the implications to the Federal government of the availability of dialysis and renal transplantation. The recommendations of that committee were to have far-reaching implications, for they recommended that a National Treatment Benefit Program be established that would entitle victims of end-stage renal disease under the Social Security Act (29). The committee report was released in the fall of 1967 and was widely read. In 1970 the reauthorization of the heart disease, stroke, and cancer funding included, for the first time, kidney disease as a target for federal support.

In late 1971 at the beginning of the 92nd Congress, the Nixon administration proposed sweeping changes in the Social Security Act. These changes primarily related to welfare reform. However, during hearings by the Ways and Means Committee of the House, a patient representing the National Association of Patients on Hemodialysis and Transplantation was hemodialyzed in the Hearing Room before members of the Committee. This exhibition apparently had an emotional impact on the Committee, for independent legislation, not part of what was subsequently to become HR-1, was introduced that would establish patient care financing for chronic renal disease. None of this proposed legislation in 1971 reached fruition. The End-Stage Renal Disease Program, however, became part of the legislative history and content of HR-1 in September, 1972. Following a protracted debate on welfare reform, Senator Vance Hartke (D-IN) prepared an amendment to HR-1 that would create a federally financed End-Stage Renal Disease Program within the Social Security Administration. The discussion on the Senate floor of the Hartke Amendment was brief, only 30 minutes in total, but significant in its content. Congress was, for the first time, to provide access to these new life-giving therapies of dialysis and transplantation despite the fact they were considered "expensive therapies." Senator Hartke said in discussion of the amendment:

> In what must be the most tragic irony of the 20th century, people are dying because they cannot get access to proper medical care. We have learned to treat or to cure some of the diseases which have plagued mankind for centuries, yet these treatments are not available to most Americans because of their cost . . . Mr. President, we can begin to set our national priorities straight by undertaking a national effort to bring kidney disease treatment within the reach of all those in need (33).

This same position was repeated by Senator Henry Jackson (D-WA):

> I think it is a great tragedy, in a nation as affluent as ours, that we have to consciously make a decision all over America as to the people who live and the people who will die. We have a committee in Seattle, when the first series of kidney machines were put in operation, who had to pass judgment on who would live and who would die. I believe we can do better than that . . . so I would hope that we would make an effort here, at least the beginning, to approve the amendment, so that we can do better than we have done heretofore (33).

After only 30 minutes of discussion, with no debate or any public hearings, the amendment was passed by the Senate and 2 weeks later adopted by the Joint Conference Committee of the House and Senate. The ESRD provision of the Hartke Amendment, Section 2991, became one small part of the larger and complex welfare reform bill, HR-1, which was signed into law by President Nixon in November, 1972.

Section 2991 provided for a major extension of Medicare coverage. Entitlement was extended to all those individuals who suffered from chronic renal failure and who require dialysis or transplantation to stay alive. Coverage also included their spouses and dependents. The government for the first time had embarked on a broad, Federally-funded health care program for a specific disease, and ensured access to therapy for all social security participants. By 1986, Medicare reimbursement to ESRD patients totalled over $2,260 million (Table 1).

Table 1. Medicare reimbursements by year for ESRD patients

	MEDICARE REIMBURSEMENT FOR ESRD PATIENTS PER YEAR (IN MILLIONS)*
1974	$ 184
1975	327
1976	481
1977	654
1978	835
1979	1,037
1980	1,268
1981	1,532
1982	1,661
1983	1,988
1984	1,994
1985	2,073
1986	2,260

*Includes transplant recipients who remain Medicare-eligible.

The original concepts of treatment of ESRD as articulated in the Bureau of Budgets Select Committee Report of 1967 viewed transplantation as the ultimate therapy for end-stage renal disease, with chronic dialysis as more a support therapy and "bridge" (in contemporary terms) to renal transplantation. This was not the result of the implementation process of the ESRD Program. In 1979 the Rand Corporation reviewed the first 5 years of the ESRD Program (29). Table 2 demonstrates the allocation of expenditures in the ESRD Program going to transplantation and to dialysis as therapies for treatment. With the implementation of the Medicare-funded ESRD Program, clinical treatment emphasis had shifted away from transplantation, as had been originally suggested, and the ESRD became predominantly a dialysis program. In 1974, 18% of the total ESRD funding went to transplantation with 82% to dialysis. By 1978 transplantation accounted for 9% of the total funding with 91% supporting dialysis. The reasons for the shift in treatment emphasis are complex and multifactorial. Also, opinions vary. To be sure, the supply of cadaveric kidneys was not sufficient to satisfy the demand with an increasing population of dialysis patients due to the new entitlement provisions of the ESRD Program. In addition, the enthusiastic expectations for renal transplantation prevalent in the late 1960s were not fully realized in the 1970s.

Table 2. Number of kidney transplants and kidney dialysis patients by year

YEAR	NUMBER OF KIDNEY TRANSPLANTS	NUMBER OF PATIENTS ON DIALYSIS
1963	163	
1964	239	
1965	305	300
1966	338	NK
1967	448	NK
1968	676	800
1969	838	1,000
1970	1,460	2,456
1971	2,909	3,482
1972	2,852	10,000
1973	3,017	11,000
1974	3,190	18,875
1975	3,730	22,000
1976	3,504	30,131
1977	3,973	32,435
1978	3,949	36,463
1979	4,189	45,565
1980	4,697	53,364
1981	4,883	58,770
1982	5,358	65,765
1983	6,112	71,987
1984	6,968	78,483
1985	7,695	84,797
1986	8,976	90,886

NK = not known.

Graft and patient survival throughout the 1970s showed gradual improvement, but enough caution was presented by the ESRD provider community to engender a "selectivity" of recipient selection, thereby limiting, by medical criteria, the number of patients referred to transplantation. This happened despite major advances in renal transplantation during the cyclosporine era later to come.

This trend toward selectivity based on medical criteria has persisted up to the present and has reflected in recent statistics from Health Care Financing

Administration. During 1986, 90,886 patients were being dialyzed in the ESRD Program. There were 8,976 renal transplantations performed in that year. At first look, this disparity between the number of patients transplanted vs. the number of patients on chronic dialysis appears to be solely a function of availability of donor kidneys for transplantation. This is not entirely the case; according to recipient registry information provided by UNOS (United Network for Organ Sharing), which lists all potential kidney recipients on all transplant waiting lists in the United States, only 10,986 patients were listed as of October, 1987. Less than 12% of the entire national dialysis pool was represented as awaiting a transplant, clearly implying that 88% of the dialysis population had undergone the process of selectivity and were considered not medically suitable for transplantation. Clearly, the implementation of the ESRD program had a dramatic impact on the practice patterns and therapeutic choices in treating end-stage renal disease. The role of transplantation in this therapy had been greatly influenced by the implementation of the ESRD Program.

The Cyclosporine Era — Foundation for Explosive Growth

The 1970s had seen steady progress in transplantation medicine and in the basic understanding of immune mechanisms underlying the rejection phenomenon. Immunosuppressive agents and protocols had changed little, but clinical experience in kidney transplantation had defined the unique clinical problems associated with immunosuppression, and thereby significantly reduced mortalities. Some of the most significant clinical contributions are listed in Table 3. With an improved understanding of the clinical subtleties, limitations, and occasionally bizarre side-effects of chronic immunosuppression (used in this unique setting to block in vivo alloreactivity), techniques were refined to the point that both long-term and short-term success rates for renal transplantation were encouraging and predictable.

Table 3. Advances in transplantation in the 1970s

Transfusion Effect

DR Typing

ALG Prophylaxis

ALG Rejection Therapy

Infectious Complications

- Better Diagnosis

- Improved Management

By 1980 most centers were reporting overall 1-yr graft survival rates for cadaveric transplantation of approximately 60%. For living donor transplants, this was considerably improved, with haplo-identical living donor renal transplants achieving 75% 1-yr graft survival and HLA identicals 85%. With cadaveric transplantation by the use of pretransplant blood transfusions, DR matching, and the use of anti-lymphocyte preparations for prophylaxis against rejection, it was clear that results in the 70% 1-yr range could be achieved for first cadaveric transplants. By 1980 renal transplantation was being done in approximately 140 centers performing about 4,200 transplantations yearly. This represented transplantation as therapy for only 9% of the total ESRD population. At this same time, heart and liver transplantation was considered experimental and limited. By 1980 there were only eight institutions performing approximately 80 heart transplantations in the United States during that year. The success rates were remarkably close to those achievable with renal transplants, i.e., 55% to 60% 1-yr patient and graft survival. In 1980 liver transplantation was not as successful as either cardiac or renal transplant. There were six centers performing about 50 hepatic transplants that year with an overall 1-yr survival rate of only approximately 35%.

In 1980, cyclosporine was introduced into the United States in selected centers for preclinical trials in renal, cardiac, and hepatic transplantation. Enthusiasm and promise were returned to the field of transplantation with the introduction of cyclosporine.

The early experience with cyclosporine in England and Europe had caused cautious optimism. In renal transplantation it had been clearly demonstrated that cyclosporine was a superior immunosuppressant in the preclinical trials. By the early 1980s, there had been dramatic increases in graft survival. For cadaveric renal transplant 1-yr graft survivals of 80% to 85% were expected, a 25% to 30% increase over that achievable in the late 1970s.

For cardiac transplantation, similar increases were reported. Eighty-three percent of the patients at Stanford were surviving at 1 yr when treated with a cyclosporine-based immunosuppressive protocol compared to 63% treated with conventional therapy, a significant 20% increase. For hepatic transplantation, the progress was even greater. At Pittsburgh, the 1-yr graft survival was over 70% when cyclosporine was used compared to only 35% with conventional therapy of historical controls transplanted in the late 1970s.

The remarkable feature about cyclosporine as a staple of immunosuppressive therapy was that not only were graft and patient survivals increased, but morbidity was decreased. The incidence of acute rejection episodes dramatically decreased in all organs, and the number and severity of infectious complications significantly decreased as well. This reduction in morbidity/mortality and increase in successful engraftment resulted in an overall reduction in the cost of all procedures and an increased public awareness and enthusiasm for transplantation as a viable therapeutic option. The introduction of cyclosporine was a major force in the advancement of transplantation medicine. With its efficacy proven, transplantation of multiple solid organs became not only an acceptable, but indeed a desirable program for many institutions that previously had been cautious and tentative about such a therapeutic approach to end-stage organ failure.

Rapid Growth — The Government Transplantation Interface

In the fall of 1983, cyclosporine was approved by the FDA for general use in solid organ transplantation. The general availability of cyclosporine and the attendant improved results accompanying its use in *all* organ transplants caused a veritable flurry of activity in the United States. A large number of centers began new transplantation programs primarily focused on cardiac transplantation. At this same time, the long-standing debate concerning reimbursement for heart and liver transplantation took a new turn. Both private and public insurers became positively inclined to cover hepatic and cardiac transplantation services. Considering heart and liver transplantation as reasonable therapy and not as experimental procedures implied several features of the health care financing industry. First, the insurers and payors of medical services were comfortable with the improved success rates. Second, there was sufficient evidence that the services were being delivered in a cost-effective enough manner to ensure some predictability of cost and benefit (outcome). This created a situation whereby the insurance industry was hard pressed to rationalize denying payment for either a heart or a liver transplant. By 1985, most private insurers paid for (treated as covered services) both heart and liver transplantation (Table 4).

Table 4. Insurance coverage for organ transplantation

	Commercial Insurer (%)	State Medicaid (%)
Kidney	97	96
Liver	80	66
Heart	85	80
Heart/Lung	69	26
Pancreas	57	6

With improved success rates and reimbursability established, the stage was set for expansion and growth in both the number of procedures performed and the number of providers. This did indeed prove to be the case. As depicted in Figures 1-3, the increase in centers and transplants performed has been explosive. The growth can be expressed a different way when one views calendar year 1986. In that year, 44% of all the heart transplants ever done in the United States were performed. Likewise, 43% of all liver transplants ever done were done in 1986. This rapid proliferation of centers and teams engaging in transplantation occurred at a unique time in the changing environment of health care delivery and reimbursement. Partly because of this unique timing, we are currently faced with a series of perplexing and complex issues regarding the delivery of transplantation services. There are, however, several other reasons.

Society has traditionally looked favorably upon the advancement of medical technology, and its relationship to transplantation has been for the most part a positive one. Yet, society has received mixed messages about transplantation that has created a certain public ambivalence. On the one hand, transplantation is perceived as life-giving therapy, surely something that deserves access to all in need. On the other hand, it is expensive, applicable to only a few, and is a medical therapy that necessitates the death of one human being for the life of another. It is this last point, the fact that only out of one family's personal tragedy can another receive the hope of continued life, that is at the core of the public ambivalence and perplexing complexity of contemporary transplantation. It is also this same issue of organ availability that in 1968 led the National

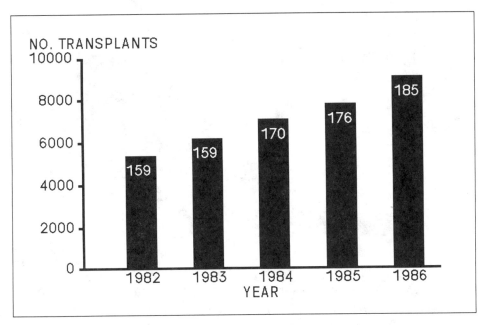

Fig. 1. Total number of kidney transplants performed in each yr (bar) and the total number of approved US transplant centers performing kidney transplants (number on bar).

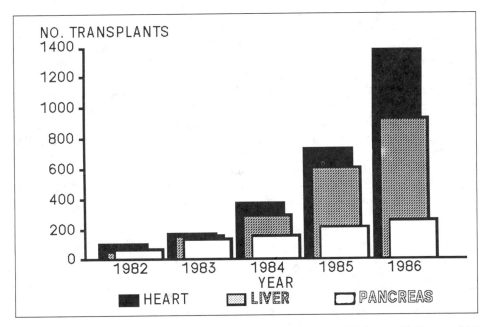

Fig. 2. Growth of nonrenal organ transplants each yr. In 1982, 103 heart, 62 liver, and 74 pancreas transplants were performed. In 1986, there were 1,368 heart, 924 liver, and 260 pancreas transplants performed.

13

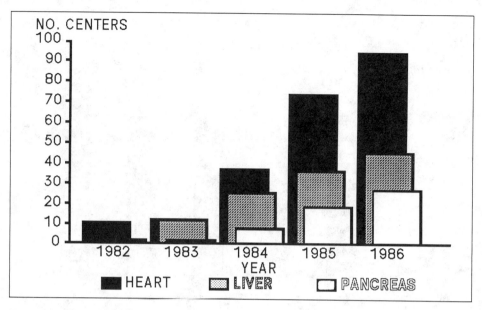

Fig. 3. Growth of nonrenal transplanting institutions by organ. For example, in 1982 there were ten heart transplant centers. By 1986 that number had risen to 94.

Conference on Commissions on Uniform State Laws to propose the Uniform Anatomical Gift Act (UAGA). The purpose of the UAGA was to regulate bodies after death in the interest of public health and safety and to dispel concern over potential liability for organ removal for transplantation. The UAGA was enacted by all states in 1973 and provides the underlying authority for all cadaveric organ retrieval in the United States. A further documentation of public ambivalence is provided by a national survey on public attitudes toward organ donation as reported in the National Heart Transplantation Study. While 93.7% of all respondents were aware of transplantation and organ donation, only 14% indicated they had signed an organ donor card. Those that had not signed a card were asked whether they were prepared to do so. Only 27.8% said yes while 53% were undecided. Clearly, there is an uncertain public sense about organ donation that will require a strong future effort in public education to ameliorate. The most frequently cited reasons for hesitancy toward organ donation are three: first, a denial of death, second, a fear of premature termination of care, and lastly, personal beliefs that contradict organ donation. In the past the public educational efforts of organ procurement agencies have traditionally centered on the need for organs and the benefits of donation and do not directly address the source of public ambivalence. If effective progress is to be made in decreasing the donor supply, those issues central to the "public ambivalence" must be directly addressed.

The issue of organ donation is a crucially important one for, as has been implied, it is the central focus of the majority of controversy in contemporary transplantation. Four key examples provide evidence of this and also demonstrate the national response. The issues are: a) equitable and publicly stated policies concerning allocation of organs, b) assurance of equal access to therapy for all those in need, c) lack of adequate supply of donor organs to meet the recipient demand, and d) competition between transplanting institutions.

The issue of organ allocation became highly visible and politicized in the early 1980s. Individual patients and institutions creatively explored forums and means by which to secure donor organs. One example of this utilized the national electronic and print media to make public pleas for individual cases. Another example used congressional representatives, senators, or governors to make public and political pleas in an attempt to use political channels to secure donor organs for individuals. The White House created a special office to facilitate individual efforts to secure donor organs. While these overtures were initiated for well meaning and altruistic motives, the end result was a process that favored those that could get to the media or politicians first! This created a great inequity in access to transplantation services among patients, and led to a heightened public interest in the entire field of transplantation. With increasing success in transplantation and numbers of patients undergoing the procedures, in particular heart and liver transplants, the question of patient access and organ allocation became a political rather than a medical issue. The political solution was a series of public hearings and eventually the passage in 1984 of the National Organ Transplant Act (P.L. 98-507). The act contained four major provisions. First, it prohibited the purchase and sale of organs for profit. Second, it provided for grants to organ procurement organizations directed at streamlining efficiency and increasing organ procurement activities. Third, it mandated the creation of a national organ procurement and transplantation network. Fourth, it established a 25-member National Task Force of Organ Transplantation. The Task Force was convened in February of 1985 and consisted of members representing a diversity of expertise and interest. The fields of medicine, law, theology, ethics, allied health, and health insurance, in addition to various government agencies, were all represented. The Task Force held eight public sessions and two public hearings prior to the publication in April, 1986 of their report and recommendations. Of the 60 recommendations put forth by the Task Force, nearly two-thirds dealt specifically with organ donation, organ procurement, or organ distribution. An additional 15 recommendations dealt specifically with patient access and its insurability.

Congress seriously read the Task Force recommendations; as a result, the Consolidated Omnibus Budget Reconciliation Act of 1988 (COBRA) contained two sections pertinent to organ transplantation. First, the Senate recommended to the Secretary that Medicare should reimburse patients for liver transplants performed that were reasonable and medically necessary. This section was merely a directive and was not binding on the Secretary. Secondly, COBRA required states to provide written standards regarding Medicaid coverage of organ transplants that would promote equal access to such services. If a state failed to provide such standards, it would be denied Medicaid payments for organ transplants.

In 1986, Congress incorporated many more of the Task Force recommendations into the Omnibus Budget Reconciliation Act of 1986 (OBRA). The intent of this legislation was to improve opportunities for obtaining organs. To add teeth to the organ procurement legislation, Congress tied three major procurement provisions to Medicare/Medicaid funding. First, as a condition for participation in Medicaid or Medicare programs, hospitals would have to establish written protocols to identify potential organ donors, make families aware of this option, and notify organ procurement agencies of these potential donors. If organ transplants were performed in the hospital, such a hospital had an additional requirement of being a member of the organ procurement and transplantation network established by the National Organ Transplant Act of 1984. The second procurement provision tied Medicare and Medicaid funding to organ procurement organizations (OPO). There were specific statutory requirements that must be met by an OPO to receive such funding. One example of such a requirement is that the OPO must be a member and abide by the policies of the Organ Procurement and Transplantation Network. The third major procurement provision of OBRA authorized Medicare reimbursement for kidney transplantation and procurement only if the procedure was performed in facilities that met prescribed federal regulations and were members of the Organ Procurement and Transplantation Network. In an attempt to implement the Task Force's recommendation concerning organ procurement, the Federal government had linked Medicare and Medicaid reimbursement to specific provisions that in essence created a national required request program applicable to all Medicare-participating hospitals in the United States. In addition, membership in the National Organ Procurement and Transplantation Network was also linked to Medicare reimbursement for all organ procurement organizations and hospitals performing transplantation procedures.

In an attempt to oversee and improve the quality of transplantation and organ procurement services in the United States, Congress had mandated the creation of a National Organ Procurement and Transplantation Network (OPTN). The Health Care Financing Administration had issued a request for applications for organizations that would qualify, and in the fall of 1987 a 3-yr contract was issued to the United Network for Organ Sharing (UNOS). As per the contract at OPTN, UNOS had in effect become the information and communication center for all solid organ transplantation services in the United States, including kidney, heart, heart/lung, liver, and pancreas. All institutions performing these procedures must maintain membership in UNOS and abide by its bylaws and policies. In addition, all OPOs providing organs for transplanting institutions must also maintain membership. UNOS, as the OPTN, also had the mandate and authority to set policy concerning several important factors including: a) criteria for membership of transplanting institutions and organ procurement organizations, b) setting national policy on organ distribution and allocation, and c) establishing a national database able to define and track all potential transplant recipients of all organs transplanted and all donor organs harvested in the United States.

To accomplish these tasks, UNOS has a governing board with broad representation of both professional and public interests. In addition, there are 11 standing committees advisory to the board, also composed of broad representations. These committees are Membership and Professional Standards, Organ Procurement and Distribution, Scientific Advisory Committee, Education, Ethics, Finance, Foreign Relations, Communications, Heart Transplantation, Transportation, and Histocompatibility.

National policy decisions have already been decided and implemented by UNOS and include such critical areas as the UNOS membership criteria for transplanting institutions and organ-procurement organizations. In addition, a national UNOS policy on organ allocation of kidneys, hearts, livers, pancreases, and hearts/lungs has been established and must be adhered to by all member institutions. A third major and complex area is data submission requirements for a complex national transplant information system. All transplanting institutions and programs must abide by these policy decisions.

The expanding nature of transplant services in the current health care delivery environment where cost-efficiency seems predominant will surely produce a lively and controversial future. The OPTN is less than 1-yr old and the implications for setting these national policies and what influence they will have on the direction transplantation takes are yet to be determined. The forces potentially influencing the field of transplantation are considerable and well beyond the control of any single transplant program. In addition to the federal regulatory, as well as UNOS, policy decision, and state regulatory agencies, one additional force is the competitive marketplace itself. Many institutions are anxious to embark on establishing their own transplant programs. The reasons for this are numerous, but invariably the need to provide accessible transplant services to their patient population is present. This need is also invariably defined as potential recipients usually in need of heart or liver transplants. This perceived need, however, is never balanced by the necessary supply of organs required to support an ever-expanding number of programs and, therefore, recipients. Inevitably, this leads to a competitive posturing of institution against institution. The competition, however, is misplaced. It is not competition for potential recipient pool that is the focus. It is, in fact, the scarce donor supply. Whether regulation, at both the state and federal level, can control the growth of both the demand (the recipient pool and number of transplanting institutions) and the supply (the available number of organs for transplantation) and keep these equitably balanced in the best interest of the patients being served remains to be determined.

To be sure, transplantation has become the most highly regulated field in medicine. The reason, however, is simple. All that practice transplantation surgery and medicine have been delegated the responsibility of stewardship of what has been called a scarce national resource — those organs donated for transplantation. As such, we must be responsible and accountable stewards if we are to maintain the public trust. It is also clear that the nationalization of transplantation and organ procurement services is an experiment of large proportion and an experiment that has just begun. The legal and administrative precedents now being set have far-reaching implications. The legal challenges have not had time to develop, the public response is yet to be heard, and the impact on the quality and availability of transplantation services to the public has yet to be defined.

Acknowledgment

The author wishes to thank Roger W. Evans, PhD, at the Battelle Human Affairs Research Center in Seattle, WA for supplying the data shown in Tables 1, 2, and 4.

References

1. Najarian JS, Simmons RL: Preface. *In:* Transplantation. Najarian JS, Simmons RL (Eds). Philadelphia, Lea & Febiger, 1972, p vii

2. Veith I: Huang Ti Nei Ching Su Wen - The Yellow Emperor's Classic of Internal Medicine. Baltimore, Williams & Wilkins Co, 1949, p 3

3. MacKinney L: Medical Illustrations in Medieval Manuscripts. Berkeley, University of California Press, 1965, p 87, fig 90

4. Hunter J: Collected Works, Volume II. London, 1835, p 161

5. Corner GW: The Hormones in Human Reproduction. Princeton, University Press, 1942

6. Bert P: Experiences et considerations sur la greffe animale. *J de l'Anat* 1864; 1:69

7. Carrel A: La technique operatoire des anastomoses vasculaires et la transplantation des visceres. *Lyon Med* 1902; 99:859

8. Carrel ME, Morell A: Anatomose bout a bout de la veine jugulaire et de l'artere carotide. *Lyon Med* 1902; 99:114

9. Guthrie CC: Applications of blood vessel surgery. *In:* Blood Vessel Surgery. New York, Longmans, Green & Co, 1912, p 113

10. Landsteiner K, Miller CP: Serological studies on the blood of the primates. III. Distribution of serological factors related to human isoagglutinogens in the blood of lower monkeys. *J Exp Med* 1925; 42:863

11. Landsteiner K: Cell antigens and individual specificity. *J Immunol* 1928; 15:589

12. Gorer PA: The genetic and antigenic basis of tumor transplantation. *Journal of Pathology and Bacteriology* 1937; 44:691

13. Gorer PA: The antigenic basis of tumor transplantation. *Journal of Pathology and Bacteriology* 1938; 47:231

14. Carrel A: The surgery of blood vessels, etc. *Johns Hopkins Hospital Bulletin* 1907; 18:18

15. Medawar PB: The behavior and fate of skin autografts and skin homografts in rabbits. *J Anat* 1944; 78:176

16. Jaboulay M: Greffe de reins au pli du coude par soudures arterielles et veineuses. *Lyon Med* 1906; 107:575

17. Unger E: Uber Nierentransplantationen. *Berliner Klinische Wochenschrift* 1909; 1:1057

18. Voronoy YY: Sobre el bloqueo del aparato reticuloendotelial del hombre en algunas formas de intoxicacion por el sublimado y sobre la transplantacion del rinon cadaverico como metodo de tratamiento de la anuria consecutiva a aquella intoxicacion. *El Siglo Medico* 1936; 97:296

19. Moore FD: Give and Take of the Development of Tissue Transplantation. Philadelphia, WB Saunders Co, 1964, p 14

20. Hume DM, Merrill JP, Miller BF, et al: Experiences with renal homo-transplantation in the human: Report of nine cases. *J Clin Invest* 1955; 34:327

21. Dubost C, Oeconomos N, Vaysse J, et al: Note preliminarie sur l'etude des functions renales de reins greffes chez l'homme. *Bull Soc Med Hop Paris* 1951; 67:1372

22. Murray JE, Merrill JP, Demmin GJ, et al: Study on transplantation immunity after total body irradiation: Clinical and experimental investigation. *Surgery* 1960; 48:272

23. Schwartz R, Dameshek W: Drug induced immunological tolerance. *Nature* 1959; 183:1682

24. Murray JE, Merrill JP, Harrison JH, et al: Prolonged survival of human-kidney homografts by immunosuppressive drug therapy. *N Engl J Med* 1963; 268:1315

25. Goodwin WE, Mims MM, Kaufman JJ: Human renal transplantation III. Technical problems encountered in six cases of kidney transplantation. *Trans Am Assoc Genitourin Surg* 1962; 54:116

26. Starzl TE, Marchioro TL, Waddell WR: The reversal of rejection in human renal homografts with subsequent development of homograft tolerance. *Surg Gynecol Obstet* 1963; 117:385

27. Deusset J: Iso-leuco-anticorps. *Acta Haematol* 1958; 20:156

28. Terasaki PI, Marchioro TL, Starzl TE: *In:* Histocompatibility Testing. Washington, DC, National Academy of Sciences, 1965, pp 83-95

29. Rettig RA: Implementing the End-Stage Renal Disease Program of Medicare. (Prepared for HCFA/HEW). Santa Monica, CA, Rand Corporation, 1980, pp 25-27

30. Starzl TE, Groth CG, Brettschneider L, et al: Orthotopic homotransplantation of the human liver. *Ann Surg* 1968; 168:392

31. Barnard CN: The operation. *S Afr Med J* 1967; 41:1271

32. Baumgartner WA, Reitz BA, Oyer PE, et al: Cardiac homotransplantation. *In:* Current Problems in Surgery. Chicago, Year Book Medical Publishers, 1979

33. 118 Congressional Record. 1972; p 33003

Chapter 2

Liver Transplantation

*Peter G. Stock, MD, John S. Najarian, MD,
and Nancy L. Ascher, MD, PhD*

Outline

Educational Objectives

In this chapter the reader will learn:

1. which critical care patients are potential organ donors.

2. the proper management of the donor prior to organ donation.

3. which critical care patients are appropriate candidates for hepatic transplantation.

4. the essential preoperative evaluation of the liver transplant recipient.

5. the management of the hepatic transplant recipient prior to transplantation.

6. the general principles of anesthesia and the operative procedure.

7. the immunosuppressive regimens during the critical postoperative period.

8. the essential postoperative care following liver transplantation.

9. the potential complications following liver transplantation, and their appropriate management.

Introduction

Orthotopic liver transplantation has become an accepted therapeutic modality for many end-stage liver diseases (1). Several advances in the surgical techniques and medical treatment of hepatic transplant recipients have facilitated patient management and resulted in markedly improved results. These advances include improved surgical techniques with special emphasis on superior methods of biliary drainage (2), meticulous donor hepatectomy utilizing slow in situ organ flushing (3), the introduction of cyclosporine into the immunonsuppressive regimens (2, 4, 5), and prompt recognition of infection and rejection (2, 6).

The increased acceptance of liver transplantation which has occurred in conjunction with improved results has resulted in a proliferation of active liver transplant centers. More than 600 transplants were done in 1985, and over 40 centers are currently active (7). The widespread interest in liver transplantation will require a broader range of critical care specialists familiar with the management of both the donor and recipient aspects of liver transplantation. In this brief review, an attempt will be made to identify the essential points of both donor and recipient selection and management during the critical perioperative time.

Cadaver Organ Donation

General Aspects

The most frequent source of organs for transplantation remains cadaveric donors, and they are obviously the only source of organs for liver transplantation. Most cadaveric organ donors are young individuals who have sustained closed-head injuries, have intact circulations, and are maintained on a respirator. The vast majority of cadaveric donors are maintained in the ICU, where the organ functions of the neurologically brain-dead donor must be maintained to avoid unnecessary loss of organs. For this reason, critical care specialists need to be cognizant of which patients represent potential donors, and the proper maintenance of the donor prior to organ procurement.

Criteria of Brain Death

The universal acceptance of the concept of brain death has allowed for normal organ perfusion prior to and throughout the donor operation. The criteria for brain death endorsed by the American Academy of Neurology dictate that there must be irreversible cessation of all functions of the entire brain, including the brain stem (8). Cessation of brainstem function can be demonstrated by a standard battery of clinical testing including: pupillary light reflex, corneal reflex, oculocephalic reflex, oculovestibular reflex, oropharyngeal reflex, and apneic reflex (9). It is important to note that the definition of brain death requires that cerebral and brainstem function are irreversibly absent. Therefore, conditions which could mask underlying intact function must be ruled out (Table 1).

Table 1. Conditions masking underlying intact cerebral function in the potential organ donor

Condition	Examples	Clinical Testing
Drug Intoxication	Barbiturates Benzodiazepines Meprobamate Methaqualone Trichlorethylene	Toxicology Screening
Total Paralysis	Exposure to drugs such as neuromuscular blocking agents or aminoglycoside antibiotics Diseases such as myasthenia gravis	Careful review of history
Surgically Correctable Lesion	Subdural or Epidural Hematoma	Computerized Tomographic Scan (CAT)
Hypothermia	——	Continuous re-evaluation during rewarming

Confirmatory studies include electroencephalography, cerebral angiography, and radionuclide brain scans. If irreversible brain death can be determined by simpler means, these tests need not be performed. Definite diagnostic criteria for irreversible brain death, which are useful in less clearcut cases, include total electrical silence maintained for 6 to 24 hours or total absence of blood flow. In the absence of these confirmatory tests, an observation period of 12 h is recommended once an irreversible condition has been established. In the case of anoxic brain damage, in which the extent of damage may be more difficult to determine, an observation period of 24 h is recommended (9). Caution must be taken in the diagnosis of brain death in the child; conditions for irreversible cessation of function are less clearly defined than in the adult.

Evaluating the Potential Function of the Donor Organ for Liver Transplantation

Although this discussion focuses on the potential utility of the liver from a given donor, it should be stressed that the short supply of all organs dictates an integrated approach to obtain maximal use of all organs. Every donor should be considered a multiple organ donor. The absolute and relative contraindications for use of the donor liver are listed in Table 2.

Donor liver function is frequently difficult to assess, as a short period of shock may result in transient elevation of liver enzymes without permanent damage to the donor organ. These enzymes should return toward normal within 12 to 24 h if the patient has been properly maintained and the liver has not sustained permanent damage. On occasion there isn't sufficient time to measure repeat enzymes; the decision to use a particular donor must be based on an assessment of potential for recovery.

23

Table 2. Contraindications to organ utilization in hepatic transplantation

Absolute Contraindications

Age > 65 yr

Infection involving the liver

Disseminated malignancy

History of liver disease

Irreversible ischemic injury to the liver

Relative Contraindications

Traumatic damage to the liver

Systemic infection (inadequately treated)

Current preservation techniques allow for successful hepatic transplantation for up to 12 h after removal. It is perceived (but not proven) in the human that the length of preservation is inversely related to hepatic function following transplantation. Utilizing cold preservation, a distance of up to 1200 miles can be travelled (using jet transportation) and allow adequate time for transplantation.

Maintenance of the Donor Prior to Organ Donation

Following the pronouncement of death, the donor needs to be carefully maintained to avoid unnecessary losses of valuable organs. The basic principles of intensive care management need to be closely adhered to prior to the donor operation. This includes frequent monitoring of vital signs; proper ventilatory management followed closely by arterial blood gases; and cardiovascular monitoring including ECG, central venous pressure, arterial pressure, and urine volume. Insertion of a pulmonary artery catheter may aid in the management of hemodynamically labile patients.

Fluid administration in the donor needs to correct a general state of volume depletion, manifest by decreased BP, oliguria, and hemoconcentration. This situation is especially prevalent in the donor with a closed-head injury, when fluid administration often has been minimized to prevent cerebral edema. Adequate fluid resuscitation can usually be accomplished with D5 1/3 normal saline plus 20 mq KCl/L. Diabetes insipidus frequently follows closed-head injury, and its presence requires the administration of a more concentrated saline solution. In general, fluid is administered to establish a urinary output of >.5 ml/kg·h. Diabetes insipidus may dictate the use of vasopressin at a dose of 1 to 5 units IM to be repeated every 4 to 5 h.

Antibiotic management during the maintenance period consists of a third-generation cephalosporin administered in therapeutic doses. In the presence of a local infection (i.e., urinary tract infection), antibiotics may need to be altered to provide the appropriate coverage. Perioperative antibiotic coverage should be administered prior to the donor operation, utilizing a drug to which neither the donor nor recipient is allergic. Special problems encountered in the maintenance of the donor prior to the donor operation are listed in Table 3.

Table 3. Frequent problems encountered in donor maintenance

Problem	Management
1. Hypotension	Rapid infusion of iv fluid. Synthetic colloid solutions or fresh frozen plasma may be used. Hypotension following adequate fluid resuscitation dictates the use of dopamine (or other pressors) to maintain BP.
2. Hypertension	Hypertension secondary to fluid overload is treated with diuretic therapy. Reflex hypertension may be managed with iv vasodilating agents such as hydralazine.
3. Diabetes Insipidus	Pitressin 2 to 5 U IM every 4 to 5 h (adult dose)
4. Electrolyte Imbalance	Appropriate alteration in iv fluid administration
5. Oliguria	Oliguria following adequate fluid resuscitation dictates use of diuretics

Care of the Liver Transplant Recipient

Recipient Selection

Indications in Adults

Liver transplantation is an appropriate procedure for any patient whose liver disease is certain to progress to end-stage liver disease. Due to the expense, high morbidity, and limited availability of organs, this procedure should be limited to those patients in which: a) progression of the liver disease is unresponsive to medical management; b) the mortality of the operative procedure is not extreme; c) the primary disease responsible for liver failure is unlikely to recur in the transplanted liver; and d) the patient has an opportunity for a normal lifestyle following the procedure.

In the adult population, diseases responsible for end-stage liver disease in which transplantation has been utilized include chronic active hepatitis, alcoholic cirrhosis, primary hepatic malignancy, primary biliary cirrhosis, secondary biliary cirrhosis, sclerosing cholangitis, alpha-1-antitrypsin deficiency, hemochromatosis, Budd-Chiari syndrome, and acute Hepatitis B. The most frequent etiology of liver failure requiring transplantation is chronic active hepatitis, although the frequency of disease culminating in the transplantation varies from center to center. The appropriate time in the progression of the disease at which transplantation should be performed is frequently difficult to determine in diseases such as primary biliary cirrhosis and chronic active hepatitis, as these diseases remit or deteriorate in an unpredictable manner. With future analysis of patients with these diseases, it may become possible to determine at which point in time the disease will progress to end-stage failure. A better understanding of the time course of these diseases will allow for a more accurate determination of the timing of transplantation, so that deterioration has not progressed beyond the point at which the operative mortality is prohibitive.

Indications for Transplantation in Children

The most common indication for transplantation in the pediatric population is biliary atresia (10). This disease occurs at a frequency estimated between 1 in 8,000 to 1 in 25,000 live births in the United States (11, 12). The vast majority of patients with this disease have had previous surgery, usually one or more Kasai procedures. This procedure, which utilizes a portoenterostomy via a Roux-en-Y jejunal limb to drain small ducts within the porta of the liver, is successful in approximately 30% of all cases (13, 14). In patients with failed Kasai procedures, 90% will die before they reach 5 years of age. For this reason, early transplantation following failed Kasai procedures is considered appropriate management for these children. Other indications for transplantation in the pediatric age group include chronic active hepatitis, hepatoma, neonatal hepatitis, congenital hepatic fibrosis, secondary biliary fibrosis, fulminant hepatitis, and the inborn errors of metabolism. The inborn errors of metabolism include alpha-1-antitrypsin deficiency, Wilson's disease, tyrosinemia, and type IV glycogen storage disease. In these patients, transplantation reverses the enzyme deficiency that was responsible for the end-stage hepatic failure (15).

Contraindications to Liver Transplantation

Strict contraindications to hepatic transplantation include widespread malignancy, irreversible infection not confined to the liver, concurrent disease that would make the risks of surgery prohibitive or impair postoperative survival, or high likelihood of disease recurrence in the transplanted organ (16).

Although hepatic malignancy which has not metastasized is not a strict contraindication to transplantation, experience has demonstrated that hepatic malignancy recurs following transplantation. One notable exception is the lamellar type of hepatic cancer, the recurrence of which has been prolonged after orthotopic liver transplantation in several instances (17). Additionally, a few pediatric patients have survived after resection of cirrhotic livers in which incidental hepatomas were found (18).

Recurrence of active hepatitis following transplantation is common, and survivors are rare. For these reasons, transplantation is a relative contraindication when HB(s)Ag or HB(e)Ag antigenemia are present (2, 19). Pichlmayr et al. (20) have revealed the frequent recurrence of disease in the transplanted organ.

Alcoholic cirrhosis is a relative contraindication to transplantation, primarily because of the risk of recurrent alcoholism. However, abstinence from alcohol for at least 6 months with completion of a treatment program qualifies a patient for potential transplantation. Patients with Budd-Chiari syndrome require anticoagulant medication after transplantation to prevent recurrent thrombosis. Previous reports of recurrent primary biliary cirrhosis probably represent chronic rejection rather than reoccurrence of the primary disease.

Patients with sclerosing cholangitis associated with ulcerative colitis probably should not be transplanted in the presence of active colonic disease. Previously active disease with or without colonic resection does not contraindicate transplantation. Postoperative evaluation of the colon must be done at frequent intervals. Finally, revascularization in patients with portal vein thrombosis may be difficult, although Shaw et al. (21) reported various techniques to circumvent this problem.

In the pediatric population, the lower age limit of a patient undergoing hepatic transplantation has yet to be defined; neonatal transplantation has been performed in a small number of infants. Transplantation is usually limited to patients whose dry weight is greater than 5.5 kg due to the prohibitively small size of the portal vein anastomosis. Hepatic transplantation for fulminant hepatitis represents a special problem. Patients who survive the acute liver failure occasionally develop aplastic anemia, which can be fatal. It is unclear whether the immunosuppression following transplantation will exacerbate the development of aplastic anemia. Future experience with transplantation of patients with aplastic anemia may demonstrate that liver transplantation is too risky to justify its use or that bone marrow transplantation should be considered as a concomitant procedure (22).

Preoperative Evaluation of the Recipient

The preoperative evaluation has three major functions: a) determine if the transplant is technically feasible via anatomical studies, b) determine if the transplant is feasible by ruling out occult infection and malignancy, and c) evaluate defects in other organ systems in order to maximize management during the perioperative period to provide the patient the best opportunity for survival following transplantation. In addition to a thorough history and physical examination, Table 4 lists the tests and laboratory studies which should be performed in the preoperative evaluation and their significance for further management of the patient.

Preoperative Management

Preoperative management consists of optimizing the function of the organ systems found to be suboptimal in the preoperative evaluation of the recipient. In patients with end-stage liver disease, frequent attention needs to be directed toward the respiratory function and nutritional status.

All recipients are begun on intensive programs of pulmonary toilet and exercise. Attention to respiratory function is necessary for four reasons: a) patients are ventilatory-dependent in the postoperative period, and optimization of function will facilitate earlier extubation; b) postoperative ascites contributes to postoperative atelectasis; c) an oversized donor liver may compromise respiratory function in the postoperative period; and d) the potential complication of phrenic nerve injury, though temporary, can exacerbate postoperative atelectasis secondary to right-sided diaphragmatic paralysis. Obviously, recipients must stop smoking prior to the procedure. Patients with chronic lung infections or bronchitis may require postural drainage. Broad-spectrum antibiotics should be administered to treat bacterial infections.

In order to minimize the detrimental effects of ascites on respiratory function, cautious diuretic therapy should be administered. The use of diuretics needs to be weighed against the potential of exacerbating renal insufficiency, particularly in those patients with evidence of the hepatorenal syndrome. Maximization of blood volume utilizing colloid may optimize the cardiac output and effectively treat the prerenal component of the hepatorenal syndrome. The use of a pulmonary artery catheter may facilitate fluid administration in these patients with labile fluid balance.

Nutritional support is guided by transferrin levels and serum amino acid analysis (23). Serum ammonia levels are carefully monitored while administering dietary protein.

Table 4. Preoperative evaluation of recipients for hepatic transplantation

Tests to Evaluate Anatomic Feasibility

Test	Significance
CAT scan, ultrasonography, celiac angiography	CAT scanning may be necessary to show portal vein patency and size if ultrasonography fails to demonstrate the portal vein.
Upper GI endoscopy	Detect location of esophageal varices and treat with sclerotherapy if bleeding.

Tests to Rule Out Occult Infection or Malignancy

Chest x-ray; blood, urine, throat, feces, ascites cultures	Contamination in any of these major sites is a relative contraindication to transplantation.
Baseline titers to cytomegalovirus, herpes and Epstein-Barr virus	Important for following the development of new infection with virus in the postoperative period.
Hepatitis screen	Assesses whether viral infection is likely to recur in the transplanted liver.
Dental consultation	Eliminate dental infections as a possible etiology of post-transplantation infections.
Hepatic ultrasound CAT scanning, alpha-fetoprotein levels, ascitic fluid cytology	Screen for occult malignancy. Malignant cells in the ascitic fluid is a strict contraindication to transplantation.

Review of Organ Systems

Cardiac - chest x-ray, ECG, formal cardiology consult, stress test if indicated	Congestive heart failure and associated fluid overload treated with fluid restriction, diuretics, and digoxin.
Pulmonary - chest x-ray, arterial blood gases, pulmonary function tests	Knowledge of respiratory reserve facilitates patient management in the early postoperative period when patients are respiratory-dependent. Preoperative pulmonary toilet or enhancement of accessory muscle function may be necessary in compromised patients.
Hepatic-liver function tests, coagulation profile	Indicates the functional capacity of the liver and the potential requirement for vitamin K, factor replacement, or preoperative exchange transfusion in the decompensated patient.
Renal - urinalysis, BUN, serum creatinine, 24-h creatinine, clearance	Evaluates the presence of hepatorenal syndrome, frequently associated with hepatic dysfunction. If cardiac output demonstrates low perfusion, cardiac stimulation may correct the problem. Hepatorenal syndrome has been reversed following successful liver transplantation (24).

Table 4. (continued)

Immunologic - tissue typing including cytotoxic antibody determinations, blood type (ABO)	No evidence as to beneficial effect of HLA matching in liver transplantation, although typing performed for retrospective analysis. Preoperative cross-matching not routinely performed due to inadequate time and unknown advantage. ABO blood group matching preferred, although successful transplants have been performed across ABO barriers (25).
Nutrition - transferrin, prealbumin, serum amino acid analysis	Specific nutritional support guided by these tests, and serial measurements of these parameters indicate efficacy of this support.

In the immediate preoperative period, the patient's overall condition is reassessed. Blood is sent to immunology for the final crossmatch, as well as to the blood bank. Large volumes of blood, platelets, fresh frozen plasma, and cryoprecipitate must be available for the operative procedure. Preoperative exchange transfusion should be considered in all patients with impaired coagulation parameters. Recent experience at the University of Minnesota suggests that the exchange transfusion may be performed in the operating room during the early stages of the operation to minimize operative bleeding. Prophylactic antibiotics/antiviral agents are administered to provide protection against herpes virus infection, minimize wound infection, and reduce colonization of the GI tract.

Anesthesia and the Operative Procedure — General Principles

This discussion will provide a brief overview of the general anesthetic and surgical principles underlying the transplant procedure. A basic understanding of these principles is necessary for proper management of the patients during the critical postoperative period. Due to the limited scope of this chapter, this discussion will provide only the essential information necessary for recognizing postoperative complications, as well as providing proper postoperative management. Several detailed descriptions of anesthesia and the operative procedure are referenced for in-depth coverage of these topics (2, 26-28).

Principles of Anesthesia

Experience at the University of Minnesota has shown that the basic principles underlying successful anesthetic management centers on the ability of the anesthesia team to deal with excessive blood loss and the associated instabilities in hemodynamic and metabolic parameters (29). Previous studies have demonstrated that patients with hepatic failure undergoing major operative procedures maintain a hyperkinetic state (30). This hyperkinetic state needs to be maintained during the transplant procedure in order to prevent a shock syndrome. The anesthesia team at the University of Minnesota utilizes a roller pump, which has the capacity to deliver 5 L of blood products per minute via a central line. This permits the anesthesiologist to infuse blood/blood products at a rate sufficient to keep left-sided filling pressures and cardiac output at a level equal to postinduction levels, and consequently prevent the shock syndrome.

In addition to the roller pump, the anesthesia team has developed a safer technique for the rapid infusion of large volumes of blood. The rapid infusion technique utilizes specially prepared blood that prevents the severe coagulopathies and hyperkalemic state normally seen when infusing massive amounts of blood. The blood is prepared for transfusion by resuspending saline-washed packed RBCs in fresh frozen plasma and Plasmolyte to obtain a Hct of 30% and a serum potassium of 4.5 ± .5 mEq/L. The blood is reoxygenated by means of a standard membrane oxygenator (Po_2 355 torr, Pco_2 35 torr), filtered (40-μ blood filter), and rewarmed to 37°C prior to infusion. Platelets and cryoprecipitate are administered to the blood infusate to maintain platelet counts > 250,000 and fibrinogen levels > 0.35 mg/dl. The blood infusate is administered at a rate sufficient to maintain cardiac output at the hyperkinetic postinduction levels. Since the initiation of the rapid-infusion technique at the University of Minnesota, there have been no intraoperative deaths during the transplantation procedure. This has been attributed to the absence of severe coagulopathies and hyperkalemia during the transplant procedure (31).

Veno-venous bypass has not been used in any patients at our institution, and several other groups have reported excellent results in the absence of the veno-venous bypass (32). Nonetheless, most groups routinely use veno-venous bypass with excellent results (33). Bypassing the inferior vena cava and portal vein into the axillary vein offers several theoretical advantages, including less renal damage secondary to decompression of the IVC, and less damage to the bowel secondary to decompression of the portal vein. We hypothesize that cyclosporine absorption in the postoperative period is superior in patients in whom bowel edema is avoided using the veno-venous bypass. As yet the specific patient in whom veno-venous bypass is indicated is unknown. Future prospective studies comparing use of the veno-venous bypass to other techniques may identify a patient population which greatly benefits from the use of veno-venous bypass.

Principles of the Operative Procedure

The standard orthotopic liver transplant procedure is a straightforward procedure (1, 16, 28). In addition to the coagulopathies associated with end-stage liver disease, the frequently associated portal hypertension with extensive portosystemic collaterilization contributes to making the recipient hepatectomy the most difficult aspect of the transplant procedure. Residual scarring from previous operations (e.g., portosystemic shunts in the adult population and Kasai procedures in the pediatric population) accentuates the difficulty of the recipient hepatectomy. If severe coagulopathies exist, a preoperative exchange transfusion may be indicated, although recent experience suggests that a more effective exchange may be accomplished in the operating room following induction of anesthesia and placement of the intravascular cannulations. The basic steps in the recipient hepatectomy involve isolating and placing vessel loops around the suprahepatic vena cava, infrahepatic vena cava, portal vein, and hepatic artery at the level of the gastroduodenal artery. In addition, it may be necessary to isolate the distal aorta at the level of the inferior mesenteric artery. The common bile duct is isolated and ligated distally (toward the liver), leaving a long proximal segment for the transplant procedure. In patients with previous Kasai procedures, a jejunal limb drains the porta hepatis. This limb needs to be taken down and either prepared for biliary drainage post-transplant, or resected if it is not to be used for biliary drainage. Following resection of the host liver, it is particularly important to achieve meticulous hemostasis, with particular attention to the retroperitoneal area where exposure is difficult following the transplant procedure.

The basics of the donor hepatectomy involve dissection and skeletonization of the major vessels around the liver, including the celiac trunk and its branches, the portal vein, and the inferior vena cava (both the supra and infrahepatic cava). The common bile duct is transected proximal to the ampulla, thus obtaining maximal length of the duct for use in transplantation. Cool saline is used to flush the bile out of the biliary tree and protect the biliary mucosa; access is via a cholecystostomy. Initial cooling of the liver is accomplished using a slow in situ flush of cold heparinized lactated Ringer's solution into the portal vein. Subsequent simultaneous flush of cold heparinized Collin's solution into the portal vein and distal aorta completes cooling of the liver. The suprahepatic cava is transected at the level of the right atrium, and the infrahepatic cava is divided at the level of the renal veins. The portal vein is divided at the confluence of the splenic vein and superior mesenteric vein. The entire thoracic aorta is incised and the lumbar arteries are ligated; this portion may be used as an aortic conduit in the recipient operation if necessary. The liver is packed in Collin's solution and can be stored on ice for up to 12 h.

After meticulous hemostasis has been achieved following the recipient hepatectomy, the first anastomosis is made to the donor suprahepatic vena cava. This is followed by the posterior wall of the infrahepatic vena cava. The anterior wall anastomosis is left incomplete for venting purposes during the flushing phase. Next, the portal vein anastomosis is completed, and the liver is reperfused after the vascular clamp on the recipient portal vein is removed. In this way, the liver is rewarmed and the hyperkalemic preservation solution is vented through the defect in the anterior infrahepatic caval anastomosis. Blood which has been stagnant within the splanchnic circulation during occlusive clamping of the portal vein is also flushed. After completion of the flush, the anterior wall anastomosis of the infrahepatic cava is completed and both caval clamps are removed. Systemic venous and portal blood are returned to the systemic circulation. This may be associated with transient hyperkalemia and a significant hemotologic disturbance characterized by prolongation of all clotting parameters. This effect is attributed to heparin contained in the preservation fluid as well as "heparinoid" products released from the ischemic liver. This reperfusion coagulopathy is occasionally reversed by treatment with protamine sulfate, although large doses of cryoprecipitate, fresh frozen plasma, and platelets are frequently necessary to reverse this coagulopathy. Amicar may be necessary during this stage of the transplant operation (34).

Following reperfusion of the liver, the arterial supply to the transplant is reestablished. This is accomplished using a celiac axis or hepatic artery-to-hepatic artery whenever possible. In a few cases in the pediatric population, the vessel size was inadequate. In these patients, an aortic conduit was utilized and an aorto-aortic anastomosis was performed at the level of the recipient inferior mesenteric artery. Finally, biliary drainage is accomplished using a choledochocholedochostomy whenever possible, or a choledochojejunostomy when the small size or absence of a recipient common duct necessitates this procedure.

Immunosuppression and Postoperative Management

Immunotherapy

The introduction of cyclosporine into immunosuppressive regimens has been associated with marked improvement of results following hepatic transplanta-

31

tion (1, 35). Improved survival following hepatic transplantation cannot, however, be singularly attributed to cyclosporine, as several groups have shown good results using conventional immunotherapy (36). Survival following transplantation is clearly the result of a combination of factors, including the experience of the group performing the transplant (31).

At the University of Minnesota, a triple immunosuppressive regimen (cyclosporine, prednisone, and azathioprine) is utilized to prevent rejection. Prior to transplantation, a 1-mg/kg dose of methylprednisolone is administered iv. Following transplantation, all patients are immediately started on the following immunosuppressive regimen: a) azathioprine 1.5 mg/kg·day iv, b) prednisone 2 mg/kg·day iv, and c) cyclosporine administered initially at a dose of 3 mg/kg·day by continuous iv infusion and an additional 10 mg/kg·day by the enteral route. Following return of bowel function, all three drugs are switched to oral administration. The azathioprine dose is adjusted to keep the patient's white blood count > 3000/mm³. The prednisone dose is tapered to 0.1 mg/kg by 3 to 6 months post-transplant. The cyclosporine dose is altered to maintain trough whole blood levels of cyclosporine between 250 and 350 ng/ml, as assessed by high-pressure liquid chromatography. With return of bowel function, this generally required 5 to 15 mg/kg·day in two divided doses in adults and 10 to 50 mg/kg·day in divided doses for children.

In order to rapidly diagnose and treat rejection, routine weekly percutaneous biopsies are utilized. Mild rejection is initially treated with steroids; moderate to severe rejection is treated using antilymphoblast globulin or OKT3 depending on selection in a prospective randomized trial comparing the efficacy of these two agents. Although the incidence of histologically proven rejection was high in both adults (74%) and children (73%), the rejection was easily reversed by individualized treatment based on the severity of rejection noted on the biopsy. In a series of 58 consecutive patients who received orthotopic liver transplants using this immunosuppressive regimen, only two patients went on to irreversible rejection and required retransplantation. Of equal importance, fatal infections using this immunosuppressive regimen were extremely rare. Additionally, none of the patients in this series developed renal insufficiency as a consequence of cyclosporine therapy. The 1-yr actuarial survival was 82% for adult recipients and 65% for pediatric patients (6).

Postoperative Care Following Liver Transplantation

Immediately following the transplant procedure, liver recipients receive management in the ICU until they no longer require ventilatory support. Patients generally require respiratory support for 24 to 48 h post-transplantation. Hypokalemic metabolic alkalosis is frequent following liver transplantation secondary to the large volumes of blood given during the transplant procedure and the liberal use of furosemide diureses. An HCl drip is occasionally required to return the blood pH to normal levels. If the HCl drip is not utilized in the face of metabolic alkalosis, it is difficult to wean the patient from ventilatory support as spontaneous respirations are decreased.

Following extubation and a hemodynamically stable postoperative course, the patient may be returned to a regular nursing ward. Nasogastric suction is continued until normal bowel function resumes. Nutritional support is provided by intravenous hyperalimentation until patients are able to take an adequate amount of oral calories. If the transplanted liver is functioning normally, the metabolic abnormalities secondary to end-stage liver disease should be reversed and standard nutritional support will be sufficient in the postoperative period (18). Chest x-rays are performed daily for 5 days following the transplant, and whenever the patient becomes febrile. This is necessary to rapidly diagnose atelectasis, pneumonia, diaphragmatic paralysis, and pleural effusion, so that prompt treatment may be initiated. Daily determinations of the following levels are made: blood urea nitrogen, creatinine, electrolytes, calcium, phosphate, white blood count, Hgb levels, coagulation parameters, and arterial blood gases.

Antibiotic coverage consists of a broad-spectrum antibiotic (i.e., cefotaxime) until the patient is extubated, and intravenous bactrim (trimethoprim sulfate) until it can be tolerated orally. As with all transplant patients, Candida prophylaxis consists of nystatin administered via the nasogastric tube until it can be tolerated orally. Herpes prophylaxis consists of acyclovir 5 mg/kg·day iv for 5 postoperative days. Daily cultures of the throat, sputum, urine, blood, and all drainage tubes are obtained for 3 days, then as indicated. All cultures are sent for aerobes, anaerobes, viruses, and fungi.

Hepatic function is evaluated by chemical determinations performed at frequent intervals. Although changes in bilirubin, transaminase, and alkaline phosphatase levels are useful in suggesting alterations in hepatic function, the specific etiology of hepatocyte malfunction is difficult to differentiate, e.g., rejection, ischemia, viral infection, cholangitis, or mechanical obstruction (37). A percutaneous liver biopsy permits differentiation between these possibilities. Rejection is characterized by lymphocytic infiltrates in the portal tract and central veins with varying degrees of bile duct epithelial and central vein endothelial damage. Treatment depends on the severity of the rejection, as previously mentioned. Herpes viral infection is treated with intravenous acyclovir, while cytomegalovirus (CMV) is effectively treated with gancyclovir. Patients with concomitant rejection and CMV infection have been successfully treated with a combination of OKT 3 or ALG and gancyclovir. The presence of polymorphonuclear leukocytes in the portal tracts is suggestive of cholangitis, and the patient is begun on the appropriate antibiotics. Fever following percutaneous biopsy is suggestive of biliary infection; blood culture at the time of fever (or liver biopsy culture) may reveal the infecting organism. Cholangitis is frequently associated with mechanical obstruction, and a search is made for evidence of biliary obstruction as an etiologic factor.

Liver function is further evaluated by a radionuclide excretory cholangiogram performed on postoperative day 1 and at weekly intervals. The normal period of time necessary for extraction of the radioisotope by the liver with subsequent excretion into the small bowel is <45 min. Prolonged extraction may be indicative of problems related to an improperly preserved donor liver, a prolonged preservation period, vascular compromise of the transplanted organ, or rejection. Delayed excretion into the biliary system may reflect hepatocellular damage secondary to rejection, ischemia, or viral infection. Finally, delayed passage of the radioisotope into the small bowel may reflect obstruction of the biliary tree and/or breakdown of the biliary anastomosis. A T-tube cholangiogram (performed with low pressures) or a transhepatic cholangiogram (in the absence of a T-tube) will provide the necessary information on the condition of the biliary tree. Right upper quadrant ultrasonography may reveal dilated intrahepatic ducts indicative of mechanical obstruction. A transcutaneous cholangiogram may be used to diagnose obstruction, and the placement of a percutaneous transhepatic tube can be used to treat biliary obstruction.

Postoperative Complications in the Liver Transplant Recipient

Immediately following liver transplantation, the patient is respiratory-dependent and placed in the ICU. There are several potential complications in the immediate postoperative period about which the critical care specialist needs to be aware. This will facilitate strategies for resolution of the problem(s). The potential complications include: bleeding, occlusion of vascular anastomoses, respiratory complications, renal failure, infections, and rejection.

Bleeding

Due to the large blood volume which may require replacement during the liver transplant operation, severe coagulation defects frequently exist in the immediate postoperative period. Postoperative hemorrhage is suggested by decreasing Hgb, deteriorating cardiovascular status, and increasing intraperitoneal pressure. Initial management should consist of a combination of blood transfusion, factor replacement and blood replacement, and platelet transfusion. A continued increase in the intraperitoneal pressure in the face of normal coagulation parameters with compromised renal function and/or respiratory function is an indication for re-exploration. Immediate function of the transplanted liver is indicated by normalization of coagulation parameters. In particular, high Factor V levels predict a lower frequency of bleeding complications (38).

Occlusion of the inferior cava presents with lower-trunk edema and renal insufficiency. A vena cavogram can confirm the diagnosis if severe operative repair must be undertaken. Milder degrees of stenosis of the suprahepatic vena cava anastomosis in children, manifest by an elevation of bilirubin and hepatic enzymes and persistent ascites, can occasionally be corrected by balloon angioplasty. Mild stenosis of the infrahepatic cava may result in mild lower extremity edema and may not warrant further therapy.

Respiratory Complications

Several problems frequently seen in liver transplant recipients can predispose to respiratory complications. Predisposing factors include: preoperative and postoperative ascites, paralysis of the diaphragm, pleural effusions, a transplanted liver which is larger than the native liver, and atelectasis exacerbated by operative pain and abdominal spasm. These predisposing problems lead to poor respiratory movement, a scenario in which pneumonia may easily develop in the immunosuppressed patient. Prevention of this complication is accomplished by vigorous pulmonary toilet in the postoperative period. Preoperative training in the use of accessory respiratory muscles may also benefit the patient during this critical period.

Despite rigorous pulmonary care in the postoperative period, some patients will require extended periods of ventilatory support, a few requiring several weeks. Bronchoscopy should be liberally utilized to re-expand atelectatic lung segments, as well as to remove and culture purulent material. Diaphragmatic pacing has not been used for the management of patients with phrenic nerve paralysis. Patients often return from the transplant operation with severe metabolic alkalosis secondary to the citrate administered in the transfused blood. This metabolic situation will decrease the spontaneous rate of respirations, which in turn prolongs the period of ventilatory support. A cautiously administered HCl drip reverses this metabolic imbalance.

If high intra-abdominal pressures generated by ascites are inhibiting normal respiratory movement, ascites can be drained via peritoneal dialysis catheters. These catheters are routinely placed during the operative procedure. If the catheters are used for this purpose, care must be taken to maintain sterility. Cautious administration of diuretics is also utilized to decrease the ascites.

Renal Failure

Compromised renal function is frequent prior to and following hepatic transplantation. Post-transplant renal insufficiency may be minimized by maintaining blood volume and cardiac output intraoperatively and in the postoperative period. The use of the introperative rapid infusion technique has permitted the anesthesiologist to maintain a constant level of perfusion during the operation, and hence avoid renal problems related to intraoperative hypovolemia. Several institutions have employed veno-venous bypass to reduce renal vein pressure during the anhepatic phase.

Intravenous cyclosporine administered in the postoperative period may cause renal insufficiency, and strict attention must be directed toward maintaining cyclosporine below nephrotoxic levels. Cyclosporine infusion should be stopped with the first sign of renal compromise and patients should be temporarily protected with conventional immunotherapy. Other nephrotoxic agents, such as aminoglycosides, should also be avoided. Finally, removal of ascites reduces intra-abdominal pressure, in turn increasing renal perfusion.

Prophylactic broad-spectrum antibiotics should be used during the perioperative period. If the GI tract is opened during the transplant procedure, such as when the jejunum is utilized for biliary drainage, topical amphotericin B (5 mg per L of irrigation) should be used as well as topical antibiotic irrigation. All patients are placed on prophylactic trimethoprim sulfamethoxazole to reduce the postoperative incidence of *pneumocystis carinae* and Nocardia infections. Following discharge, the patients remain on this drug, as it has provided very effective long-term prophylaxis in renal transplant recipients.

Viral infections are a frequent problem following transplantation, especially herpes virus and CMV. Due to the high incidence of both of these infections, patients receive postoperative acyclovir prophylaxis (5 mg/kg·day × 5 days) for herpes. Evidence of herpes simplex infection is immediately treated with additional acyclovir at a dose of 10 mg/kg·day. In a given patient, the beneficial therapeutic effects of this drug need to be weighed against its potential nephrotoxic effects, particularly in the presence of renal insufficiency. The recent addition of the anti-CMV agent gancyclovir has greatly facilitated the treatment of CMV infections.

Fungal infections are a common postoperative problem; some groups report a 25% frequency of fungemia or fungal abscess (39). The incidence of these infections has been decreased by utilizing high-dose oral, esophageal, and gastric nystatin. Any evidence of candidosis is an indication for prompt initiation of systemic amphotericin B.

Improved biliary drainage technique has decreased the incidence of cholangitis. Nonetheless, it is still common. Liver biopsy may provide tissue for culture, and in turn may provide information regarding the appropriate choice of antibiotic therapy.

Finally, central venous lines have had an extremely high rate of bacterial contamination (6), stressing the necessity for sterile technique in their placement. These lines should be removed promptly if they are not essential for management in order to avoid bacterial colonization.

Rejection

The incidence of biopsy-proven rejection is extremely high following liver transplantation (approximately 75% in both children and adults). In our series, these rejection episodes occurred between 3 and 70 days post-transplant. The average time to first rejection was 23 days in the pediatric population and 15 days in the adult population (6). The only reliable diagnostic test is percutaneous biopsy, which should be performed weekly in the post-transplant period. Non-specific findings suggestive of rejection include elevated temperature, elevated bilirubin, elevated liver enzymes, loss of sensorium, change in the serum amino acid profile, and decreased uptake or concentration on the nuclear radioisotope scan (40). We treat mild rejection initially with steroids; moderate to severe rejection is treated using anilymphoblast globulin or OKT 3. This approach has provided safe and effective immunotherapy following liver transplantation. Although the incidence of primary rejection episodes is high, the great majority can be reversed with appropriate immunotherapy guided by serial routine biopsies.

References

1. Starzl TE, Iwatsuki S, Van Thiel DH, et al: Evolution of liver transplantation. *Hepatology* 1982; 2:614

2. Iwatsuki S, Shaw BW, Starzl TE: Biliary tract complications in liver transplantation under cyclosporin-steroid therapy. *Trans Proc* 1983; 15:1288

3. Rosenthal JT, Shaw BW, Hardesty RL, et al: Principles of multiple organ procurement from cadaver donors. *Ann Surg* 1984; 198:617

4. Borel JF: The history of cyclosporin A and its significance. *In:* Cyclosporin A. White DJG (Ed). Oxford, Elsevier Biomedical Press, 1981, pp 5-17

5. Starzl TE, Iwatsuki S, Shaw BW, et al: Liver transplantation. Presented to the First International Congress on Cyclosporine, Houston, TX, May 16, 1983

6. Stock PG, Snover D, Payne W, et al: Biopsy-guided immunosuppressive therapy in the treatment of liver transplant rejection: An individualized approach. *Clin Trans* 1987; 1(4):179

7. American Council on Transplantation Newsletter. Chevy Chase, MD, July-August, 1986

8. Medical Consultants on the Diagnosis of Death: Guidelines for the determination of death. *JAMA* 1981; 246:2184

9. Ascher NL, Bolman RM, Sutherland DER: Multiple organ donation from a cadaver. *In:* Manual of Vascular Access, Organ Donation, and Transplantation. Simmons RL, Finch ME, Ascher NL, et al (Eds). New York, Springer-Verlag, 1984, pp 105-143

10. Malatack JJ, Zitelli J, Gartner JC: Pediatric liver transplantation under therapy with cyclosporin A and steroids. *Trans Proc* 1983; 15:1292

11. Shim WKT, Kasai M, Spencer MA: Racial influence in the incidence of biliary atresia. *Progressive Pediatric Surgery* 1974; 6:53

12. Alagille D: Extrahepatic biliary cirrhosis. NIH Consensus Development Conference on Liver Transplantation, 1982, pp 17-36

13. Kasai M, Watarabe I, Oni R: Follow up studies of long term survivors after hepatic portoenterostomy for "noncorrectable" biliary atresia. *J Pediatr Surg* 1975; 10:173

14. Barkin RM, Lilly JR: Biliary atresia and the Kasai operation: Continuing care. *J Pediatr* 1980; 96:1015

15. Ascher NL, Najarian JS: Liver transplantation in children. *In:* Surgery of the Liver and Biliary Tract. Blumgart LH (Ed). Edinburgh, Churchill Livingstone, In Press

16. Ascher NL, Simmons RL, Najarian JS: Host hepatectomy and liver transplantation. *In:* Manual of Vascular Access, Organ Donation, and Transplantation. Simmons RL, Finch ME, Ascher NL, et al (Eds). New York, Springer-Verlag, 1984, pp 255-284

17. Craig JR, Peters RL, Edmondson HA, et al: Fibrolameller carcinoma of the liver: A tumor of adolescents and young adults with distinctive clinicopathologic features. *Cancer* 1980; 46:372

18. Van Wyk J, Halgrimson CG, Giles G, et al: Liver transplantation in biliary atresia with concomitant hepatoma. *S Afr Med J* 1972; 46:885

19. Corman JL, Putnam CW, Iwatsuki S, et al: Liver allograft: Its use in chronic active hepatitis with macronodular cirrhosis, hepatitis B surface antigen. *Arch Surg* 1979; 114:75

20. Pichlmayr R, Ringe B, Luchart W, et al: Liver transplantation. *Trans Proc* 1987; 19:103

21. Shaw BW, Iwatsuki S, Bron K, et al: Portal vein grafts in hepatic transplantation. *Surg Gynecol Obstet* 1985; 161:66

22. Stock PG, Steiner M, Freese D, et al: Hepatitis associated aplastic anemia after liver transplantation. *Transplantation* 1986; 43:595

23. Weisdorf SA, Lysne J, Cerra FB: Total parenteral nutrition in hepatic failure and transplantation. *In:* Total Parenteral Nutrition: Indications, Utilization, Complications, and Pathophysiological Considerations. Leventhal E (Ed). New York, Raven Press, 1986, pp 463-475

24. Iwatsuki S, Carman J, Popoutzer M, et al: Recovery from hepatorenal syndrome after successful orthotopic liver transplantation. *Surg Forum* 1973; 24:348

25. Putnam CW, Starzl TE: Transplantation of the liver. *Surg Clin North Am* 1977; 57:361

26. Estrin JA, Buckley JJ: Anesthetic management during liver transplantation. *In:* Manual of Vascular Access, Organ Donation, and Transplantation. Simmons RL, Finch ME, Ascher NL, et al (Eds). Springer-Verlag, New York, 1984, pp 285-291

27. Calne RY, Williams R: Liver transplantation. *Curr Probl Surg* 1979; 16:1

28. Calne RY (Ed): Liver Transplantation. New York, Grune & Stratton, 1983

29. Estrin JA, Belani K, Karnavas AG, et al: A new approach to massive blood transfusion during pediatric liver resection. *Surgery* 1986; 99:64

30. Fath JJ, Estrin J, Belani K, et al: Lactate metabolism during hepatic transplantation: Evidence for a perfusion-sensitive patient population. *Trans Proc* 1985; 17:284

31. Stock PG, Estrin JA, Fryd DS, et al: Early factors influencing early survival following liver transplantation. *Am J Surg,* In Press

32. Wall WJ, Grant DR, Duff JH, et al: Liver transplantation without venous bypass. *Transplantation* 1987; 43:251

33. Shaw B, Martin D, Marquez J, et al: Advantages of venous bypass during orthotopic transplantation of the liver. *Semin Liver Dis* 1985; 5:344

34. Kang Y, Lewis JH, Navalgund A, et al: Epsilon aminocaproic acid for treatment of fibrinolysis during liver transplantation. *Anesthesiology* 1987; 66:766

35. Krom RA, Gips CH, Newton D, et al: A successful start of a liver transplantation program. *Trans Proc* 1983; 15:1276

36. Pichlmayr R, Broelsch C, Newhaus P, et al: Report on 68 human orthotopic liver transplantations with special references to rejection phenomenon. *Trans Proc* 1983; 15:1279

37. Snover DL, Sibley RK, Freese DK: Orthotopic liver transplantation: A pathologic study of 63 serial liver biopsies natural history of rejection. *Hepatology* 1984; 4:1212

38. Stock P, Estrin JA, Payne W: Prognostic perioperative factors in outcome following liver transplantation. *Trans Proc* 1987; 19:2427

39. Dummer JS, Hardy A, Poosatter A, et al: Early infections in kidney, heart and liver transplant recipients on cyclosporine. *Transplantation* 1983; 36:259

40. Snover DC, Sibley RK, Freese DK: Orthotopic liver transplant rejection: A sequential liver biopsy study. *Transplantation* 1985; 17:272

Self-Assessment Questions

1. The criteria for brain death dictate there must be *irreversible* cessation of all functions of the entire brain. Which of the following potential conditions could mask underlying intact cerebral function?
   A. drug intoxication
   B. hypothermia
   C. subdural hematoma
   D. all of the above

2. Absolute contraindications to the organ utilization in hepatic transplantation include all of the following *except:*
   A. disseminated malignancy
   B. history of liver disease
   C. lung infection in patient receiving antibiotics
   D. hypoperfusion with rising liver enzymes

3. Frequently encountered problems in the maintenance of the closed-head injured donor include which of the following?
   A. hypotension
   B. hypertension
   C. diabetes insipidus
   D. hypoxemia
   E. all of the above

4. Transplantation for which of the following diseases has a high risk for reoccurrence in the transplanted organ?
   A. acute hepatitis B
   B. Wilson's disease
   C. tyrosinemia
   D. alpha$_1$-antitrypsin deficiency

5. The most frequent indication for transplantation in the pediatric population is:
   A. biliary atresia
   B. hepatoma
   C. neonatal hepatitis
   D. alpha$_1$-antitrypsin deficiency

6. Hepatic malignancy which has the best chance of long-term survival following liver transplantation is:
   A. primary hepatoma
   B. Klatskin tumor
   C. metastatic colon cancer
   D. fibrolamellar liver cancer

7. Pediatric patients transplanted for which of the following diseases are at increased risk for developing aplastic anemia?
   A. alpha-1-antitrypsin deficiency
   B. extrahepatic biliary atresia
   C. fulminant hepatitis
   D. tyrosinemia

8. Which of the following represents a strict contraindication to liver transplantation?
   A. small portal vein
   B. hepatorenal syndrome
   C. Budd-Chiari syndrome
   D. none of the above

9. Reperfusion coagulopathy may be managed with:
   A. protamine sulfate
   B. cryoprecipitate
   C. amicar
   D. all of the above

10. A severe metabolic alkalosis post-transplantation secondary to citrate in transfused blood is best managed by:
    A. HCl drip
    B. NaCl infusion
    C. K^+ supplement
    D. no intervention necessary

11. The most reliable diagnostic test for diagnosing rejection of the transplanted liver is:
    A. elevated temperature
    B. elevated bilirubin
    C. biopsy of the transplanted liver
    D. elevated liver function tests

Self-Assessment Answers

1. D	5. A	9. D
2. C	6. D	10. A
3. E	7. C	11. C
4. A	8. D	

Chapter 3

Pulmonary Transplantation

Thomas R. J. Todd, MD, FRCS(C)

Outline

Educational Objectives

In this chapter the reader will learn:

1. to understand the development of single lung transplantation and the rationale for its current success.

2. to appreciate the problems with the organ donor process.

3. to understand the criteria for donor lung acquisition.

4. to understand the care both pre and postoperatively of the lung transplant recipient.

Introduction

Following the first attempt at single lung transplantation in 1963 by Hardy et al. (1), considerable interest was not accompanied by appreciable success. In fact, despite some 44 transplants attempted prior to 1983, only one patient managed to be discharged from the hospital and that was for an extremely short period. The majority of patients succumbed within the first 30 days. Of those who survived the initial operative trauma, the most common cause of morbidity and subsequent mortality was bronchial anastomotic dehiscence or stenosis. It was assumed that this complication was the result of bronchial ischemia, in that the lung is transplanted without an oxygenated blood supply. Several other problems were identified as experience with the procedure grew. It was clear that sepsis in the contralateral native lung should preclude transplantation. In addition, it was felt that patients with emphysema should not undergo single lung transplantation, as ventilation/perfusion mismatching would be assured via maximal blood flow to the low-resistance transplanted lung and maximal ventilation to the compliant native lung. The frequency of postoperative complications dictated that the transplant team should have available all forms of respiratory support such as extracorporeal membrane oxygenation (ECMO) and high-frequency ventilation. As this decade arrived, interest in pulmonary transplantation had waned.

Our first experience with single lung transplantation in 1977 resulted in a fatal outcome on the 19th postoperative day secondary to bronchial anastomotic dehiscence. At autopsy, however, it became evident that the atrial suture line also demonstrated poor healing. It was thus felt that there might be a general impairment of wound healing. This then led to the hypothesis that the bronchial complications were related to: a) inadequate bronchial blood supply and b) poor wound healing induced by corticosteroid immunosuppression.

Experiments conducted by Lima and Cooper (2) demonstrated that in dogs receiving autotransplants, bronchial anastomotic healing could be successfully completed if steroids were not utilized. Autotransplanted dogs receiving cyclosporin immunosuppression had satisfactory healing of the bronchial anastomosis while those receiving corticosteroids not only had a greater incidence of bronchial complications, but also demonstrated a marked reduction in anastomotic breaking strength.

Further experiments in homografted dogs investigated the ability of pedicled omental grafts to re-establish bronchial artery blood flow when wrapped about the bronchial anastomosis. Within 4 days of transplantation, it was evident that the omental vessels had established a rich anastomotic communication with the bronchial circulation of the donor lung (3).

Successful human transplantation followed shortly thereafter. A single right lung transplant was performed on a 59-yr-old man with idiopathic pulmonary fibrosis. This recipient was O_2 dependant at rest and desaturated markedly and quickly on minimal exercise despite receiving 6 L/min of supplemental O_2. Corticosteroid administration was avoided for the first 3 wk and a pedicled omental graft was employed about the bronchial anastomosis. Four years later, this initial successful patient is alive and well, fully functional despite a ruptured abdominal aortic aneurysm that occurred 1 yr following his transplantation. Despite this and subsequent successes, there remained several problems in the expansion of the program.

As noted, single-lung transplantation was considered a viable option for patients with pulmonary fibrosis. However, for reasons noted above, patients with septic lung disease (bronchiectasis and cystic fibrosis), patients with emphysema, and patients with right ventricular failure were not considered eligible. Thus, an operation that would allow for transplantation of both lungs seemed desirable. Heart-lung transplantation did present a viable alternative; yet, it appeared unwarranted to transplant a heart into a recipient whose heart was normal, particularly when there was a considerable demand for donor hearts. In addition, the incidence of bronchiolitis obliterans following heart-lung transplantation is significant (4). The ability to transplant both lungs without the heart would allow patients with pulmonary sepsis and emphysema to undergo transplantation, while at the same time providing a donor heart for a second recipient requiring cardiac transplantation. Lastly, it had been observed that successful lung transplant recipients at 1 yr did not show signs of bronchiolitis obliterans.

Following several series of animal experiments (5), double-lung transplants seemed technically feasible. The first double-lung transplant was successfully undertaken in December, 1986.

Indications

It should be emphasized that the following statements reflect the state-of-the-art in September, 1987. All aspects of pulmonary transplantation are in a state of flux and will no doubt provide for many changes over the next several years.

The indications for single-lung transplantation are outlined in Table 1. At present, intubation and ventilation are considered to be contraindications for transplantation as associated tracheobronchitis, colonization of the airway, and pulmonary sepsis would likely lead to overwhelming sepsis in the immunocompromised recipient. As success with pulmonary transplantation continues, the role of double-lung transplantation in this group of patients will be assessed. Candidates must be O_2 dependent at rest and, despite supplemental O_2, must demonstrate desaturation with exercise. Their disease process must no longer be responsive to corticosteroids. The latter is particularly important so that prednisone may be avoided in the preoperative and immediate postoperative period. As one is contemplating single-lung transplantation, the disease process must first have resulted in pulmonary noncompliance without superimposed sepsis. It is wise to avoid the risk of leaving sepsis behind in the native lung postoperatively and to avoid the possibility of ventilating an overly compliant native lung instead of the transplanted lung. The latter precludes the role of single-lung transplantation in patients with emphysema.

Table 1. Indications for single-lung transplantation

Oxygen dependence at rest

Desaturation with exercise despite supplemental O_2

Unresponsiveness to corticosteroids (hence, ability to discontinue the drug)

No evidence of pulmonary sepsis

Right ventricular ejection fraction greater than 25%

Potential recipients enter a program of respiratory and nutritional rehabilitation. Respiratory muscle training is considered to be important to ensure a smooth postoperative course. Patients transplanted within days of entering the program have been more difficult to wean from ventilatory support despite excellent function of the graft. Most of the potential recipients are debilitated at the time of approval and have developed considerable loss of lean body mass.

The indications for double-lung transplantation involve the same degree of O_2 dependence in patients who have pulmonary sepsis or emphysema (Table 2).

Table 2. Indications for double-lung transplantation

O_2 dependence at rest

Desaturation with exercise despite supplemental O_2

Avoidance of corticosteroids

Pulmonary sepsis

Emphysema

Right ventricular ejection fraction less than 25%

Donor Criteria

Once brain death has been declared, donor lungs deteriorate rapidly. Not only is neurogenic pulmonary edema common, but pulmonary sepsis onsets rapidly and aggressively. In addition, cardiac dysfunction is common following brain death. Our own experience with young multiple-organ donors has revealed a significant incidence of impaired cardiac performance on 2-D echocardiography. There is experimental evidence to suggest that coronary artery vasospasm may occur with marked rises in intracranial pressure (6).

As a result, the criteria for accepting donor lungs must be scrupulous. A corollary to the above is that donor assessment should proceed rapidly to ensure that lung harvesting occurs before pulmonary dysfunction supervenes. Portable x-rays are obtained and must be clear. X-rays are repeated every 2 h while awaiting organ extraction. The vertical and horizontal measurements of the lungs are obtained from the portable chest film. The vertical dimension is taken somewhat obliquely from the apex of the thoracic cage to the dome of the diaphragm. The horizontal diameter is measured at the level of the diaphragmatic dome. If the diaphragms are not at the same level, the horizontal dimension is taken twice. These measurements are compared to similarly obtained values in the recipient, as the transplanted lungs must fit in a rigid box. Initially, it seemed imperative to ensure that the lungs were well matched size wise to prevent postoperative pleural spaces or, alternatively, to ensure that the donor lung was not compressed within the recipient thorax. If the donor lung is larger (greater than 3 cm in both dimensions) it is suggested that the single lung be transplanted into the left hemithorax. Any problems with proper fit can be overcome by the ability of the left hemidiaphragm to descend. The lungs of individuals waiting for single-lung transplantation are contracted, and the thoracic cage is smaller than predicted for the patient's height and weight. Thus, it is acceptable for the donor lung to be larger. As illustrated in Figures 1 and 2, the recipient readily adapts. However, caution should be exercised if the donor lung dimensions are 5 cm or greater in both vertical and horizontal dimensions.

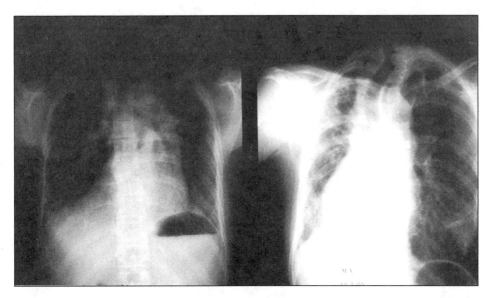

Fig. 1. The pre and postoperative x-rays of a patient receiving a single left lung transplant. Note how the chest has increased in size and how the diaphragm has descended to accommodate the oversized lung.

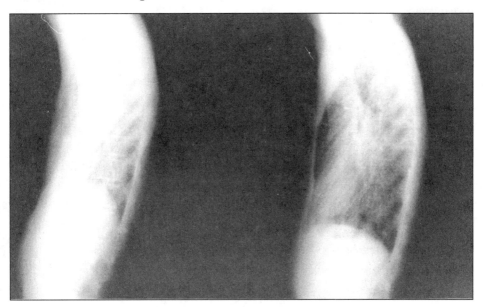

Fig. 2. The pre and postlateral film of the patient receiving a single left lung transplant. This patient had a markedly scaphoid chest with a pectus deformity. The chest has accommodated to the large lung.

Candidates for double-lung transplantation have expanded chest volumes. Smaller lungs are not only acceptable but desirable to ensure that the diaphragms may reassume a more normal and efficient contour. The rapid adjustment of the chest wall to smaller donor lungs is noted in Figure 3. Again, a note of caution — we do not, as yet, know the limitations imposed by the thoracic cavity; in general, one should be careful to secure lungs within 5 cm of the recipient measurements.

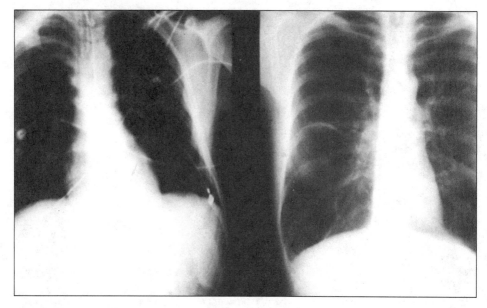

Fig. 3. The pre and postoperative chest x-rays of a patient receiving a double-lung transplant. Postoperatively, the chest has decreased in size and the diaphragm has ascended to accommodate the smaller lung.

Probably the most important assessment of the donor lungs is that obtained through arterial blood gases. The assessment is made on an F$_{IO_2}$ of 100% and 5 cm H$_2$O of PEEP. PaO$_2$ of 300 torr or greater is required. Arterial blood gas determinations are repeated frequently to ensure that function is maintained. We have witnessed PaO$_2$ fall from 375 torr to 75 torr within one hour due to the pulmonary complications associated with elevated intracranial pressure.

Bronchoscopy is routine. Visual assessment is more important in approving the donor for transplant than actual culture data. The presence of significant tracheobronchitis is a relative contraindication given the concerns over bronchial anastomotic healing. Secretions should be obtained for Gram stain and culture. Antimicrobial agents are administered to the donor and recipient based on the initial Gram stain. A bronchus blocker is passed through the glottis beside the endotracheal tube and under bronchoscopic guidance manipulated into the left main bronchus down to the lobar bifurcation. This is performed to facilitate lung preservation as will be noted below.

Lung Graft Preservation

The scarcity of organ donors has demanded that organ extraction be undertaken in hospitals distant from the transplant hospital. This has resulted in an increase in ischemic time and emphasizes the need for improved means of lung preservation. There are currently two methods employed for the preservation of lung grafts. The first involves external cooling of the lung with ice-cold Collins solution. External coolings should be facilitated by atelectasis and hence, the bronchus blocker in the left main bronchus is inflated prior to extraction. Cold Collins solution is instilled into the hemithorax and the lungs are transported in ice-cold Collins solution. We have preserved 16 lungs in this manner (7).

The second method of preservation involves the flushing of the pulmonary circulation with a cold solution that possesses either an intracellular or extra-cellular electrolyte mix. There is experimental evidence to suggest that various chemical substances such as PGE_1 or Verapamil may be of adjunctive value in preventing reperfusion lung injury. To date we have employed pulmonary flush with 3 to 4 L of cold Collins solution preceded by 500 μg PEG_1 in five cases. Each of these cases were also exposed to atelectasis and external cooling of the left lung as noted above.

Ischemic times in our experience have ranged from 2.5 to 5.5 h. Initial pulmonary dysfunction has occurred in three of our 21 patients. Two of these had short ischemic times as the lungs were locally extracted. One experienced a hyperacute rejection and the other (obtained from a drowning victim) developed overwhelming pseudomonas pneumonia. The third patient developed bilateral air space disease within 48 h, requiring maximum mechanical ventilatory support. In the latter case, the donor lungs were extracted at a distant site with the longest ischemic time of 5.5 h. Of these three patients, one succumbed (the patient receiving the graft from the drowning victim).

Postoperative Care

Immunosuppression

The mainstay of early immunosuppression has been antilymphocyte globulin (ALG). The patient is skin-tested against horse serum and, if nonreactive, ALG is commenced at an initial dose of 10 to 15 mg/kg body weight infused constantly over 24 h. The dose is monitored by daily determinations of the absolute lymphocyte count. The end-point of therapy is an absolute lymphocyte count of 75 to 110 × 10/mm. Values above or below this figure have demanded an adjustment of dose. The ALG is usually employed for 7 to 8 days, at which point cyclosporin levels are predictably in the therapeutic range.

Immuran is administered in an initial daily dose of 2 mg/kg body weight and thereafter in a dose of 1 mg/kg. A fall in leucocyte counts below 4,000 suggests that the dose should be reduced or the medication temporarily eliminated.

Cyclosporin is begun within 24 h of the patient returning to the ICU, usually in a dose of 300 mg twice daily via a nasogastric tube. All of these patients have undergone a small laparotomy in order that an omental pedicle might be mobilized into the chest. The incision and possible traction on the stomach have resulted in gastric ileus and stasis that may last for some 3 to 4 days. Thus, the development of adequate serum levels of cyclosporin is delayed. If therapeutic levels are delayed beyond the 4th day, Erythromycin (250 mg three times daily) administered either intravenously or orally accelerates the increase in cyclosporin levels by inhibiting the metabolism of the drug (8). Serum levels of 160 to 250 mg are desirable during the first 3 wk until corticosteroids are begun.

As indicated, corticosteroids are avoided during the first 3 wk in an effort to improve bronchial healing. By the end of the third week, prednisone (30 to 40 mg/day) is commenced and gradually decreased over the ensuing weeks to a maintenance dose of 10 to 15 mg daily. As noted above, immunosuppression is not without its complications. As a result, it is important to monitor absolute lymphocyte counts, total white cell counts, platelets, and serum cyclosporin levels. The onset of azotaemia should suggest a decrease in the dosage of cyclosporin irrespective of the serum level.

47

Table 3. Signs of pulmonary rejection

Fever

Hypoxemia - desaturation

Radiographic changes:

— Peri-hilar flare

— Homogeneous infiltrate

— Appearance of or increase in pleural effusion

The diagnosis of rejection is difficult and is often based more on clinical experience than on sound scientific data. In our experience, rejection onsets at least twice in the first 3 wk, usually around days 5 to 7 and/or days 11 to 14. This, along with the characteristics noted in Table 3, lead one to institute treatment with high-dose methylprednisolone in pulse therapy. The fever is usually low grade. When accompanied by a fall in O_2 saturation, a temperature of 37.4°C should alert the physician to the possibility of rejection. The desaturation and hypoxemia are occasionally out of keeping with the lack of radiographic evidence of parenchymal disease in the transplanted lung. However, the chest x-ray is usually abnormal, characterized by a hilar flare and/or a homogenous low-density interstitial infiltrate. Pleural effusions appear rapidly. Clearly, all these signs are also possible in pneumonia, although the hilar flare is not characteristic of infection. Nonetheless, this constellation of findings at the appropriate time has led us to administer 1 g methylprednisolone followed by 500 mg the following day. The administration of the steroid is not only therapeutic but is also diagnostic, as hypoxemia and infiltrates disappear within hours of initiating therapy. Quantitative perfusion scans are obtained by days 3 or 4 and subsequently every 5 days. The perfusion to the transplanted lung increases over the first month. A sudden decrease in perfusion, even without the signs noted in Table 3, is another indication for steroid administration; this usually results in a prompt restoration of flow to the transplanted lung.

Antibiotic Selection

As previously noted, the donor and recipient receive antibiotics based on the initial Gram stain of the donor bronchial secretions. These are discontinued 72 h later and further antimicrobials are added only upon the diagnosis of pneumonitis and the appropriate culture data.

Ventilation

Jet ventilation and ECMO are kept in reserve but are rarely (n = 2) necessary unless significant reperfusion injury becomes evident. The FIO_2 is kept as low as possible with the addition of PEEP and the initial of diuresis to return the patient to his or her preoperative weight. Depending on anesthetic reversal, graft preservation, fluid administration, and preoperative conditioning, weaning and extubation times will vary. In our experience, this usually occurs between days 2 and 5. The end-points of ventilatory support are the same as in any intensive care patient, i.e., to achieve the lowest FIO_2 and peak airway pressure (PAP) compatible with sufficient ventilation and oxygenation. FIO_2 should be less than .50. This can be achieved by several maneuvers. PEEP has been the mainstay of ventilatory support for 15 yr. However, excessive levels of PEEP may be deleterious to bronchial anastomotic healing if PAPs are elevated. As a result, it is important to recognize the role of diuresis in these volume-overloaded patients who also have impaired capillary permeability. Third, and particularly when single-lung transplantation has been performed, one should take advantage of the regional disparities in pulmonary artery flow distribution produced by postural changes. Depending on the adequacy of graft preservation, the native or the transplanted lung may participate more effectively in oxygenation. Thus, lying the patient on his or her side with the good lung dependent may improve ventilation/perfusion matching and allow one to lower the FIO_2. Similarly, the redirection of pulmonary artery flow can be achieved by pulmonary artery balloon catheters. Figure 4 demonstrates such a balloon catheter in place in the left pulmonary artery in a patient who has received a right lung transplant.

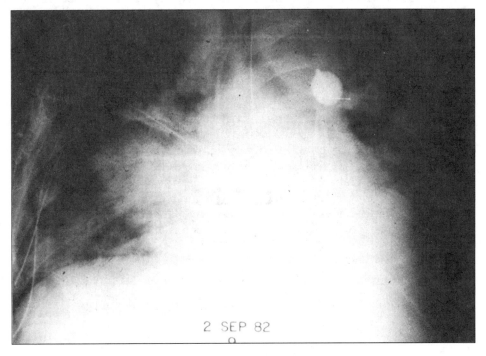

2 SEP 82

Fig. 4. A chest x-ray of a patient receiving a single-lung transplant. Note the dye in the pulmonary balloon catheter. The latter was used to divert pulmonary arterial blood flow to the appropriately functioning right lung.

PAP should be kept below 50 cm H_2O to prevent anastomotic damage and hemodynamic embarrassment. Minute ventilation can be maintained by increasing the rate and decreasing the tidal volume. Such maneuvers will lower the PAP and allow for the institution of further PEEP.

Hemodynamic Management

Inotropes (dopamine) are frequently required in the initial post-operative period, but are reduced to minimal doses (less than 5 μg/kg·min) by 24 h. Fluids are required in the first 24 h to keep abreast of third-space loses; if oliguria remains a problem, dopamine is maintained in order to favor renal cortical blood flow.

Double-lung transplantation requires cardiopulmonary bypass; yet, in our experience with 14 single-lung transplants, only three have required the support of partial femoral-femoral bypass. When bypass and concomitant anti-coagulation are required, three potential problems emerge. The first involves significant postoperative hemorrhage. Although usually controlled with reversal of heparinization (protamine) and transfusion of clotting factors (FFP, platelets, cryoprecipitate), the problem may be more severe than that encountered following heart or heart-lung transplantation (when the latter is undertaken for cardiac disease). Pulmonary disease frequently leads to the presence of numerous vascular adhesions which may become problematic when anti-coagulation ensues.

The second problem is the potential for cardiac tamponade should the chest drains become obstructed with fibrin or clot. Thus, careful and frequent monitoring of preload is essential. The third difficulty lies in the fact that following complete bypass (double-lung transplantation) left ventricular function may deteriorate either due to poor myocardial preservation or air embolism. For all these reasons, pulmonary artery catheterization is an integral part of postoperative management. This allows for frequent assessment of right ventricular and left ventricular preload, cardiac output and systemic vascular resistance.

After the first 24 h, the overriding objective is the maintenance of urine output with forced diuresis in an effort to return the patient to his or her preoperative weight. As pulmonary microvascular permeability will be altered for an indefinite amount of time, the reabsorption of third-space fluids results in continued pulmonary edema. This limits one's ability to wean the patient from mechanical assistance. As long as metabolic alkalosis is not problematic, oliguria beyond 24 h should be managed with furosemide unless the patient has already regained his or her preoperative weight and/or the preload is low (less than 18 torr).

Renal Function

Careful monitoring of BUN and creatinine are required in order that the combination of forced diuresis and cyclosporin therapy does not result in impaired renal function. A rise in serum creatinine dictates a re-evaluation of cyclosporin requirements and of intra-vascular volume.

Weaning

As indicated above, most patients have been involved in a rehabilitation program prior to transplantation. Those who have not have weaned slowly despite excellent graft function. An interesting observation in single-lung recipients has been the subjective sensation of dyspnea despite satisfactory tidal volume, muscle strength, and arterial blood gases. We have speculated that the subjective sensation is the result of abnormal afferent fiber traffic from stretch receptors in the native lung. The noncompliant native lung is poorly ventilated and becomes progressively atelectatic. The denervated transplanted lung provides no neural afferent information of sufficient ventilation. We have found that prior education of patients and their awareness of the phenomenon decreases the anxieties of early weaning. This hypothesis is supported by the fact that the phenomenon has not been witnessed in patients undergoing double-lung transplantation where both lungs are denervated.

Weaning is commenced as soon as possible. If negative inspiratory force is greater than −30 cm H$_2$O and vital capacity is greater than 700 ml we proceed immediately to a continuous positive airway pressure wean. If these values are less than ideal an intermittent mandatory ventilation wean is first attempted. Strong psychological support of these patients is important. Whether for the reasons noted above or because of the nature of their surgery, insomnia, agitation, and noncompliance are frequent. Constant reassurance and frequent explanation of procedures and progress has been a prerequisite for the successful weaning process. The insomnia has been particularly problematic. Lorazepam and Triazolam appear to offer the best and least complicated form of sedation.

Results

To date (September, 1987), we have performed 21 transplants (14 single and seven double). The mortality and long-term survival are noted in Table 4. There were three deaths in the single-lung group. One died of pseudomonas pneumonia 1 wk after receiving a donor lung from a drowning victim. The second died at 3 wk of inadvertent air embolism during the removal of a central venous line. The third developed early pulmonary artery hypertension and respiratory failure. A biopsy of the transplanted lung revealed typical features of primary pulmonary hypertension. The donor was 53 years of age, above the age recommended by our program. The single death following double-lung transplantation was the result of necrosis of the tracheal bronchial tree. A second desperate transplant was unsuccessful.

Table 4. Results of pulmonary transplantation

	No	Hospital Deaths	Strictures	Survival (months)
Single-lung	14	3	2	1-48
Double-lung	7	1	1	1-11

Long-term complications have fortunately been minimal. Two single recipients and one double recipient have bronchial strictures. All have been readily handled with the insertion of indwelling silicone stents. The patient with bronchial stenosis following double-lung transplantation is particularly interesting, as the strictures in the left main bronchus is some distance from the tracheal anastomosis. This has been observed by others following heart-lung transplantation and suggests that the left main bronchus may be the site of bronchovascular watershed. This observation will clearly require further observation and experimentation.

Bronchiolitis obliterans has yet to be observed. Two patients developed a vascular form of rejection proven at open lung biopsy. The first died of septic complications during augmented immunosuppression. The same patient was the only one unable to tolerate prophylactic septra and developed *Pneumocystis carinii*. The second patient is undergoing treatment. Lastly, one patient succumbed to generalized lymphoma at 1 yr following transplantation.

Interest in pulmonary transplantation has grown considerably. To our knowledge there have been successful single-lung transplants performed in Mississippi (n = 1), Houston (n = 2), Chicago (n = 2) and Birmingham, England (n = 1). With further improvement in surgical technique and immunosuppression long-term results should improve. The small donor pool is currently the rate-limiting step. Recently, we have developed techniques for simultaneous extraction of a heart for one recipient and a double-lung block for a second recipient. Thus, two patients may benefit from a single donor. The future, however, lies in the development of improved means of preservation of donor lungs. The latter will enable the donor pool to increase further so that fewer potential recipients will succumb to their disease while on waiting lists.

References

1. Hardy JD, Webb WR, Dalton ML, et al: Lung homotransplantation in man. *JAMA* 1963; 186:1865

2. Lima 0, Cooper JD, Peters WJ, et al: Effects of methylprednisolone and azathioprine in bronchial healing following lung autotransplantation. *J Thorac Cardiovasc Surg* 1981; 82:211

3. Dubois P, Choiniere L, Cooper JD, et al: Bronchial omentopexy in canine lung allotransplantation. *Ann Thorac Surg* 1984; 38:211

4. Burke CM, Slanville AR, Theodore J, et al: Lung immunogenecity, rejection and obliterative bronchiolitis. *Chest* 1987; 92:547

5. Patterson GA, Cooper JD, Goldman B, et al: Technique of successful clinical double lung transplantation. *Ann Thorac Surg* (In Press)

6. Shanlin RS, Sole MJ, Rahimifar M, et al: Increased intracranial pressure elicits hypertension, increased sympathetic activity, ECG abnormalities and myocardial damage in rats. *J Am Coll Cardiol* 1987 (Submitted)

7. Todd TRJ, Menkis AH, Koshal A, et al: Simultaneous extraction of heart and lungs for separate transplant recipients. *J Thorac Cardiovasc Surg* (Submitted)

8. Freeman DJ: Cyclosporin/erythromycin interaction in normal subjects. *Br J Clin Pharmacol* 1987; 23:776

Chapter 4

Heart-Lung Transplantation

Riyad Y. Tarazi, MD,
Robert S. Bonser, MB, BCh, MRCP(UK), FRCS(Eng),
and Stuart W. Jamieson, MB, BS, FRCS(Eng)

Outline

Educational Objectives

In this chapter the reader will learn:

1. the historical basis of heart-lung transplantation and the advances leading to the clinical reintroduction of this procedure.

2. to understand the basis of recipient and donor selection and the methods of maintaining donor organs in optimal condition prior to organ harvesting.

3. the principles of the donor and recipient operations and the controversies regarding preservation of the heart-lung bloc.

4. an understanding of early and late complications of heart-lung transplantation, their prevention, manifestations, and treatment.

Introduction

Heart-lung transplantation now provides a therapeutic option for patients with end-stage lung and heart disease. Its reintroduction into clinical practice has been predominantly due to the successful development of a primate model and the utilization of cyclosporin A as an immunosuppressive agent (1, 2). Cyclosporin A reduces the requirement for steroid therapy and its inherent problems in relation to tissue healing and infection. Cardiopulmonary transplantation is an evolving procedure; it is anticipated that improvements in perioperative mortality and overall clinical outcome will occur. Although long-term prognosis awaits further clinical experience, preliminary results are encouraging.

Historical Review

Experimental heart and lung transplantation was first performed by Demikhov in Russia in 1946 (3). Transplants were performed on dogs without the use of hypothermia or cardiopulmonary bypass by a careful sequence of anastomoses, allowing surgery to be accomplished with only a very short period of cerebral ischemia. Although only two of a total of 67 animals survived for a maximum of 5 days, this represented a remarkable achievement.

Further work in the canine model using central cooling and circulatory arrest led to survival periods of up to 22 h following the implantation (4, 5). In 1963 it was demonstrated that the denervation of both lungs was compatible with a normal respiratory pattern in primates, whereas in dogs complete pulmonary denervation led to an abnormal respiratory pattern incompatible with survival (6). This ability of primates but not dogs to survive bilateral lung denervation was confirmed by Nakae et al (7). Subsequently, Castaneda et al. (8, 9) were able to perform heart-lung autotransplantation in baboons with prolonged survival.

The first human heart-lung transplant operation was performed in 1968 by Cooley (10) in a 2-month-old infant with complete atrioventricular canal. Although it was observed that the child had spontaneous respiration postoperatively, the patient died 14 h after implantation due to respiratory insufficiency. In 1970 Lillehei (11) performed the second clinical heart-lung transplant in a 43-yr-old emphysematous patient who subsequently died of respiratory failure 8 days postoperatively.

In 1971, Barnard and Cooper (12) in Cape Town performed heart-lung transplantation in a patient with chronic obstructive airway disease with a survival period of 23 days. The disappointing early clinical experience with both lung and heart-lung transplantation confined further developmental work to the laboratory (13). A simplified operative method limiting the number of anastomoses performed was then developed, thus reducing the technical difficulties (14).

The discovery of cyclosporin A and investigation of its use as an immunosuppressive agent in heart transplantation allowed a reduction in the amount of steroids needed to prevent rejection and helped reduce tracheal anastomotic complications (2, 15). In addition, the demonstration of a collateral circulation originating from the coronary arteries, feeding the carinal region of the trachea via the adventitia of the great vessels, further reduced tracheal anastomotic problems (16). In single and double-lung transplantation, this collateral circulation is not preserved and further measures such as omental wrapping are necessary to secure tracheal or bronchial healing (17).

In 1980 Reitz et al. (1) reported successful auto and allo-heart-lung transplantation with extended survival in primates. Following these developments, clinical heart-lung transplantation was reintroduced at Stanford University in 1981 (18, 19).

Selection of Recipients

The major experience with heart-lung transplantation has been in end-stage cardiopulmonary disease (20). Pulmonary hypertension of either primary origin or secondary to the development of Eisenmenger's syndrome constitutes the largest recipient group (21). More recently, heart-lung transplantation has been successfully undertaken in patients with chronic parenchymal lung disease. Recent developments in single and double-lung transplantation may allow the application of these procedures in patients with chronic pulmonary conditions where right ventricular failure has not occurred (22, 23).

Recipients for heart-lung transplantation must have a severely restricted effort tolerance (New York Heart Association Class III or IV) leading to a poor quality of life, or a life expectancy < 1 yr. Apart from cardiopulmonary impairment, the general physical condition of the recipient should be well maintained without evidence of concurrent systemic disease. Younger patients (<45 yr) without secondary renal or hepatic dysfunction are likely to have a lower morbidity and mortality, and more successful rehabilitation.

Previous extensive thoracic or cardiac surgery is associated with a higher mortality because of the increased risk of intra and postoperative bleeding. Other contraindications include poorly controlled diabetes mellitus, collagen vascular disease, active peptic ulceration, systemic sepsis, or a bleeding diathesis not reversed by blood product administration. Careful psychologic assessment should be performed prior to acceptance of patients onto the transplant waiting list to ensure that potential recipients can cope with the prolonged hospitalization and intensive follow-up required. The presence of a supportive family structure is also important.

Donor Selection, Donor-Recipient Matching, and Donor Management

Selection of Donors

Clinical application of heart-lung transplantation is currently limited by the availability of suitable donors. Most organ donors are the victims of severe cranial trauma, or a catastrophic vascular or tumor-related cerebral insult. During the necessary period of ventilatory support, the lungs are susceptible to a number of complications including neurogenic pulmonary edema, fat embolism, infection, and atelectasis, thus making them unacceptable for transplantation. This susceptibility to lung injury reduces the number of potential donors to a fraction of those used for liver, kidney, and heart donation. More significant than this donor organ scarcity is the lack of reliable methods of long-term protection of the heart-lung bloc, thus limiting the use of distant organ procurement (24).

Donors must meet the criteria of brain death and be free of cardiac or pulmonary impairment by available history and physical examination. Currently, donor acceptance criteria include an age <35 yr, without evidence of a penetrating chest injury or lung contusion. The chest x-ray must show a normal heart size and clear lung fields, and the ECG should be normal. Ideally, shorter periods of ventilator support are desirable in order to reduce the possibility of exogenous bacterial and fungal contamination of the trachea and bronchi. There should be minimal nonpurulent tracheal aspirate. Peak inflation pressures should be <30 cm H_2O with a minute ventilation of 15 ml/kg at 8 breath/min. Adequate gas exchange is mandatory, with a Pa_{O_2} >100 torr on an F_{IO_2} of .40. If these criteria are fulfilled, attention is directed at matching the potential recipient to donor weight and size.

Matching of Donor and Recipient

Measurement of maximal thoracic diameter and the height of the thoracic cavity are compared between the donor and ABO-compatible recipients. Final matching will be performed by the donor harvesting team by superimposing donor and recipient chest x-rays comparing, albeit subjectively, thoracic cavity shape, and size. Ideally, the donor thorax should be slightly smaller than that of the recipient to avoid postoperative atelectasis secondary to size discrepancy. Retrospective recipient serum-donor lymphocyte cross-matching is performed for recipients without antileukocyte antibodies to pooled donor lymphocytes. Prospective cross-matching is necessary for antibody-positive recipients.

Donor Management

Once the potential donor is provisionally accepted for heart-lung donation, close liaison between the donating hospital and the transplant unit is continued in order to maintain the donor organs in optimal condition. The potential heart-lung recipient is admitted to the hospital and prepared for surgery. In addition, a size-matched ABO-compatible heart transplant recipient is also admitted in case the lungs are found by the harvesting team to be unsuitable for transplantation and only cardiac transplantation can be performed. Central venous and arterial pressure lines are inserted into the donor, who is placed on a warming blanket to prevent hypothermic deterioration of cardiac function. Every effort is made to keep the CVP as low as possible by fluid restriction and diuresis, as long as hemodynamic stability is maintained. Intravenous fluid administration is kept to a minimum in order to minimize any hydrostatic contribution to the development of neurogenic pulmonary edema. If excessive urine output occurs due to diabetes insipidus, vasopressin or desmopressin administration may be required. Fluid replacement should consist of Ringer's lactate at a volume to replace the previous hour's urine output plus 30 to 50 ml to cover insensible losses. Hemodynamic instability due to diuresis-induced hypovolemia should be partly corrected by fluid replacement and partly by manipulation of the peripheral vascular resistance using the alpha-adrenergic agonists phenylephrine or metaraminol.

In order to prevent spillover of gastroesophageal contents or oropharyngeal secretions into the airways, a nasogastric sump tube is inserted and connected to low-pressure wall suction. Careful attention is directed to clearing pulmonary secretions with regular gentle aspiration via the endotracheal tube. Retrieved aspirate is sent for culture and direct examination, and the results are communicated to the recipient unit when they become available.

The donor should be intubated with a large-bore, low-pressure cuff, endotracheal tube connected to a volume cycle ventilator. Tube position should be confirmed by x-ray. A PEEP of 3 to 5 cm H_2O is maintained to help prevent atelectasis, and the FIO_2 is kept at .40 or lower to maintain a PO_2 >100 torr.

With careful attention to the above details, potential donor organs can be maintained in satisfactory condition for several days, although the likelihood of pulmonary complications increases with the total period of ventilation. The final decision regarding the suitability of donor organs rests with the harvesting team. If thoracic size matching is satisfactory and acceptance criteria are fulfilled, the lungs are inspected directly via a median sternotomy for pleural adhesions, consolidation, or other pathology. If satisfactory, the recipient hospital is contacted, and donor and recipient operations are coordinated in order to minimize total ischemic times.

The Donor Operation

The donor operation is coordinated with other organ procurement teams. Following inspection of the heart and lungs via a median sternotomy, circumferential mobilization of the innominate vein, aorta, and superior and inferior vena cava is performed. The thymic fat pad is removed, and the pericardium is resected down to the level of the pulmonary veins including removal of the phrenic nerves. The trachea is exposed between the superior vena cava and ascending aorta. Following this, other organ procurement teams will mobilize the abdominal organs for transplantation. At the time of harvesting, heparin (3 mg/kg iv) is administered, and infusion lines for the pulmonary artery flushing solution and for cardioplegia are placed in the main pulmonary artery and aorta, respectively. Following heparinization, the innominate vein and superior vena cava are ligated and divided. The inferior vena cava is clamped above the diaphragm and the heart is allowed to empty. The distal ascending aorta is cross-clamped and cold cardioplegia solution (1000 ml) is instilled into the aortic root. Pulmonary artery flushing is commenced with 60 ml/kg of modified Collins solution infused into the main pulmonary artery over a period of 3 to 4 min. This is facilitated by the use of a single roller pump. Once pulmonary artery flushing and cardioplegic instillation are begun, the tip of the left atrial appendage is removed and the inferior vena cava is divided above the clamp to adequately vent the heart. Additional topical cooling with copious amounts of 4°C cold Ringer's lactate solution aids the induction of hypothermia. Occasional manual ventilation is continued during pulmonary artery flushing using unheated room air. After completion of infusion, the aorta is transected below the cross-clamp. The trachea is mobilized and stapled with the lungs held in the position of 50% inflation. Heart-lung harvesting is then completed by division of the posterior pleural reflections and pulmonary ligaments anterior to the esophagus. The organs are transferred to a container containing cold Ringer's solution which is then sealed and stored in a similar sterile container. These are then transferred into an insulated, sealed transportation box containing 4°C cold electrolyte solution mixed with ice.

Recipient Operation

Removal of Recipient Heart and Lungs

The diseased heart and lungs are excised separately in order to protect the phrenic nerves (25). The operation proceeds via a median sternotomy. Pleural and pericardial adhesions are divided prior to heparinization and the thymic fat pad excised, avoiding injury to the phrenic nerves, to expose the great vessels. Following the administration of heparin (300 U/kg body weight), cardiopulmonary bypass is established using bicaval cannulation and high ascending aortic return. The caval tapes are then snared, the aorta is cross-clamped, and the heart is allowed to fibrillate. The excision of the heart is performed at the level of the atrioventricular junction and just above the arterial valves. A substantial atrial cuff is left in situ, the left atrial remnant of which is later excised during the bilateral pneumonectomy. Attention is next directed to the left lung which is exposed following an incision in the pericardium just anterior to the pulmonary veins and posterior to the phrenic nerve. The lung is drawn into the middle of the chest behind the phrenic nerve and the pulmonary artery is divided, leaving a button of pulmonary artery wall in the region of the arterial ligament. The left atrium is divided vertically in the oblique sinus, allowing removal of the left pulmonary veins. The left main bronchus is identified, the bronchial arteries are controlled by cautery or clips, the bronchus is stapled and divided, and the lung is removed. The right lung is excised in a similar manner, leaving the tracheobronchial junction, aorta, and right atrium for subsequent anastomoses. Most of the posterior pericardium is preserved to reduce postoperative bleeding. Meticulous hemostasis of the posterior mediastinum is performed at this time, avoiding damage to the vagus nerve.

Implantation of Donor Organs

The donor organs are removed from their storage container and transferred to the operative field. Specimens for culture are aspirated from donor and recipient trachea. The recipient trachea is trimmed one ring above the carina and the bronchial stumps are excised. The donor trachea is divided at a similar level and anastomosed using a single continuous suture technique. The lungs are then placed in their respective cavities below the phrenic nerve pedicles. During implantation, the heart and lungs are protected by continuous irrigation with cold electrolyte solution. The right atrial and aortic anastomoses are next performed after trimming the donor aorta to a suitable length and opening the donor's right atrium to accommodate the anastomosis.

Following completion of the anastomoses, the heart is de-aired, ventilation restarted, and the aortic cross-clamp removed. Upon completion of the rewarming and resumption of cardiac action, cardiopulmonary bypass is discontinued with the patient ventilated on an F_{IO_2} of .40, with 5 cm H_2O of PEEP and an isoproterenol infusion to maintain the heart rate at 100 to 120 beat/min. Following satisfactory hemostasis, the chest is closed with mediastinal and pleural drainage.

Heart-Lung Preservation

Satisfactory protection of donor hearts has been achieved using cardioplegic arrest with topical cooling; this is found to be suitable for distant procurement and medium-term preservation (26). In experimental attempts to preserve donor heart-lung blocs, attention has been directed predominantly to the ischemic and reperfusion damage to the lungs, as they appear to be more sensitive than solid organs. Injury to the lungs may occur as a consequence of denervation, loss of lymphatic drainage, surgical manipulation, ischemia, and reperfusion injury of the ischemic organ. During donor organ removal, surgical manipulation is kept to a minimum but little can be done about the effects of denervation and lymphatic division. During harvesting and implantation, O_2 concentrations are kept to the minimum necessary to maintain adequate tissue O_2 delivery in order to reduce possible O_2 toxicity to the donor lungs. Prolonged warm ischemia of the lung or other inadequate preservation technique results in interstitial and intra-alveolar edema, rupture of the alveolar-capillary membrane, and hemorrhage into the interstitium and alveoli (27).

Methods of donor lung preservation have been developed in two ways, first by metabolic maintenance and second by metabolic inhibition. An autoperfusing working heart-lung preparation has been used by some workers (28, 29). This system utilizes the beating heart as a pump for perfusing the lungs during storage. In addition, cyclic ventilation via the trachea is used to maintain oxygenation. A heat exchanger is necessary within the circuit, which must be constantly observed to monitor any deterioration. In addition, nutrients may be added to the heparinized circuit to maintain aerobic metabolism of the organ bloc. This technique has been used successfully in some clinical cases but is clearly complex and cumbersome, and is no longer in active use.

The majority of centers have concentrated on the inhibition of metabolism by the induction of hypothermia during transport and storage. Surface cooling alone appears unsatisfactory as a preservation method, as the lung is an excellent thermal insulator (30). Hypothermic flushing of the lungs via the pulmonary artery has produced good protection for over 4 h in primates and has been used successfully clinically at our institution (31, 32).

The optimal composition of the pulmonary artery perfusate remains unclear (33). Certainly, cardioplegic-type solutions, although satisfactory for myocardial preservation, yield very poor results in experimental lung preservation, and attention has centered around the use of a modified Collin's solution that was used successfully in renal allograft preservation. This solution, which has an intracellular-type composition, is modified by the addition of 50% dextrose (65 ml/L of solution) and magnesium sulfate (8 mEq) added to increase osmolarity and preserve membrane integrity. This solution has been used clinically as a cold pulmonary artery flush with successful results for ischemic times of up to 4 h.

Whole-donor cooling using cardiopulmonary bypass is a second way of achieving lung hypothermia with or without pulmonary artery flushing (34). Once cardiopulmonary bypass is established, cooling to around 12°C may be achieved within 18 to 48 min of the onset of bypass. At this temperature, the organs are harvested and stored in cold donor blood without further preparation. Preservation times of up to 4 h again appear to be satisfactory using this method. This core cooling technique is attractive because experimental work suggests that cooling with normokalemic whole blood results in satisfactory lung preservation for over 12 h (35). Unfortunately, the technique is noticeably more cumbersome than a simple pulmonary artery flush, and requires more personnel in the harvesting team and additional equipment. In addition, the effect of core cooling on other organs to be harvested remains unknown. A further concern is that cardiopulmonary bypass may itself lead to some degree of lung injury mediated by the complement system, which is activated by the polymers of the extracorporeal circuit (36). Complement activation leads to the stimulation of circulating neutrophils which subsequently sequester within the pulmonary circulation and may lead to lung injury (37).

Currently, both simple hypothermic pulmonary artery flushing and core cooling techniques are in clinical usage, and allow limited periods for organ transport and storage. The simplicity of hypothermic flushing of the lungs via the pulmonary artery has led to the routine use of this technique at our institution.

Postoperative Care

Immediate Postoperative Management

This consists essentially of care similar to that routinely used after cardiac surgery. Ventilation is maintained with a low FIO_2 (less than .40). The patient is allowed to wake from anesthesia and is weaned from the ventilator within the first 24 to 48 h postoperatively. The chronotropic actions of isoproterenol are often required immediately after surgery to maintain the heart rate at 100 to 120 beat/min. Postoperative hypertension is controlled by sodium nitroprusside infusion. During surgery, pump priming volumes and intravenously administered fluids are kept to a minimum. In the early postoperative period, fluid maintenance is carefully monitored and a diuresis is induced using intravenous furosemide. Chest drains are usually kept in place for at least 48 h because of the increased drainage associated with posterior mediastinal dissection.

Antibiotics

Broad-spectrum systemic antibacterial coverage, currently using cephamandole and nafcillin, is commenced at anesthetic induction. Antibiotics are continued until the chest drains are removed. Following extubation, oral "swish and swallow" nystatin and low-dose cotrimoxazole are commenced in order to provide prophylaxis against oral candida and pulmonary pneumocystis infestation.

Precautions are taken to avoid opportunistic infection. Reverse-barrier nursing, ideally in specially constructed cubicles with a bacterially filtered positive-pressure system, is continued while the patient remains in the ICU. Subsequently, protection is afforded by restricting patient visiting to close relatives and attending personnel. When the patients are fully ambulatory, they are allowed out of their rooms and need only to wear a protective mask while walking around the hospital. Careful surveillance for infection continues throughout their postoperative course (38).

Pulmonary Care

While intubated, pulmonary toilet is performed using soft suction catheters. Sputum accumulation in the denervated lung will not excite coughing and chest physiotherapy is required to aid expectoration. Early extubation, within the first 24 to 48 h, is aimed for; following this, vigorous physiotherapy and breathing exercises are commenced as soon as the patient is able to cooperate. Once ambulant, the patients begin a structured rehabilitation program including increasing distances of walking and cycle ergonometry. Self-administered breathing exercises and expectoration procedures are continued after discharge.

Immunosuppressive Management

The immunosuppressive protocols for heart-lung transplantation continue to evolve. It is our current practice to use cyclosporin A and azathioprine beginning preoperatively. A single dose of cyclosporin A (6 mg/kg) is given before transfer to the operating room; this is continued in the postoperative period in two divided doses. The cyclosporin A dose is adjusted according to whole-blood trough levels, which are measured daily, until a level of 200 ng/ml is maintained. Cyclosporin monitoring is continued on a twice-weekly basis for the first month and less frequently thereafter. Renal and hepatic dysfunction must be closely monitored to limit drug-induced toxicity. Azathioprine (2.5 mg/kg orally) is also administered prior to surgery; this dose is continued postoperatively. Adjustment may be necessary if the WBC count falls below 5,000/mm³.

In contrast to our heart transplant immunosuppressive protocol, oral steroids are not commenced until 2 wk postoperatively. Methylprednisolone (500 mg iv) is given prior to reperfusion of the implanted organs and a further 375 mg is administered in three divided doses over the first 24 h. Oral prednisone is introduced 2 wk postoperatively at a dose of 0.2 mg/kg·day.

Early Postoperative Complications

Rejection

The mainstay of rejection diagnosis following heart-lung transplantation is by radiologic examination of the lungs. Initial impressions that lung and heart rejection occurred simultaneously and that rejection could be monitored by endomyocardial biopsy have not been proven (39). Asynchronous rejection may occur with pulmonary rejection preceding myocardial changes. Therefore, the endomyocardial biopsy may not have an important role in rejection surveillance. The typical features of pulmonary rejection include fever, hypoxia, and increasing (sometimes asymmetrical) opacification of the lungs on chest x-ray (40). The general condition of the patient may remain extremely satisfactory during rejection and appear inconsistent with the radiographic changes. The diagnosis is confirmed by exclusion of pulmonary infection, by negative bacterial, viral and fungal cultures of expectorated sputum or bronchoscopically obtained specimens, and by the response to antirejection therapy.

Treatment of rejection must be individualized for each patient. Concern regarding tracheal healing and the effects of steroids argue against large-dose bolus steroid therapy in the early postoperative period. Initially, attempts are made to optimize nonsteroidal immunosuppression by increasing the dose of cyclosporin to ensure adequate circulating levels. Low-dose prednisone administration (0.2 mg/kg) may be begun. If these measures are not accompanied by rapid clinical improvement, bolus methylprednisolone (1 g iv daily for 3 days) is administered. In refractory cases, antilymphocyte globulin may be added, with the aim of reducing the T-lymphocyte count to 5% of total lymphocytes.

Implantation Response

A second cause of a diffuse pulmonary infiltrate in the postoperative period is the so-called implantation response (41). This is believed to be due to the effects of denervation and loss of lymphatic drainage, and is associated with an afebrile illness accompanied by tachypnea, loss of compliance, impaired gas exchange, and elevated pulmonary vascular resistance. This response usually occurs within the first 3 days postoperatively and may be related to inadequate preservation.

The clinical picture is difficult to differentiate from infection or rejection, requiring intensive investigation to exclude these including, on occasion, a trial of antirejection medication. Management of this condition hinges on the production of dehydration by aggressive diuresis, which may be limited by renal impairment and hypovolemic low cardiac output. Hemofiltration to reduce fluid overload may be necessary. During this period, adequate nutrition and maintenance of serum protein levels may help reduce edema.

Renal Failure

Some degree of renal dysfunction perioperatively is seen in the majority of patients. Severe renal dysfunction requiring hemofiltration or hemodialysis is seen in up to 30% of recipients. This high renal complication rate is due to a combination of factors including the use of high-dose cyclosporin, postoperative dehydration to prevent the implantation response, and the use of nephrotoxic agents such as aminoglycoside antibiotics. Careful attention to urinary output and serum creatinine levels, and adjusted doses of potentially nephrotoxic agents may deter renal dysfunction, but occasionally a period of reversible renal dysfunction has to be tolerated in order to salvage a patient from pulmonary edema due to any cause.

Bleeding

The presence of large collateral bronchial vessels and a coagulopathy in cyanotic patients potentiates the risk of postoperative bleeding. A previous thoracotomy with its consequent adhesions is a relative contraindication to heart-lung transplantation. These potential problems are anticipated during surgery and every effort made to secure primary hemostasis. All dissection is performed with electrocautery; the majority of the posterior pericardium is preserved to reduce the amount of dissection. Fresh frozen plasma, cryoprecipitate, and platelets are transfused after discontinuation of bypass and the administration of protamine to correct abnormalities in the coagulation profile. Reoperation is occasionally necessary, although inspection of the posterior mediastinum may be impossible once the donor organs have been implanted.

Nerve Injury

The phrenic, vagus, and left recurrent laryngeal nerves are at risk during the procedure and special care is taken to protect them. The phrenic nerves are maintained on ribbons of pericardium but a transient injury may occur as a consequence of nerve stretching during removal or reimplantation of the lungs beneath the phrenic pedicle. A button of pulmonary artery wall is left in situ in the region of the arterial ligament to protect the recurrent laryngeal nerve. The vagus nerve, lying on the esophagus, is identified and protected during cautery hemostasis of the posterior mediastinum. In addition, preservation of the posterior pericardium reduces vagal trauma.

Tracheal Anastomotic Problems

Bronchial healing is a major source of concern following single or double-lung transplantation; additional techniques such as bronchial omentopexy are required to secure healing (17). In heart-lung transplantation, tracheal anastomotic dehiscence is far less common although no less serious. Improved healing of the tracheal anastomosis in heart-lung transplantation is thought to be due to the reduced use of steroids and the presence of coronary-bronchial collaterals supplying the carinal region of the donor trachea.

Late Postoperative Management

Following discharge from the hospital, patients are reviewed twice weekly in order to adjust immunosuppression and to provide continued surveillance for infection and rejection. Frequent chest x-rays, and hematological and biochemical profiles are performed along with serial pulmonary function tests. This intensive follow-up is gradually eased after the first month; by 1 yr postoperatively, only 3 monthly clinic visits may be necessary.

By 3 months, patients tend to be well rehabilitated and if stable, will be allowed to return to their homes. In the early post-transplant period, pulmonary function tests show a restrictive ventilatory defect which improves slowly over the first 12 months. More ominously, a mixed obstructive and restrictive airway picture may develop at any time between 6 wk and 2 yr post-transplant; this signifies the development of a panbronchitis which can progress to an obliterative bronchiolitis and bronchiectasis (42). This condition, which is also a complication of bone marrow transplantation but not other organ grafts, is of unknown etiology but may represent an abnormal response to viral infection, chronic rejection, or another host-versus-graft reaction. Once established, the condition tends to deteriorate inexorably although early diagnosis and treatment by high-dose steroids may lead to its reversal or arrest (43). Symptomatically, patients present with a new cough or dyspnea. Examination reveals audible coarse crackles and occasional rhonchi. Investigation demonstrates hypoxemia and a mixed obstructive-restrictive ventilatory defect on pulmonary function tests. Chest radiography and sputum culture allow infection to be excluded. The x-ray is usually clear, although peribronchial thickening and lower zone micronodular opacities may be seen. Treatment is by augmentation of oral steroids and subsequently by more intense monitoring of possible infectious complications. In late irreversible disease, retransplantation may be necessary. Other late complications in common with heart transplantation include hypertension, weight gain, opportunistic infection, and progressive cyclosporin nephrotoxicity. Hypertension is managed by careful control of cyclosporin levels, diuretics, and vasodilator therapy. Beta blockade is avoided because of its bronchospastic effects, and negative chronotropy and inotropy.

Clinical Results

Perioperative Mortality

Of the initial 28 patients undergoing heart-lung transplantation at Stanford University, 28% died within the first 30 postoperative days (44). More recently, the International Registry of Heart Transplantation has collated data from 14 world centers regarding 163 heart-lung transplant recipients (Kaye MP, personal communication). World-wide, an early operative mortality of 40% has been experienced. Early death is associated with prolonged periods of cardiopulmonary bypass and extensive hemorrhage. Previous extensive cardiac or thoracic surgery has a particular increased risk because of the presence of pleural and pericardial adhesions responsible for major blood loss. Additional deaths are related to opportunistic infection, predominantly bacterial, leading to systemic sepsis and multiple organ failure. Distant organ procurement appears to be associated with an increased mortality; this is related to difficulty in ensuring adequate lung preservation.

Late Results

One-year survival in the original Stanford series was 64%, falling to 55% at 3 yr (44). Data from the International Registry for Heart Transplantation has shown an actuarial 1-yr survival world-wide of 55.4%, falling to 51.9% at 2 yr (Kaye MP, personal communication). Comparison of results between centers is difficult because the patient populations are not homogenous. There is no standardization of patient selection, organ procurement and preservation protocols, operative techniques, and postoperative management. Detailed analysis of results from each center is awaited.

Of the patients surviving the perioperative period in the Stanford series, nearly one-third developed late disability as a consequence of obliterative bronchiolitis (42). As previously indicated, the etiology of this condition remains obscure. It follows an unremitting downhill course over a period of 6 months to 2 yr unless detected early and treated with high-dose steroids, which may lead to partial or complete reversal. In patients free of this condition, a restrictive ventilatory defect persists which is probably related to postoperative chest-wall splinting rather than interstitial lung disease (45). Exercise is encouraged and is associated with normal ventilatory changes.

The cardiac response to exercise is limited, as it is in heart transplantation, by the dependance of the denervated heart on circulating catecholamines and increased venous return to increase cardiac output in response to exertion (46). These changes are fully compatible with a physically active life in the rehabilitated recipient. Progressive intimal proliferation occurs in the coronary and pulmonary arteries of the heart-lung transplant. Eventually, cardiac failure and myocardial infarction can be anticipated in some recipients (47, 48).

Future

Following successful heart-lung transplantation, the quality of life of recipients is greatly improved. The technique offers great promise as a treatment of end-stage lung and heart disease. Further progress is necessary in a number of areas in order to reduce postoperative morbidity and mortality, and to increase the application of this form of therapy.

Careful recipient selection will help reduce perioperative mortality by excluding patients with previous extensive cardiothoracic surgery and with severe concurrent systemic disease. Wider application of the technique will depend upon the supply of donors. Increasing public awareness may increase the number of donors available; more importantly, improvement in protection methods for the heart-lung bloc will enable maximal utilization of the present donor pool. The diagnosis of rejection and its differentiation from an infection or implantation process remains difficult. Studies of bronchial-alveolar lavage cell content are not sufficiently sensitive or specific at present, and further research is required into the diagnostic differentiation of the postoperative pulmonary infiltrate (49).

Alternatives to cyclosporin A are required for maintenance immunosuppression to prevent the long-term nephrotoxic consequences of the use of this drug.

Further investigation is also needed into the prevention and treatment of obliterative bronchiolitis. In addition, long-term survival can be anticipated to be adversely affected by coronary arterial intimal proliferation in common with heart transplant recipients; as yet, no answer to this has been found. If some of these problems can be overcome, the outlook for heart-lung transplantation is extremely encouraging.

References

1. Reitz BA, Burton NA, Jamieson SW, et al: Heart and lung transplantation: Auto-and allo-transplantation in primates with extended survival. *J Thorac Cardiovasc Surg* 1980; 80:360

2. Borel JF, Feurer C, Gubles HU, et al: Biological effects of cyclosporin A: A new antilymphocytic agent. *Agents and Action* 1976; 6:468

3. Demikhov VP: Some essential points of the techniques of transplantation of the heart, lungs and other organs. Medgiz State Press for Medical Literature in Moscow 1960, p 29. Translated from Russian by Basil Haigh, Consultant's Bureau, New York, 1962

4. Neptune WB, Cookson BA, Bailey CP, et al: Complete homologous heart transplantation. *Arch Surg* 1983; 66:174

5. Webb WR, Howard HS: Cardiopulmonary transplantation. *Surg Forum* 1957; 8:313

6. Haglin J, Telander RL, Muzzal RE, et al: Comparison of lung autotransplantation in the primate and dog. *Surg Forum* 1963; 14:196

7. Nakae S, Webb WR, Theodorides J, et al: Respiratory function following cardiopulmonary denervation in dog, cat and monkey. *Surg Gynecol Obstet* 1967; 128:1288

8. Castaneda AR, Arnar O, Schmidt-Habelman P, et al: Cardiopulmonary autotransplantation in primates. *J Cardiovasc Surg* 1972; 37:523

9. Castaneda AR, Zamora R, Schmidt-Habelman P, et al: Cardiopulmonary autotransplantation in primates (baboons): Late functional results. *Surgery* 1972; 72:1064

10. Cooley DA, Bloodwell RD, Hallman GL, et al: Organ transplantation for advanced cardiopulmonary disease. *Ann Thorac Surg* 1969; 8:30

11. Lillehei CW: In discussion of Wildevuur CRH, Benfield JRA. A review of 23 human lung transplantations by 20 surgeons. *Ann Thorac Surg* 1970; 9:495

12. Barnard CN, Cooper DKC: Clinical transplantation of the heart: A review of 13 years personal experience. *J R Soc Med* 1981; 74:670

13. Wildevuur CRH, Benfield JRA: A review of 23 human lung transplantations by 20 surgeons. *Ann Thorac Surg* 1970; 9:489

14. Reitz BA, Pennock JL, Shumway NE: Simplified operative method for heart and lung transplantation. *J Surg Research* 1981; 31:1

15. Oyer PE, Stinson EB, Jamieson SW, et al: Cyclosporine A in cardiac allografting: A preliminary experience. *Transplant Proc* 1983; 18:1247

16. Ladowski JS, Hardesty RL, Griffith BP: Pulmonary artery blood supply to the supracarinal trachea. *Heart Transplantation* 1984; 4:40

17. Lima O, Goldberg M, Peters WJ, et al: Bronchial omentopexy in canine lung transplantation. *J Thorac Cardiovasc Surg* 1982; 83:418

18. Jamieson SW, Stinson ER, Oyer PE, et al: Heart-lung transplantation for irreversible pulmonary hypertension. *Ann Thorac Surg* 1984; 38:554

19. Jamieson SW, Reitz BA, Oyer PE, et al: Combined heart and lung transplantation. *Lancet* 1983; i:1130

20. Starnes VA, Jamieson SW: Current status of heart and lung transplantation. *World J Surg* 1986; 10:442

21. Kaye MP: The Registry of the International Society for Heart Transplantation: Fourth Official Report - 1987. *J Heart Transplant* 1987; 6:63

22. Cooper JD, Pearson FG, Patterson GA, et al: Technique of successful lung transplantation in humans. *J Thorac Cardiovasc Surg* 1987; 93:173

23. Dark JH, Patterson GA, Al-Jilaihawai AN, et al: Experimental en-bloc double-lung transplantation. *Ann Thorac Surg* 1986; 42:394

24. Jamieson SW, Starkey T, Sakakibara N, et al: Procurement of organs for combined heart-lung transplantation. *Transplant Proc* 1986; 18:616

25. Jamieson SW, Stinson EB, Oyer PE, et al: Operative technique for heart-lung transplantation. *J Thorac Cardiovasc Surg* 1984; 87:930

26. Thomas FT, Szenpeterey SS, Mammana RE, et al: Long distance transportation of human hearts for transplantation. *Ann Thorac Surg* 1978; 26:344

27. Veith FJ, Crane R, Torres M, et al: Effective preservation and transportation of lung transplants. *J Thorac Cardiovasc Surg* 1976; 72:97

28. Ladowski JS, Kapelanski DP, Teodori MF, et al: Use of autoperfusion for distant procurement of heart-lung allograft preservation prior to heart-lung transplantation. *Heart Transplantation* 1985; 4:330

29. Teodori MF, Stevenson WC, Ladowski JS, et al: Autoperfusing heart-lung preparation for preservation in heart-lung transplantation. *Surg Forum* 1985; 36:331

30. Scheuler S, Warnecke H, Hetzer R, et al: The limits of cold ischemia for preservation of the lung. *Heart Transplantation* 1984; 4:70

31. Starkey TD, Sakakibara N, Hagberg RC, et al: Successful six-hour cardiopulmonary preservation with simple hypothermic crystalloid flush. *J Heart Transplant* 1986; 8:291

32. Reichart BA, Novitzky D, Cooper DK, et al: Successful orthotopic heart-lung transplantation in the baboon after five hours of cold ischemia with cardioplegia and Collin's solution. *J Heart Transplant* 1987; 6:15

33. Haverich A, Scott WG, Jamieson SW: Twenty years of lung preservation - A review. *Heart Transplantation* 1985; 4:234

34. Hardesty RL, Griffith BP: Procurement for combined heart-lung transplantation: Bilateral thoracotomy with sternal transection, cardiopulmonary bypass and profound hypothermia. *J Thorac Cardiovasc Surg* 1985; 89:798

35. Modry DL, Walpoth BW, Cohen RG, et al: Heart-lung preservation in the dog followed by lung transplantation: A new model for the assessment of lung preservation. *Heart Transplantation* 1985; 2:287

36. Kirklin JK, Westaby S, Blackstone EH, et al: Complement and the damaging effects of cardiopulmonary bypass. *J Thorac Surg* 1983; 8:45

37. Till GO, Johnson KJ, Kinkel R, et al: Intravascular activation of complement and acute lung injury. *J Clin Invest* 1982; 69:1126

38. Brooks RG, Hofflin JM, Jamieson SW, et al: Infectious complications of heart-lung transplant recipients. *Am J Med* 1985; 79:412

39. McGregor CGA, Baldwin JC, Jamieson SW, et al: Isolated pulmonary rejection after combined heart and lung transplantation. *J Thorac Cardiovasc Surg* 1985; 90:623

40. Reitz BA, Gaudiani VA, Hunt SA, et al: Diagnosis and treatment of allograft rejection in heart-lung transplant recipients. *J Thorac Cardiovasc Surg* 1983; 85:354

41. Siegelman SS, Sinha SB, Veith FJ: Pulmonary reimplantation response. *Ann Surg* 1973; 177:30

42. Burke CM, Theodore J, Dawkins KD, et al: Post-transplant obliterative bronchiolitis and other late lung sequelae in human heart-lung transplantation. *Chest* 1984; 86:824

43. Griffith BP, Hardesty RL, Trento A, et al: Heart-lung transplantation: Lessons learned and future hopes. *Ann Thorac Surg* 1987; 43:6

44. Dawkins KD, Jamieson SW, Hunt SA, et al: Long-term results, hemodynamics and complications after human heart-lung transplantation. *Circulation* 1985; 71:919

45. Theodore J, Jamieson SW, Burke CM, et al: Physiological aspects of human heart-lung transplantation: Pulmonary status of the post-transplanted lung. *Chest* 1984; 86:349

46. Schroeder S: Haemodynamic performance of the human transplanted heart. *Transplant Proc* 1979; 11:304

47. Griepp RB, Wexler L, Stinson EB, et al: Coronary arteriography following cardiac transplantation. *JAMA* 1972; 22:147

48. Griepp RB, Stinson EB, Bieber CP, et al: Control of graft arteriosclerosis in human heart transplant recipients. *Surgery* 1977; 81:262

49. Gryzan S, Paradis IL, Hardesty RL, et al: Bronchoalveolar lavage in heart-lung transplantation. *Heart Transplantation* 1985; 4:414

Self-Assessment Questions

1. Advances allowing the reintroduction of clinical heart-lung transplantation include:
   A. the use of azathioprine and high-dose steroid suppression
   B. cyclosporin
   C. bronchial omentopexy
   D. tracheal anastomosis

2. Acceptable potential indications for heart-lung transplantation include all but the following:
   A. primary pulmonary hypertension
   B. Eisenmenger's syndrome in uncorrected ventricular septal defect
   C. cyanotic congenital heart disease following bilateral Blalock shunts

D. chronic, sterile interstitial lung disease

E. 50-yr-old female with primary pulmonary hypertension and diabetes mellitus

3. Donor acceptance criteria include:
   A. Pao_2 >100 torr on 1.00 Fio_2
   B. pneumothorax
   C. left bundle branch block
   D. Age <35 yr

4. Matching criteria for donor and recipient always includes:
   A. size
   B. sex
   C. prospective donor-recipient cross-matching
   D. ABO compatibility
   E. rhesus compatibility

5. Appropriate interventions to maintain stability in a hypotensive potential heart-lung donor would include:
   A. increasing PEEP to 10 cm H_2O
   B. adequate volume replacement to achieve a CVP of 15 cm H_2O
   C. adequate volume replacement to accommodate urinary losses
   D. increasing pulmonary vascular resistance
   E. increasing systemic vascular resistance

6. In the donor operation which one of the following is not performed?
   A. protection of the phrenic nerves
   B. topical cooling of donor organs
   C. mobilization of the inferior vena cava
   D. pulmonary artery flushing

7. Which of the following achieve adequate short-term lung preservation?
   A. cold cardioplegic flushing
   B. cold extracellular-type solution flushing
   C. cold intracellular-type solution flushing
   D. cooling on cardiopulmonary bypass

8. In the recipient operation the phrenic, vagal, and left recurrent nerves are protected by:
   A. leaving the phrenic nerve on a ribbon of pericardium
   B. removal of the posterior pericardium
   C. leaving a cuff of pulmonary artery at the level of the arterial ligament
   D. avoidance of cautery hemostasis

9. The mainstay of pulmonary rejection diagnosis in the early stages of heart-lung transplantation is:
   A. serial pulmonary function tests
   B. serial arterial blood gases
   C. measurement of pulmonary vascular resistance
   D. serial chest x-rays

10. Obliterative bronchiolitis is:
    A. an acute implantation response
    B. found in renal, liver, and bone marrow transplants
    C. a chronic complication, common with heart transplantation

D. inevitably fatal and irreversible

E. due to chronic infection with staphylococcus epidermis

F. detected by changes in pulmonary function tests

11. One-year survival following heart-lung transplantation is in the region of:
    A. 28%
    B. 60%
    C. 40%
    D. 72%

12. Appropriate management of late hypertension following heart-lung transplantation would not include the use of:
    A. modulation of cyclosporin dosage
    B. diuretics
    C. propranolol
    D. vasodilators

Self-Assessment Answers

1. B, D
2. C, E
3. D
4. A, D
5. C, E
6. A
7. C, D
8. A, C
9. D
10. F
11. B
12. C

Chapter 5

Cardiac Transplantation

Bartley P. Griffith, MD

Outline

Educational Objectives

In this chapter the reader will learn:

1. to understand the current selection of cardiac transplant candidates.

2. to understand the results following cardiac transplantation.

3. to understand the postoperative management of the recipients.

Introduction

Since the world was stunned in 1967 by the drama of early cardiac transplantation (1), much has been learned about the selection of candidates, the operative procedure, cyclosporine-based immunosuppression, and long-term follow-up of survivors (2-5). Current first-year survival rates average above 80% (6), and cardiac transplantation no longer is considered an exotic remedy but a therapeutic one, now nearly universally available. More than 100 centers are involved in the United States, and more than 1,100 procedures were performed in 1986 alone (7).

Selection

Patients considered for cardiac transplantation generally suffer from congestive heart failure (New York Heart Association Class IV). In our experience, the etiology has been primarily divided between ischemic (55%) and idiopathic (45%) cardiomyopathy. Ventricular failure from end-stage valve disease and other causes, such as myocardial tumor or endocardial fibroelastosis, have been rarer indications (2). Infrequently, patients with modestly impaired ventricles and uncorrectable plus incapacitating angina have been transplanted, but those with previous life-threatening arrhythmias and adequate ventricular function have been better treated with medical management and/or an implanted automatic defibrillator. It would appear that those candidates with severe impairment of left ventricular function and frequent arrhythmia are at the greatest risk of death. Recent reviews of current medical therapy for congestive heart failure suggest that cardiac transplantation remains a far superior definitive treatment for those patients who are eligible (8, 9).

Candidates are matched to perspective donors by ABO blood group compatibility and weight. Because of the limited ex vivo life of the hypothermically stored heart, prospective histocompatibility testing and matching is impractical; in fact, retrospective testing to date has failed to show a strong influence on the results. During evaluation of a candidate, the presence of preformed cytotoxic antibodies is determined by reacting the serum of the candidate against a panel of donor lymphocytes that express all known HLA antigens. Should the candidate's serum react to more than 10% of the cells, it is thought that a similar cross-match should be performed prospectively to a specified donor in order to reduce the chance of a humorally mediated hyperacute rejection (10).

The strict criteria for selection of candidates evolved throughout the 1970s and were based upon the results with conventional immunosuppression of azathioprine, steroids, and antithymocyte globulin (Table 1) (2, 11). Recently, age barriers have expanded to infancy and beyond 60 yr, and patients with nondisabling systemic illnesses including diabetes, sarcoidosis, amyloidosis, and previously treated malignancy are often accepted as candidates (12). Those with limited pulmonary reserve from airway and parenchymal diseases continue to pose a high perioperative and postoperative risk and are avoided. Patients who

---

TABLE 1: Criteria and contraindications for transplant recipients

---

Criteria for Selection of Candidates

1. Terminal heart disease with estimated life expectancy of less than 6 to 12 mo
2. Age < 50 to 55 yr
3. Normal or reversible renal and hepatic function
4. Absence of active infection
5. Absence of pulmonary infarction in the preceding 8 wk
6. Absence of insulin-dependent diabetes mellitus or hyperglycemia requiring treatment with insulin or oral hypoglycemic agents
7. Psychosocial stability and a supportive social milieu

Contraindications

1. PVR > 6 Wood units (orthotopic transplantation)
2. Cross-match incompatibility between recipient and donor
3. Significant peripheral vascular or cerebrovascular disease
4. Active peptic ulcer disease
5. Drug addiction
6. Alcoholic cardiomyopathy and continued alcohol abuse
7. Co-existing systemic illness that may limit life expectancy or may compromise recovery from cardiac transplantation
8. Pre-existing malignant disease
9. Chronic bronchitis and chronic obstructive lung disease

---

are mortally ill with severe congestive heart failure requiring hospitalization and support of their circulation with intravenous inotropes and aortic counter-pulsation have survived comparatively as well as those less desperately ill (13). The key to success in this group has been the exclusion of those with infection and severe dysfunction of end organs. In an attempt to prevent irreversible damage from inadequate cardiac output, a number of centers have experimented with mechanical devices, such as the total artificial heart and ventricular pumps, in successful efforts to bridge dying patients to transplantation (6, 14). It appears that the right ventricle of the donor may fail when the recipient's pulmonary vascular resistance (PVR) is elevated beyond 6 Wood units. Attempts to preoperatively manipulate the elevated pulmonary vascular resistance using vasodilators have been helpful when reversibility of the PVR has been proven (15). Other measurements, including pulmonary arterial pressures above 70 systolic and transpulmonary gradients of 15 mm Hg, have been associated with poor outcomes (16). It would appear that patients chronically ill with high pulmonary arterial pressures and widened transpulmonary gradients pose the greatest risk for acute failure of the donor's right ventricle, and are better suited for heterotopic cardiac transplantation (17).

Patients with end-stage cardiac disease are at risk for pulmonary emboli and are therapeutically anticoagulated while awaiting transplantation. Should pulmonary emboli occur, there may be an undetected rise in the PVR which might cause an acute worsening of heart failure and might preclude successful orthotopic transplantation. While success has been possible following cardiac transplantation in the setting of pulmonary infarction, recipients are at an increased risk from pneumonia and lung abscess; thus, transplantation preferably should be delayed 4 to 6 wk after pulmonary emboli and infarction are noted (2, 18).

Preoperative Preparation

All candidates are reviewed to determine the severity of their illness; and if the patient is judged not likely to survive more than 1 year without cardiac replacement, a series of evaluations is made. A cardiac catheterization must be performed within 3 to 6 months to determine the PVR and the suitability for an orthotopic procedure. Renal function is judged from serum creatinine and liver disease detected by enzymes of hepatic function, including bilirubin and prothrombin times. Decisions regarding reversibility of end-organ dysfunction are based on their degrees and their chronicity. Patients should have a strong desire to live and should be able to follow the demands of postoperative follow-up. Candidates are tested preoperatively for evidence of prior exposure to tuberculosis, toxoplasmosis, cytomegalic virus, human immunodeficiency virus, Epstein-Barr virus, and hepatitis A and B. Additional blood is drawn for typing of ABO, human lymphocyte antigen, and for the presence of preformed antibodies (19).

Once a patient is selected, an entry is made on a candidate's list which prioritizes them to medical urgency and time waiting. Previously, most candidates could remain at home prior to transplantation if arrangements could be made to return to the operating center within 4 h. However, because the wait for donors has increased from 1 wk to over 4 wk for those candidates who are mortally ill, more patients have been readmitted to the hospital for augmented medical therapy of progressive congestive heart failure. In 1986, 60% of the heart transplant recipients in Pittsburgh were maintained on intravenous inotropes and 25% were maintained by aortic balloon prior to transplantation in an attempt to keep them alive and manage hepatic, cerebral, and renal impairments. In the latter group, every effort is made to lessen the risk of iatrogenic infection by avoidance of urinary and central vascular catheters.

Orthotopic Transplantation

Following median sternotomy, the transplant recipient is placed on cardiopulmonary bypass and the diseased ventricles are removed at the level of the atrioventricular groove. The aorta and main pulmonary artery are transected just above the semilunar valves. Maintenance of the right and left atrial cuffs with corresponding superior-inferior cavae and pulmonary veins permits a faster and technically easier anastomosis to be performed to the donor's atria (Fig. 1) (20). The cold, preserved donor's heart is removed from its insulated container, and its left atrium is opened through an incision uniting the orifices of the four pulmonary veins. The lateral wall of the right atrium is opened to its mid portion along the line beginning at the inferior atrial caval junction directed toward the right atrial appendage. In preparation of the donor's heart during cardiectomy, the superior vena cava is stapled closed with careful avoidance of the region of the sinal atrial node. Additionally, the aorta of the donor can be temporarily stapled proximal to the origin of the innominate artery to enable the installation of additional doses of cardioplegic solution during the implant procedure. If the aorta is not stapled, a vent can be placed in the left atrial appendage or through the right superior pulmonary vein of the recipient for the continuous installation of cold saline solution.

Each atrial anastomosis is completed with a 3-0 polypropylene suture in a continuous circumferential manner. The left atrial anastomosis is begun at the base of the left atrial appendage of the donor, and the suture line is run from within the atrium beginning first along the lateral and inferior edges. The right atrial anastomosis is begun along the inferior atrial septal junction. The aortic and pulmonary arterial anastomoses are performed with a 4-0 polypropylene suture in a continuous vertical fashion.

Following the release of the aortic cross-clamp, air is vented from the dome of the aorta via a needlehole and is suctioned from the left ventricular cavity via the previously positioned vent catheter. After rewarming from a core temperature of 28°C, either ventricular fibrillation or idioventricular rhythm generally occurs. Ventricular fibrillation can be cardioverted to an organized pattern of contraction, and at normothermia a normal sinus rhythm usually has been restored. Occasionally, atrioventricular block or sinus arrhythmia necessitates the use of temporary ventricular pacing.

Postoperative Management

Following the surgical procedure, recipients are treated similarly to any other patient who has undergone open heart surgery. An adequate preload is necessary; frequently, intravenous inotropes are required to maintain adequate function of the donor's denervated organ. When PVR is elevated and there is evidence of right ventricular failure, the vasodilatory effects of prostaglandin E_1 and isoproterenol have been quite beneficial. While humorally mediated hyperacute rejection can occur within the first 12 h, it is rare, and cell-mediated rejection generally does not cause problems for the first postoperative week. Antibiotics, usually cephalosporins, are given perioperatively but discontinued early postoperatively to prevent an emergence of serious resistant bacterial and fungal infections. Because infection is the most common cause of death after heart transplantation, every effort is made in surveillance and in minimizing immunosuppression (21). The most commonly employed strategies for immunosuppression are presented in Table 2. All recipients remain electrocardiographically monitored and in the hospital for at least 3 wk, and have weekly endomyocardial biopsies for 6 wk. While an effort is made to separate recipients from each other and the rest of the inpatient population, isolation procedures are not likely beneficial. Immunosuppression is augmented and hospital stay lengthens when histologic evidence of rejection occurs (22). Unfortunately, to date noninvasive measures, including voltage and frequency averaged ECGs, physical exams, chest x-rays, echocardiograms, nuclear ventriculography, cytoimmune monitoring of peripheral lymphocytes, and measurement of white blood cell metabolites have been unreliable when compared to the endomyocardial biopsy (12). After 2 months, the biopsy is performed monthly for 6 months and then 3 to 4 times yearly. Clinically, unsuspected myocyte necrosis is not infrequent in the early postoperative period and can occur much later as well. Recipients have generally required one to two treatments for histologic rejection in the first 3 postoperative months. Rejection is treated with pulses of methylprednisolone and, if it is recurrent or severe, antithymocyte or monoclonal antibody (OKT 3) is added. Annual coronary arteriograms have been required to detect occlusive coronary artery disease, which is not common in the first year but affects nearly 40% of the recipients by the third postoperative year (23). Unfortunately, this process is unpreventable and seems to correlate only with the number of previous episodes of rejection. Because it is an aggressive and diffuse process, it usually can only be treated by retransplantation (2).

In addition to immunosuppressive medications, recipients are prescribed aspirin and persantine in the hopes of lowering the incidence of coronary occlusion (24); these patients also require multiple antihypertensive agents to control cyclosporine-related toxicity. Most patients require combinations which include diuretics, vasodilators, and calcium channels blockers, angiotensin-converting enzymes, and beta receptors to control systolic and diastolic hypertension (25). Careful outpatient follow-up is required, not only to seek infection and rejection, but also to manage the significant hypertension and nephrotoxicity associated with cyclosporine. Elevation of serum creatinine above 2 mg% occurs frequently when the doses of cyclosporine exceed 5 mg/kg·day (5), and have been the stimulus for the use of lower doses of cyclosporine and the adoption of successful immunosuppression protocols which rely on low doses of prednisone (0.05 to 0.1 mg/kg·day), azathioprine (1.0 to 2.0 mg/kg·day), and cyclosporine (2.5 to 5.0 mg/kg·day) (3, 26).

Pediatric Transplantation

Most children referred for cardiac transplantation have idiopathic cardiomyopathy. Structural malformation considered for treatment has included pulmonary atresia, hypoplastic and univentricular heart tricuspid atresia, Ebstein's malformation, transposition of the great arteries, and tetralogy of Fallot with postoperative dysfunction of the right ventricle (5, 26). Recently,

Bailey (27) has demonstrated the remarkable success of transplantation in babies with hypoplastic left heart syndrome. His experimental and clinical experience suggests that the neonatal period might be an ideal time for cardiac transplantation. Rejection has not been a problem in five of six children treated, as neonates have survived between 6 months and 2 yr postoperatively. The recipients appear to be growing normally, and their only immunosuppressant is low-dose cyclosporine.

Between 1968 and 1983, the International Heart Transplant Registry has included 111 procedures performed in children less than 15 yr old and another 149 in those between 15 and 20 yr (4). Survival rates in children carefully selected for transplantation appear to be similar to those of adults. While children can be followed exactly as adults, babies cannot reasonably be subjected to endomyocardial biopsy; thus, a combination of noninvasive monitoring techniques is employed.

TABLE 2: Commonly employed immunosuppression strategies

DRUG	DOSE	COMMENT
	Preoperative	
Azathioprine	4.0 mg/kg/iv	
Cyclosporine	5.0-10.0 mg po	Deleted in many centers due to acute nephrotoxicity
	Intraoperative	
Methylprednisolone	500 mg	With reperfusion of the heart
	Postoperative	
Azathioprine	2.0 mg/kg·day	Dose adjusted to keep WBC >5,000
Cyclosporine	2.5-5.0 mg/kg·day	Begun when patient is stable with diuresis (24-36 h postop); adjust to 500-700 mg/ml whole blood RIA
Methylprednisolone	125 mg q8h × 3 doses	
Prednisone	0.3-0.15 mg/kg·day	Wean over 3-6 mo
Antithymocyte globulin (ATGAM, Upjohn, Kalamazoo, MI)	10 mg/kg iv qd	For in-house preparation Dose varies per potency
	Rejection	
Methylprednisolone	1 gm iv × 3 days	Mild or moderate rejection
Antithymocyte globulin	× 5-7 days	Severe or recurrent rejection
Orthoclone OKT 3 and	5 mg iv qd × 14 days	Severe or recurrent rejection
Prednisone	1 mg/kg; taper after 10 days	Steroid augmentation after OKT 3 completed
	Maintenance	
Cyclosporine	2.5-5.0 mg/kg·day	Doses adjusted based on individual history of rejection and drug toxicity
Prednisone	0.0-0.15 mg/kg·day	
Azathioprine	1.0-2.0 mg/kg·day	

References

1. Barnard CN: The operation: A human heart transplantation, an interim report of the successful operation performed at Groote Schuur Hospital, Capetown, South Africa. *S Afr Med J* 1967; 41:271

2. Baumgartner WA, Reitz BA, Oyer PE, et al: Cardiac homotransplantation. *Curr Prob Surg* 1979; 1:61

3. Griffith BP, Hardesty RL, Bahnson HT: Powerful but limited immune suppression for cardiac transplantation with cyclosporine A and low-dose steroid. *J Thorac Cardiovasc Surg* 1984; 87:35

4. Kaye MP: The Registry of the International Society for Heart Transplantation. Third Official Report. *Heart Transplantation* 1986; 5:2

5. Myers BD, Ross J, Newton L, et al: Cyclosporine-associated chronic nephropathy. *N Engl J Med* 1984; 311:699

6. Hill JD, Farrar DJ, Hershon JJ, et al: Use of a prosthetic ventricle as a bridge to cardiac transplantation for postinfarction cardiogenic shock. *N Engl J Med* 1986; 314:626

7. Kaye MP: The Registry of the International Society for Heart Transplantation. Fourth Official Report. *Heart Transplantation* 1987; 6:63

8. Stevenson LW, Fowler MB, Schroeder JS, et al: Patients denied cardiac transplantation for non-medical criteria: A control group. *J Am Coll Cardiol* 1986; 7:9A

9. Stevenson LW, MacAlpin RN, Drinkwater D, et al: Heart transplantation at UCLA: Selection and survival. *Heart Transplantation* 1986; 5:62

10. Hardesty RL, Griffith BP, Trento A, et al: Mortally ill patients and excellent survival following cardiac transplantation. *Ann Thorac Surg* 1986; 41:126

11. Pennock JL, Oyer PE, Reitz BA, et al: Cardiac transplantation in perspective for the future. *J Thorac Cardiovasc Surg* 1982; 83:168

12. Griffith BP, Hardesty RL, Trento A, et al: Cardiac transplantation: Emerging from an experiment to a service. *Ann Surg* 1986; 204:308

13. Hardesty RL, Griffith BP: Multiple cadaveric organ procurement for transplantation with emphasis on the heart. *Surg Clin North* Am 1986; 66:451

14. Griffith BP, Hardesty RL, Kormos RL, et al: Temporary use of the Jarvik-7 total artificial heart prior to transplantation. *N Engl J Med* 1987; 316:130

15. Addonizio CJ, Robbins RC, Reison DS, et al: Transplantation in patients with high pulmonary vascular resistance. *Heart Transplantation* 1987; In Press

16. Kormos RL, Thompson ME, Hardesty RL, et al: Utility of preoperative right heart catheterization data as a predictor of survival after heart transplantation. *Heart Transplantation* 1987; In Press

17. Griffith BP, Kormos RL, Hardesty RL: Heterotopic cardiac transplantation: Current status. *J Cardiac Surg* 1987; In Press

18. Young NJ, Yazbeck J, Esposito G, et al: The influence of acute preoperative pulmonary infarction on the results of heart transplantation. *Heart Transplantation* 1986; 5:20

19. Thompson ME, Dummer JS, Griffith BP, et al: Cardiac transplantation 1985: Hope, promise, reality. *In*: Progress in Cardiology. Yu PN, Goodwin JF (Eds). Philadelphia, Lea & Febiger, 1986, pp 191-233

20. Lower RR, Shumway NE: Studies on orthotopic homotransplantation of the canine heart. *Surg Forum* 1960; 11:18

21. Dummer JS, Montero CG, Griffith BP, et al: Infections in heart-lung transplant recipients. *Transplantation* 1986; 41:725

22. Billingham ME: Diagnosis of cardiac rejection by endomyocardial biopsy. *Heart Transplantation* 1980; 1:25

23. Uretsky BF, Murali S, Reddy PS, et al: Development of coronary artery disease immunosuppressed with cyclosporine and prednisone. *Circulation* 1987; In Press

24. Greipp RB, Stinson EB, Bieber CP, et al: Control of graft arteriosclerosis in human heart transplant recipients. *Surgery* 1977; 81:262

25. Thompson ME, Shapiro AP, Johnson M, et al: New onset of hypertension following cardiac transplantation: A preliminary report and analysis. *Transplant Proc* 1983; 15:2573

26. Bolman RM, Elick B, Olivari MT: Improved immunosuppression for cardiac transplantation. *Heart Transplantation* 1985; 4:123

27. Bailey L, Concepcion W, Shattuck H, et al: Method of heart transplantation for treatment of hypoplastic left heart syndrome. *J Thorac Cardiovasc Surg* 1986; 92:1

Self-Assessment Questions

1. What is the expected percentage for 1-yr survival following cardiac transplantation?

2. What is the common feature uniting the indications for cardiac transplantation?

3. What are the most common indications for cardiac transplantation?

4. What criteria are important in matching prospective donors and recipients?

5. What level of pulmonary vascular resistance represents an obstacle to orthotopic cardiac transplantation?

6. Why should candidates for cardiac transplantation be therapeutically anticoagulated?

7. Why do recipients of orthotopic cardiac transplantation frequently have two P waves evident in their ECGS?

8. Why do current postoperative immunosuppressive regimens include low doses of cyclosporine, steroids, and azathioprine?

9. What long-term problem is likely to limit survival in many recipients?

10. What is the current time limit for "ex vivo" preservation of the donor hearts.

Self-Assessment Answers

1. 80% of patients currently treated with cardiac transplantation are expected to survive 1 yr.

2. All patients suffer from New York Heart Association Class IV cardiac failure.

3. The most common indication for cardiac transplantation today is ischemic heart disease followed by idiopathic cardiomyopathy.

4. Donors and recipients are matched by ABP blood group compatibility and weight.

5. Six Wood units.

6. Because there is a high incidence of pulmonary emboli in this population of patients, and pulmonary emboli can cause elevation of pulmonary vascular resistance and, if embolic episodes evolve into pulmonary infarctions, patients might be at an increased risk for infection following cardiac transplantation.

7. Orthotopic transplantation results in preservation of recipient and donor atria, and the recipient's atrial contraction frequently can be seen marching through the ECG.

8. Postoperative immunosuppression is aimed to prevent rejection, but also to use a balance in immunosuppressive drugs so that their individual toxicities can be limited by lowering their doses.

9. Atherosclerotic coronary occlusive disease in the recipient.

10. While exceptions have existed, most believe donor hearts should be implanted within 4 h of cardiectomy.

Chapter 6

Current Topics in Renal Transplantation

*Eric S. Berens, MD, Mark W. Shelton, MD, and
Douglas W. Hanto, MD, PhD*

Outline

Educational Objectives

In this chapter the reader will learn:

1. to identify the major areas of current research in clinical renal transplantation.

2. to develop an awareness of immunosuppressive drugs and regimens, such as the use of monoclonal antibodies and triple drug therapy.

3. to understand some of the factors important in preoperative preparation of the patient: blood transfusions and HLA typing.

Introduction

The modern era of transplantation began in 1902 with the development of the technique of vascular anastomosis using sutures by Alexis Carrel, a French surgeon, who was awarded the Nobel prize for his work (1). Utilizing these techniques, Carrel (2) between 1902 and 1912 performed a large series of organ transplants in animals. Although they were the first to report technically successful organ transplants, prolonged graft survival did not occur, and would not be achieved for several decades after the basic concepts of transplantation immunity were developed. Much of the early experimental work that led to our understanding of the cellular mechanism of allograft rejection was performed by Medawar, Billingham, and Brent during the late 1940s and early 1950s. They demonstrated that viable cells transferred specific allograft immunity and established the concept of second-set rejection, i.e., an animal previously skin-grafted will reject a second identical skin graft more rapidly, reflecting "immunologic memory." During the early 1950s, human kidney transplants were performed without immunosuppression and without success. In 1954, Murray (3) performed the first successful kidney transplant between identical twins without immunosuppression. In this era before tissue typing and crossmatching, the twins' genetic identity was demonstrated pretransplant by the recipient's inability to reject a skin graft from his twin brother.

The use of immunosuppression in clinical transplantation was introduced in 1958 by Murray (3) in Boston and Hamburger et al. (4) in Paris; the latter group independently performed a series of human kidney allografts using total-body irradiation. In 1959 Schwartz and Dameshek (5) reported that 6-mercaptopurine (6-MP) blocked antibody production in rabbits. Calne (6) and Zukoski et al. (7) later showed that 6-MP prolonged canine renal allograft survival. In 1961 azathioprine (AZA), the oral preparation of 6-MP, was shown to prolong kidney allograft survival in man, thus initiating the modern era of transplantation (3). In 1963 Starzl reported that prednisone combined with AZA produced further improvements in the results of clinical kidney transplantation. This report established "conventional" immunotherapy that is still in use today (3).

In the early years of renal transplantation, the phenomenon of hyperacute rejection was often seen but not understood. In 1966 Kissmeyer-Nielsen et al. (8) demonstrated that hyperacute rejection is mediated by preformed antidonor lymphocytotoxic antibodies in the recipient's serum. Recipient serum is now routinely tested against donor lymphocytes for the presence of donor-specific alloantibodies, and a positive T cell crossmatch is a contraindication to renal transplantation. The importance of preformed antibodies against B cell antigens is still controversial (9).

More recent advances and controversies in renal transplantation will be the topics for discussion in this chapter. The observation in 1974 by Opelz et al. (10) that random pretransplant blood transfusions improved cadaver graft survival rates has recently been questioned (11). The role of donor-specific transfusions in improving the results of living related donor kidney transplantation are clear. The introduction of cyclosporine (CsA) and the monoclonal antibody OKT3 have had a major role in improving the results of organ transplantation. The role of tissue typing is less in the CsA era. Whether total lymphoid irradiation and ABO incompatible transplants play major roles in renal transplantation has not yet been established. The intention of this chapter is to highlight the importance of these current topics in renal transplantation.

Donor-Specific Transfusion (DST)

Blood transfusions are important in cadaver and living-related transplants. In 1973 Opelz et al. (12) reported that random pretransplant blood transfusions were associated with an improvement in cadaver renal allograft survival rates. Recent data suggest that this transfusion effect may not be as important in CsA-treated patients (11-13). This unresolved issue will not be discussed further. Of greater interest and importance was the first clinical report in 1973 of the beneficial effect of donor-specific transfusions in recipients of kidneys from living-related donors by Newton and Anderson (14). Four patients received three transfusions 2 wk apart from their prospective living-related donors while continuously receiving AZA immunosuppression. None of these patients became sensitized to the donor, and all subsequently underwent successful transplantation without rejection using AZA and prednisone (P). The clinical importance and usefulness of DST protocols have persisted even with the introduction of protocols using CsA in living-related transplants.

In 1980 Salvatierra et al. (15) reported a 94% 1-yr graft survival in 1-haplotype mismatched related donor-recipient pairs with DST (Table 1). These results were comparable to their results with HLA identical recipients (96%) and low-mixed leukocyte culture (MLC) pairs without DST (89%), and better than their results in high-MLC patients without DST (56%). The incidence of rejection was likewise reduced to 44%, similar to that in HLA identical recipients. AZA was not used in this series and the incidence of sensitization of the recipient to the donor was 29%, a principal disadvantage of DST. Several series since then have confirmed that sensitization rates can be lowered to 8% to 15% by administration of AZA during the period of transfusions without reducing the graft survival rate (16-18). DST are now being used with HLA-identical sibling donors, haplo-identical donors, and HLA-mismatched sibling donors with a 90% to 95% 1-yr graft survival rate (19). A major advantage is that the majority of patients will achieve excellent long-term function without rejection and without the need for CsA.

Table 1. Percent graft survival with and without donor-specific transfusions

	3-Month	1-Yr
With DST (n = 23)	100	94 ± 5
Without DST		
1-haplotype match		
high MLC (n = 34)	65 ± 8	56 ± 9
low MLC (n = 74)	90 ± 3	89 ± 4
HLA-identical (n = 69)	99 ± 1	96 ± 2

Adapted with permission from Salvatierra et al (15).
DST = donor-specific transfusion, MCL = mixed-leukocyte culture.

Donor-specific transfusions have also been used in pediatric renal transplantation. The University of California, San Francisco, reported 97% 1-yr and 93% 2 and 5-yr actuarial graft survival rates in 37 pediatric renal transplant patients treated with DST (20). In children treated with concomitant AZA during the DST protocol, 11% became sensitized compared to 26% in children treated with DST alone. Among 6 haploidentical living-related transplants performed without DST, two grafts were rejected within the first year. The University of Wisconsin has reported an overall 95% 1-yr and 90% 5-yr graft survival rate in 39 pediatric living-related transplants who received DST only (10 patients) or DST + AZA (29 patients; Fig. 1) (21). Graft survival for AZA-DST was 97% at 1 yr and 95% at 2 yr, whereas graft survival for DST-only patients was 85% at 1 yr and 80% at 2 yr. The sensitization rates were similar to the San Francisco study, 10% in the AZA-DST group compared to 21% in the DST-only group. The data from these two centers support the conclusion that living-related donor transplantation preceded by DST, with concurrent administration of AZA is the treatment of choice for children with end-stage renal disease except when an HLA-identical sibling donor is available and DST are unnecessary.

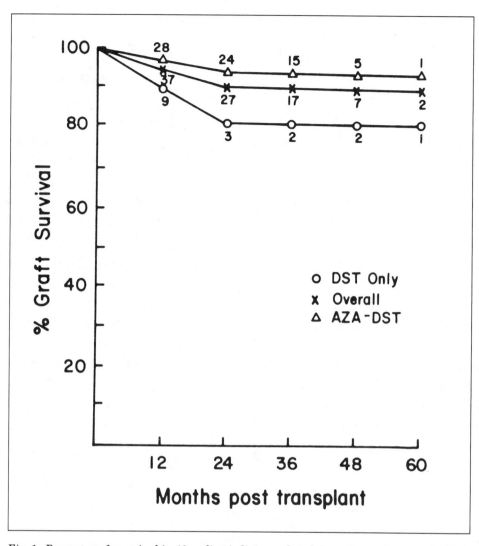

Fig. 1. Percent graft survival in 40 pediatric living-related donor transplants at the University of Wisconsin from 1981 to 1986. (○ = DST only; Δ = azathioprine + DST; and × = all patients combined. Reproduced with permission from Friedman et al (21).

The University of Minnesota has recently reported the results in 16 pediatric living-related donor recipients pretreated with DST and AZA (22). Only one of the initial 17 (5.9%) children in the protocol became sensitized (5.9%). Of the 16 patients transplanted only 12 grafts (75%) were functioning at 1 yr. The causes of graft loss were arterial thrombosis (technical), recurrent hemolytic-uremia syndrome, recurrent oxalosis, and chronic rejection. Therefore, actual 1-yr graft loss from rejection was only 6.3% (one of 16), although two patients with functioning grafts had ongoing chronic rejection at 12 and 18 months. They are less enthusiastic about DST in children because of their excellent results with standard immunosuppression (AZA, P, and antilymphoblast globulin plus low-dose CsA). So et al. (personal communication) has reported on 18 mismatched-related and 10 cadaver kidney transplants with 100% and 90% graft survival rates with a mean follow-up of 17.3 months. This protocol may be advantageous when the patient has only one living donor and where it would be preferable to avoid the risk of sensitization that would then relegate the child to a cadaver transplant.

Because of a shortage of cadaver organs and the improved results with DST, these transfusions have now been utilized in living-unrelated donor transplants (17, 23, 24). The University of Wisconsin evaluated DST with and without AZA in 31 living-unrelated donor transplants (Fig. 2). There was an overall 24% sensitization rate in the initial 41 patients entered into the protocol, but the number of patients treated with concomitant AZA was not given. The highest rate of sensitization (55%) was in the husband-to-wife combination in which the wife had two or more children by the husband. If these patients are excluded the sensitization rate was 15%, similar to their 12% sensitization rate in living-related donor-recipient combinations. Actuarial graft survival was 90% at 1 and 5 yr, comparable to HLA-identical and DST living-related transplants (Fig. 2). Although the use of living-unrelated donors has evoked some controversy, the results are excellent and more centers are performing spouse-to-spouse transplants when living-related donors are not available.

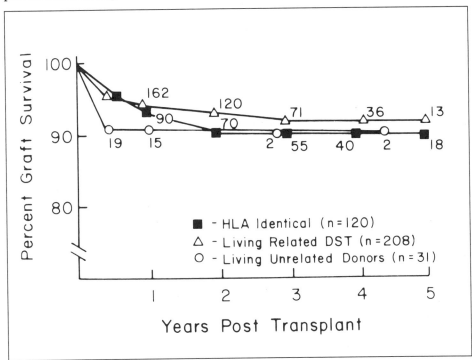

Fig. 2. *Renal allograft survival at the University of Wisconsin from 1981 to 1987. Reproduced with permission from Belzer et al (23).*

With the introduction of CsA, the advantages of DST have been questioned. Iwaki and Terasaki (25) compiled data from several centers and demonstrated 88% 1-yr graft survival in haploidentical living-donor transplants with DST compared to 85% 1-yr graft survival seen in CsA-treated non-DST patients (not a statistically significant difference). Recent reports from individual centers have yielded slightly better results with the use of CsA (26), but longer follow-up of larger numbers of patients is needed. The main advantage of CsA compared to DST is that a recipient would not be denied a kidney from the prospective donor because of DST-related sensitization. CsA, however, also has many adverse side-effects including nephrotoxicity, hypertension, and high cost. To date, no prospective randomized studies with long-term follow-up evaluating DST versus CsA have been reported.

In conclusion, there is strong evidence that donor-specific transfusions have improved kidney allograft survival in adult and pediatric HLA-mismatched and haploidentical, living-related donor transplants. Recent evidence also suggests that the traditionally high survival rates already seen in HLA-identical matches may be improved even further with the use of DST (19). In addition, evidence supports the benefit of DST in living-unrelated donor transplants, which may enlarge the prospective living donor pool for many patients in need of kidney allografts.

Use of Cyclosporine in Cadaver Transplantation

Conventional immunosuppression, consisting of antilymphocyte globulin (ALG), P, and AZA, has been modified frequently since the introduction of CsA. In 1976 Borel (27) described the immunosuppressive properties of an extract from the fungi, Tolypocladium inflatum. Cyclosporin A (CsA), one of four cyclosporins originally derived and designated as A,B,C, and D, was found to inhibit cellular and humoral immunity without bone marrow suppression. This property of CsA led to a proliferation of experimental and clinical studies investigating its mechanism of action and potential for clinical application. CsA was found to selectively inhibit the synthesis and release of interleukin-2 (IL-2) by activated T lymphocytes. In addition, it blocks the IL-2 activation of resting T lymphocytes (28). Currently, the United States Accepted Nomenclature (USAN) for "cyclosporin A" is "cyclosporine"

Calne et al. (29) first reported the clinical use of CsA in man in combination with Prednisone and Cytimum (a cyclophosphamide derivative) resulting in overimmunosuppression, and a high incidence of infectious complications and death. The encouraging results of other uncontrolled trials using less CsA in combination with P (30, 31) led to several prospective, randomized clinical studies. The European Multicenter Trial Group found an improvement in cadaver allograft survival from 52% (AZ + P) to 72% at 1 yr (CsA + P) (32). The Canadian Trial found an improvement from 67% to 84% (33), and the University of Minnesota (CsA + P vs. AZA + P + ALG) reported an improvement from 73% to 84% (34). There were also fewer infectious complications in the CsA groups while mortality rates remained comparable to conventional therapy.

The adverse side-effects of CsA have been well described. These include nephrotoxicity, hypertension, hyperkalemia, and hyperuricemia. CsA-induced neurological effects include tremors, paresthesias, muscle weakness, and seizures. Allograft thrombosis and a CsA-associated arteriopathy have also been described in CsA-treated patients (35).

The data from these studies indicated that the use of CsA was primarily limited by its nephrotoxicity which was, however, reversible. Subsequent trials have attempted to find a combination of agents which would permit a lower dose of CsA to minimize nephrotoxicity, but still preserve the improved graft survival rates and lower rates of infection.

Several triple (AZA + P + CsA) or quadruple (AZA + P + CsA + ALG) therapy regimens have been described. Simmons et al. (26) reported a prospective single-armed study that combined CsA, AZA, P, and ALG for prophylactic immunosuppression after kidney transplantation. Patients were started on AZA, low-dose P, and ALG (7 to 14 days at 20 mg/kg·day). CsA (8 mg/kg·day) was not started until the serum creatinine fell below 3.0 mg/dl and ALG was simultaneously stopped. Their preliminary results demonstrated that by reducing the baseline dosage of CsA and avoiding the use of CsA in the presence of acute tubular necrosis (ATN), they could achieve an 85% 6-month graft survival rate, reduce the incidence of CsA toxicity from 24% to 2%, lower the average serum creatinine, and shorten the hospital course when compared to results from a previous randomized trial of CsA + P vs. AZA + P + ALG.

In response to evidence that early CsA treatment prolongs the duration of ATN and predisposes to chronic CsA nephrotoxicity, other transplant centers have also delayed starting CsA until the serum creatinine falls below some arbitrary level. Light et al. (36) started CsA after the creatinine fell below 5.0 mg% and Deierhoi et al. (37), when it was below 3.0 mg%. In both studies, AZA + P + ALG were given initially for 7 to 21 days and CsA therapy was started 1 to 2 days before stopping ALG. Although they both reported excellent graft survival rates (91% and 85% respectively at 1 yr) with a low infection rate for first grafts, neither study compared their results to a control group (Table 2).

Table 2. Quadruple therapy in cadaver renal allograft recipients (35, 37, 83)

	Patient Survival 2-yr	Graft Survival 2-yr
University of Wisconsin (n = 278)		
- all grafts	91%	85%
- 2nd grafts	94%	64
Ohio State University (n = 304)		
- 1st grafts	95%	85%
- 2nd grafts	91%	72%
Washington Hospital Medical Center (n = 99)		
- all grafts	—	91% (1-yr)

Fries et al. (38) did not use prophylactic ALG and started all patients on AZA, P, and CsA immediately after transplantation. They reported acute nephrotoxic episodes in 68% of patients and average creatinines were significantly higher in the study group (134 + 49 µmol/L) compared to conventional (AZA + P) therapy (97 + 11 µmol/L) at 18 months. Half of the patients initially enrolled in the AZA + P group were eventually switched to the CsA group because of ALG-steroid resistent rejection or side-effects related to conventional therapy (i.e., osteonecrosis, diabetes, or prolonged leukopenia). Actuarial graft survival was improved, but not significantly, in the AZA + P + CsA experimental group compared to the AZA + P group (83% and 76% at 1 yr, respectively). However, patient survival was significantly better in the triple-therapy group (95% compared to 88% at 1 yr) and the incidence of serious infections was dramatically less in the triple-therapy group (4 vs. 17, $p <.002$).

Despite these good results with triple and quadruple therapy, not all centers have had equal success. Fifty-five patients were randomized to a clinical trial of CsA + AZA + P vs. CsA alone at the Royal Infirmary, Cardiff, Wales (39). Actuarial graft survival was similar for both groups (75% triple and 78% CsA at 1 yr), however patient survival was much better in the CsA group (96% vs. 78%) due to the significantly greater incidence of life-threatening infections in the triple-therapy group (10 vs. 0; $p <.01$). Jones et al. (40) from Oxford reported that triple-therapy with CsA + AZA + P produced excellent actuarial graft survival (79% at 1 yr), but not obviously better than CsA alone or CsA + P. This was not a randomized trial and data on the comparative groups were not presented. Although the degree of nephrotoxicity had been reduced with lower doses of CsA, the authors stated that renal function remained suboptimal at 6 months.

In conclusion, it appears that the use of triple therapy (AZA + P + CsA) in cadaver renal transplant recipients is associated with improved patient and graft survival and a reduction in infectious complications. This is most likely related to the lower dosages of P and CsA required and a reduction in the frequency of acute rejection episodes. The use of CsA immediately post-transplant is associated with an increased incidence of CsA nephrotoxicity, prolongation of the duration of ATN, and a decrease in graft survival. The use of ALG induction in the immediate post-transplant period has circumvented these problems and is highly recommended.

Monoclonal Antibodies for the Treatment of Allograft Rejection

Several clinical trials published during the early 1980s established the usefulness of ALG in the treatment of acute renal allograft rejection (41-43). These preparations are polyclonal antibody preparations from the sera of animals (most frequently horses, rabbits, and goats) immunized with human lymphoid cells. Their potency, specificity, and toxicity vary between batches. In addition, up to 25% of acute cadaver allograft rejection episodes are not reversible with ALG; whether ALG is any more effective than steroids has been questioned (44). As a result, the search for more potent, more specific, and less toxic reagents has continued.

In 1975 Köhler and Milstein (45) demonstrated that murine monoclonal antibodies could be produced by stable hybridomas. By 1980, researchers using hybridoma technology had developed a variety of antibodies that reacted with cell surface molecules on human T cells, B cells, monocytes, and granulocytes. In 1981, Cosimi et al. (46, 47) introduced the clinical use of one such monoclonal antibody, OKT3, as a treatment for renal allograft rejection. In subsequent years, OKT3 has been extensively studied and found to be a new and valuable addition to the current list of immunosuppressive agents. Although this section will focus on OKT3 as one well studied example, other new monoclonal antibodies, such as anti-IL-2 receptor antibody, may become equally important as this new field develops.

OKT3, a mouse monoclonal antibody, reacts with a 19 kilodalton glycoprotein, T3, that is associated with the human T cell antigen receptor complex (48). In vitro, OKT3 blocks the generation of functional effector T cells and inhibits the activity of mature cytotoxic effector lymphocytes (49, 50). In vivo, OKT3 acts as an opsonizing antibody and T3-positive cells are rapidly removed from the circulating lymphocyte pool by the reticuloendothelial system (51). Subsequently OKT3 was shown to reverse rejection episodes that were unresponsive to both steroid and ALG therapy (52). This resulted in the salvage of kidneys that would otherwise have been lost to rejection. The 6-month graft survival rate was 60% in these patients.

The side-effects associated with OKT3 administration are most severe with the first dose and include pyrexia (73%), chills (57%), vomiting (13%), nausea (11%), dyspnea (21%), chest pain and tightness (14%), and wheezing (11%) (53). This symptom complex has been attributed to mediators released as a result of T cell destruction. Severe pulmonary edema has also been reported in patients who had pre-existing fluid overload. Steroid and antihistamine administration prior to OKT3 administration can decrease the severity of these side-effects in most patients.

Early clinical trials tested the use of OKT3 as primary therapy for first rejection episodes in cadaver donor renal allograft recipients whose baseline immunosuppression consisted of AZA and P only. The Ortho Multicenter Transplant Study Group (53), reported that OKT3 reversed rejection in 94% of 63 patients, while conventional high-dose steroid treatment reversed rejection in 75% of 60 patients ($p = .009$) (Fig. 3). Although the 1-yr graft survival rate was 62% for the

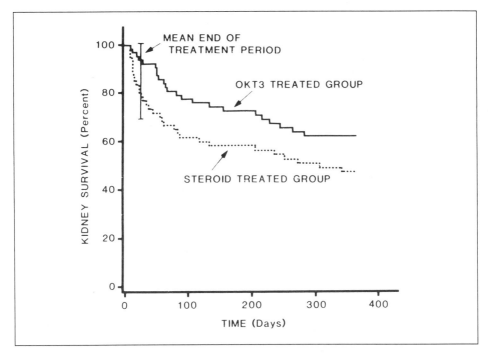

Fig. 3. Life table analysis of kidney survival in patients randomly assigned to OKT3 or steroid treatment for acute renal allograft rejection. Reproduced with permission from (53).

OKT3 group and 45% for the steroid group, the recurrent rejection rates for both groups were not significantly different (66% and 73% respectively; $p = .52$). Subsequently, OKT3 was shown to reverse rejection episodes that were unresponsive to both steroid and ALG therapy (52). This resulted in the salvage of kidneys that would otherwise have been lost to rejection. The 6-month graft survival rate was 60% in these patients.

Another significant problem is that OKT3 stimulates an immune response against the foreign mouse protein. The anti-OKT3 antibody response can be isotypic, idiotypic, or both. Anti-idiotypic antibodies inhibit the binding of OKT3 to T cells and thereby reduce its therapeutic activity whereas the anti-isotypic antibodies (anti-mouse IgG2a) do not appear to neutralize OKT3 immunosuppressive activity (54). The frequency of antibody production was approximately 73% in the early clinical series which seriously limited the ability to retreat patients with OKT3. Subsequent studies have shown, however, that with the concomitant administration of azathioprine or cytoxan during OKT3 therapy, this is reduced to less than 40% (55). Many of these responses are also low-titer, which do not preclude retreatment with OKT3. It is now common practice to measure the antibody response to OKT3 in all patients undergoing OKT3 treatment and to avoid retreatment if the patient develops a high-titer response (>1:100). It is likely that similar antibodies with different isotypic determinants will be developed and used in patients with antibodies to OKT3.

Early studies also reported a high incidence (>60%) of recurrent rejection after OKT3 therapy. Most of these patients received only AZA and P without CsA. It has now been shown that by starting CsA 2 to 3 days prior to discontinuing OKT3, the incidence of recurrent rejection is reduced to approximately 20% (56).

Other monoclonal antibodies are currently under investigation as new treatments for allograft rejection. The most promising has been anti-IL-2 receptor monoclonal antibody (anti-IL-2) which has been shown to prolong murine cardiac and skin allograft survival (57) and rat cardiac allograft survival (58). There is a sound theoretical basis for believing that an antibody to the IL-2 receptor might be effective in preventing allograft rejection. Activated T cells express a variety of plasma membrane receptors that are absent from the surface of resting T cells. The expression of cell surface IL-2 receptors is increased by exposure to alloantigens, mitogens, and interleukin 1. Once these receptors accumulate at the cell surface, interaction with its ligand, IL-2, results in clonal expansion of specifically activated T cells. Treatment with anti-IL-2 receptor antibody could theoretically prevent this clonal expansion in vivo and thereby block rejection. Whether this will hold true in further animal and human studies is unknown. Preliminary studies from France indicate that anti-IL-2 antibody may be effective in man.

Total Lymphoid Irradiation

For over 20 yr, patients with Hodgkin's disease have been successfully treated by total lymphoid irradiation (TLI) (59). TLI focuses on the major lymphoid regions of the body, while sparing vital nonlymphoid and major bone marrow regions, especially the long bones. The fields used for TLI encompass all the major supradiaphragmatic and subdiaphragmatic lymphoid regions, as well as the spleen. Patients with Hodgkin's disease who have been treated with TLI have long-lasting impairment in cell-mediated immune functions. Because of this evidence, and evidence that TLI impaired the ability of rodents to reject organ allografts, TLI was considered for use in clinical renal transplantation in the late 1970s as an alternative immunosuppressive regimen in patients who were at high risk for allograft rejection.

To date, five clinical transplant centers have reported studies utilizing pre-transplant TLI in humans. The first clinical study of TLI was begun in 1979 at the University of Minnesota in splenectomized cadaver renal transplant recipients who had previously rejected at least one transplant while on conventional immunosuppression (AZA, P, and ALG) (60). Patients received up to 4,150 rads pretransplant (in 100 to 150 rad fractions), followed by maintenance AZA and P post-transplant. Graft survival rates at 24 months were 72% in the TLI group compared with 38% in a historical control group given AZA and P without TLI (Fig. 4). This pilot study showed that optimal results were achieved with 2,500 rads delivered in 100-rad fractions followed by transplantation within 2 wk.

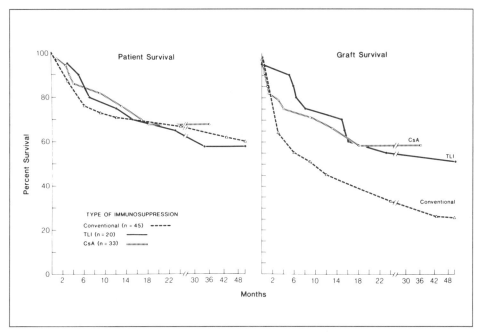

Fig. 4. Acturial patient and renal allograft survival rates according to immunosuppressive regimen after retransplantation at the University of Minnesota. Reproduced with permission from Sutherland et al (84).

Waer et al. (61) have shown that patients receiving TLI pretransplant can be managed with less steroids without a detrimental effect on graft function. Based on this clinical report and animal studies a prospective study of TLI in primary cadaver renal allograft recipients was undertaken by Levin et al (62). Patients received TLI to a total dose of 2,000 rads and were transplanted a mean of 9 days later (range 0 to 65 days). Antithymocyte globulin (ATG) was administered every other day for the first 11 days post-transplant. Low-dose P was started on the day of transplant and continued as the sole maintenance immunosuppressive drug. One-year graft survival was 77%, compared to 67% seen in primary cadaver renal transplant patients given CsA and P without TLI. These results are still inferior compared to present protocols utlizing triple (AZA + P + CsA) or quadruple (AZA + P + CsA + ALG) therapy (85%, 12-month graft survival). Furthermore, 60% of patients had at least one rejection episode requiring increased steroids and in many instances the addition of AZA. There were also two deaths (8%) from disseminated viral infections. Therefore, the advantages of TLI as a primary therapeutic modality are not yet clear. Other studies have suggested that CsA use might decrease the radiation dose necessary, and that a combination of low-dose TLI and low-dose CsA + P may be superior.

In conclusion, total lymphoid irradiation should still be considered experimental at this time. However, it is possible that the use of TLI will reduce the requirements for other immunosuppressive drugs post-transplant. Therefore, it may also have a role in patients at high risk for either allograft rejection or complications from immunosuppressive drugs.

Role of HLA Matching in the 1980s

The human lymphocyte antigen (HLA) system is made up of the gene products, or antigens, of the major histocompatibility locus (MHC) and is the major transplantation antigen system in man along with the ABO blood group system. HLA-A and HLA-B matching began to be utilized in clinical transplantation in the late 1960s in the hopes of reducing the incidence of rejection and improving graft survival. Although numerous studies were performed, the data most relevant to current issues come from the 1980s, after the introduction of HLA-DR typing.

It is clear that HLA matching in renal transplantation is beneficial when considering two-haplotype-matched living-related grafts, i.e., HLA-identical siblings. These patients have 95% long-term allograft survival, require less immunosuppression, and have fewer complications. However, since the introduction of donor specific transfusion (DST) and CsA, there has not been uniform agreement that HLA matching is beneficial in living-related, living-unrelated, or cadaver donor kidney transplants.

Early studies showed that one- or zero-haplotype-matched living-related recipients had poorer graft survival rates compared to recipients of HLA identical grafts (63). If these patients were subdivided into high and low responders based on mixed leukocyte culture (MLC) reactivity between the recipient and donor, it could be shown that low reponders had an 80% graft survival rate at 1 yr, compared to 63% in the high responders. Because the results in the high responders were not significantly different from the cadaver graft survival rates, many institutions abandoned transplantation between haploidentical donor-recipient pairs with a high MLC stimulation index. With the introduction of DST, however, the results of one-and zero-haplotype living-related and living-unrelated transplants have improved markedly and now approach those in HLA identical siblings, regardless of their MLC reactivity, as discussed above.

Most of the current HLA tissue typing controversy revolves around its usefulness in cadaver kidney transplantation. A large number of single-center and multicenter reports have been published, but with contradictory conclusions. There are several possible explanations that are important to consider when critically examining these data.

First, there are significant differences in cadaver renal allograft survival rates among different transplant centers. Cicciarelli et al. (64) pointed out that this "center effect" was "one of the strongest influences on kidney graft survival." Transplant centers with poor cadaver graft survival rates usually show a positive influence of HLA matching, whereas centers with good graft survival rates see little influence of HLA matching. A recent series of 2,670 first cadaver renal transplants at over 100 transplant centers in 1983 and 1984 identified a persistent center effect despite the widespread use of CsA (65). After discounting for statistical variation, the greatest difference between the best and the worst centers was approximately 40% to 50%.

Multicenter studies have also been criticized for combining different patient populations and treatment protocols, further enhancing the "center effect." Data collection is also more likely to be of uneven quality.

Second, single center studies have limited numbers of patients. A statistical analysis by Mickey (65) demonstrated that as many as 300 to 400 subjects may be insufficient to detect a 10% to 20% difference between treatment outcomes. The difference in 1-yr graft survival between the best and poorest matched categories has usually been approximately 10% to 15%. If one assumes a 4% difference per mismatched antigen, about 1,200 cases would be required to have a 90% chance of obtaining a statistically significant increase using a 5% test. Three hundred and fifty transplants would be required for a 50% chance. Thus, single-center studies have difficulty reaching statistically significant conclusions.

Prior to widespread CsA use, several large collaborative studies demonstrated a 10% to 15% improvement in graft function with HLA-A and HLA-B matching (66-68). In the CsA era, an improvement in graft survival with good matches is difficult to demonstrate. Cicciarelli et al. (69) compiled results from a large number of centers reporting to the UCLA Transplant Registry and could only show a 6% improvement in the best HLA-A and HLA-B matches compared to the worst matches in patients not treated with CsA. In CsA-treated patients, there was no statistically significant difference between the best and worst matches. The results for HLA-DR typing showed only a 7% improvement in both non-CsA and CsA-treated patient groups (best vs. worst matches). Several other multicenter studies have found no significant improvement in survival with HLA-A, HLA-B or HLA-DR matching when CsA is used (32, 63).

Whether matching for DR antigens is beneficial is still unclear. Single-center studies from England (70) and the United States (71) demonstrated a significant improvement in 1-yr cadaver graft survival rates from 50% with two mismatches to 80% with no mismatches. Ting (72) has emphasized that the benefit of HLA-DR matching is an "all or none" phenomenon, i.e., the improvement in graft survival rates is only seen when there are no mismatches at the DR locus. Other multicenter and single-center studies have not been able to show a beneficial effect of DR matching in CsA-treated patients (63). For example, data from the University of Minnesota failed to show a significant effect of DR matching in 208 first cadaver graft recipients with 1 and 3-yr follow-up (73). However, they were able to show a 10% improvement in graft survival in second transplants with no DR mismatches. A recent study by Gilks et al. (74) could show a beneficial effect only if there was DR identity and at most one A or B mismatch.

In conclusion it appears that there is little benefit of HLA-A or HLA-B matching in cadaver allograft recipients treated with CsA. If there is an effect of DR matching in CsA-treated patients it is small and only demonstrable when there are no DR mismatches. There may be some benefit of DR matching in second transplants or in highly sensitized patients (75).

ABO-Incompatible Transplants

It is generally accepted that ABO-compatibility between a kidney donor and recipient is necessary and that allografts between ABO incompatible individuals lead to hyperacute or accelerated acute rejection mediated by blood group isoagglutinins. There have been isolated case reports, however, of successful ABO-incompatible kidney allografts (76). Why not all ABO-incompatible allografts are not rejected is not well understood. There has been increased interest in ABO-incompatible transplants because of the recent success in ABO-incompatible bone marrow transplant recipients (77-79). Methods have been developed to remove natural anti-A and anti-B isoagglutinins by plasmapheresis using specially designed immunoabsorbent columns (80).

Using this experience Alexandre et al. (81) have performed a series of 19 ABO-incompatible kidney transplants. These included 14 living-related haploidentical donors and five living-unrelated donors (all spouses). The recipients were prepared for transplantation with a pretransplant protocol that included donor-specific platelet transfusions, plasmapheresis, splenectomy, injection of substance A or B blood group antigen, and standard immunosuppression with CsA, AZA, steroids, and antilymphocyte serum. The 2-yr graft survival rate is 83% with two grafts lost to irreversible acute rejection at 9 and 19 days, and one lost to chronic rejection at 7 months. This is slightly lower but not significantly different from the 92% graft survival rate obtained in 40 ABO-compatible living donor transplants performed during the same time period.

A related issue is whether cadaver kidneys from patients with the blood group A2 can be transplanted into group O recipients. A2 erythrocytes bear fewer A antigenic determinants and are less susceptible to isoagglutinins. Breimer et al. (82) from Sweden has reported a series of 17 cadaver renal transplants from blood group A2 donors to blood group O recipients. Ten grafts functioned long-term with the longest surviving over 5 yr at the time of the report. There were no cases of hyperacute rejection. None of these patients underwent plasmapheresis or immunoabsorption and there were no cases of hyperacute rejection. We recently transplanted a living-related A2 kidney into a group O recipient that was rejected at 9 days. We were able to document that this was a humoral rejection mediated by anti-A antibody (unpublished observation). Therefore, we would not recommend transplantation between group A2 donors and group O recipients.

Summary

Donor-specific transfusions, CsA, and OKT3 have had major impacts on living-related and cadaver donor renal transplantation. The results with donor-specific transfusions in haploidentical and HLA-mismatched living-related recipients, and now in living-unrelated recipients, approaches those in HLA-identical sibling recipients. Quadruple immunosuppression with AZA, P, ALG, and CsA has significantly improved cadaver allograft survival rates and reduced the morbidity of cadaver transplantation. OKT3 is an effective new immunosuppressive agent that has an established role in the treatment of rejection, especially those resistant to conventional therapy, and may have a role in prophylactic protocols. The role of total lymphoid irradiation is not yet clear and its use must still be regarded as experimental. HLA matching does not appear to have a strong role in living-related transplantation where donor-specific transfusions have resulted in improved results in mismatched related and unrelated patients. Similarly, HLA matching does not appear to have a major impact in cadaver transplant recipients treated with CsA. Finally, the future of ABO incompatible transplants is promising, but will require further study.

References

1. Carrel A: La technique operatoire des anastomoses vasculaires et la transplantation des visceres. *Lyon Med* 1902; 98:859

2. Carrel A: Results of the transplantation of blood vessels, organs and limbs. *JAMA* 1908; 51:1662

3. Murray JE: Remembrances of the early days of renal transplantation. *Transplant Proc* 1981; 13(Suppl 1):9

4. Hamburger J, Vaysse J, Crosnier J, et al: Renal homotransplantation in man after radiation of the recipient. *Am J Med* 1962; 32:854

5. Schwartz R, Dameshek W: Drug-induced immunological tolerance. *Nature* 1959; 183:1682

6. Calne RY: The rejection of renal homografts. Inhibition in dogs by 6-mercaptopurine. *Lancet* 1960; i:417

7. Zukoski CF, Lee HM, Hume DM: The prolongation of functional survival of canine renal homografts by 6-mercaptopurine. *Surg Forum* 1960; 11:470

8. Kissmeyer-Nielsen F, Olsen S, Peterson VP, et al: Hyperacute rejection of kidney allografts associated with pre-existing humoral antibodies against donor cells. *Lancet* 1966; ii:662

9. Morrow CE, Sutherland DER, Fryd DS, et al: Renal allograft survival in patients with positive B cell crossmatch to their donor. *Ann Surg* 1984; 199:75

10. Opelz G, Mickey MR, Terasaki PI: HLA and kidney transplants: Reexamination. *Transplantation* 1974; 17:371

11. Opelz G: Improved kidney graft survival in nontransfused recipients. *Transplant Proc* 1987; 19:149

12. Opelz G, Sengar DPS, Mickey MR, et al: Effect of blood transfusions on subsequent kidney transplants. *Transplant Proc* 1973; 5:253

13. Lundgren G, Groth CG, Albrechtsen D, et al: HLA-matching and pre-transplant blood transfusions in cadaveric renal transplantation — changing picture with cyclosporin. *Lancet* 1986; ii:66

14. Newton WT, Anderson CB: Planned preimmunization of renal allograft recipients. *Surgery* 1973; 74:430

15. Salvatierra O Jr, Vincenti F, Amend W: Deliberate donor-specific blood transfusions prior to living related renal transplantation. *Ann Surg* 1980; 192:543

16. Anderson CB, Sicard GA, Etheredge EE: Pretreatment of renal allograft recipients with azathioprine and donor-specific blood products. *Surgery* 1982; 92:315

17. Sollinger HW, Burlingham WJ, Sparks EMF, et al: Donor-specific transfusions in unrelated and related HLA-mismatched donor-recipient combinations. *Transplantation* 1984; 38:612

18. Glass NR, Miller DT, Sollinger HW, et al: Comparative analysis of the DST and imuran-plus-DST protocols for living donor renal transplantation. *Transplantation* 1983; 36:636

19. Salvatierra O Jr, Melzer J, Vincenti F, et al: Donor-specific blood transfusions versus cyclosporine — The DST story. *Transplant Proc* 1987; 19:160

20. Potter D, Garovoy M, Hopper S, et al: Effect of donor-specific transfusions on renal transplantation in children. *Pediatrics* 1985; 76:402

21. Friedman A, Deierhoi M, Chesney R, et al: Donor-specific transfusions in renal transplantation in children: Effect of azathioprine plus transfusions. *Transplantation* 1987; 44:159

22. Chavers BM, Nevins TE, Knaack M, et al: Early acute tubular necrosis, late rejection in pediatric renal transplantation with donor-specific transfusions. *Transplant Proc* 1987; 19:1526

23. Belzer FO, Kalayogly M, Sollinger HW: Donor-specific transfusion in living-unrelated renal donor-recipient combinations. *Transplant Proc* 1987; 19:1514

24. Sollinger HW, Kalayoglu M, Belzer FO: Use of the donor specific transfusion protocol in living-unrelated donor-recipient combinations. *Ann Surg* 1986; 204:315

25. Iwaki Y, Terasaki P: Donor specific transfusion. *In:* Clinical Transplants 1986. Teraski PI (Ed). Los Angeles, UCLA Tissue Typing Laboratory, 1986, p 267

26. Simmons RL, Canafax DM, Strand M, et al: Management and prevention of cyclosporine nephrotoxicity after renal transplantation: Use of low doses of cyclosporine, azathioprine, and prednisone. *Transplant Proc* 1985; 17:266

27. Borel JF: Comparative study of in vitro and in vivo drug effects on cell-mediated cytotoxicity. *Immunology* 1976; 31:631

28. Britton S, Palacious R: Cyclosporin A - Usefulness, risks and mechanism of action. *Immunol Rev* 1982; 65:5

29. Calne RY, White DJ, Thiru S, et al: Cyclosporine A in patients receiving renal allografts from cadaver donors. *Lancet* 1978; ii:1323

30. Calne RY, White DJG, Evans DB, et al: Cyclosporin A in cadaveric organ transplantation. *Br Med J* 1981; 282:934

31. Starzl TE, Weil R III, Iwatsuki S, et al: The use of cyclosporine A and prednisone in cadaver kidney transplantation. *Surg Gynecol Obstet* 1980; 151:17

32. European Multicenter Trial Group: Cyclosporine and cadaver renal transplantation: One year follow-up of a multicenter trial. *Lancet* 1983; ii:986

33. The Canadian Multicenter Transplant Study Group: A randomized clinical trial of cyclosporine and cadaver renal transplantation. *N Engl J Med* 1983; 309:809

34. Najarian JS, Fryd DS, Straud M, et al: A single institution, randomized, prospective trial of cyclosporin versus azathioprine-antilymphocyte globulin for immunosuppression in renal allograft recipients. *Ann Surg* 1985; 201:142

35. Schlanger RE, Henry ML, Sommer BG, et al: Identification and treatment of cyclosporine-associated allograft thrombosis. *Surgery* 1986; 100:329

36. Light JA, Aquino A, Ali A, et al: Quadruple drug therapy prevents graft loss from acute rejection without increasing mortality. *Transplant Proc* 1987; 19:1927

37. Deierhoi MH, Sollinger HW, Kalayoglu M, et al: Quadruple therapy for cadaver renal transplantation. *Transplant Proc* 1987; 19:1917

38. Fries D, Hiesse C, Charpentier B, et al: Triple combination of low-dose cyclosporine, azathioprine, and steroids in first cadaver donor renal allografts. *Transplant Proc* 1987; 19:1911

39. Salaman JR, Griffin PJA, Ross WB, et al: A controlled trial of triple therapy in renal transplantation. *Transplant Proc* 1987; 19:1935

40. Jones RM, Murie JA, Allen R: Immunosuppression with cyclosporine, azathioprine, and prednisolone in cadaver renal allograft recipients. *Transplant Proc* 1987; 19:1926

41. Shield CF, Cosimi AB, Tolkoff-Rubin H, et al: Use of antithymocyte globulin for reversal of acute allograft rejection. *Transplantation* 1979; 28:461

42. Filo RS, Smith EJ, Leapman SB: Therapy of acute cadaveric renal allograft rejection with adjunctive antithymocyte globulin. *Transplantation* 1980; 30:445

43. Hoitsma AJ, Reekers P, Kroeftenberg JG, et al: Treatment of acute rejection of cadaveric renal allografts with rabbit antilymphocyte globulin. *Transplantation* 1982; 33:12

44. Howard RJ, Condie RM, Sutherland DER, et al: The use of antilymphoblast globulin in the treatment of renal allograft rejection. *Transplantation* 1977; 24:419

45. Köhler G, Milstein C: Continuous cultures of fused cells secreting antibody of predefined specificity. *Nature* 1975; 256:495

46. Cosimi AB, Burton RC, Colvin RB, et al: Treatment of acute renal allograft rejection with OKT3 monoclonal antibody. *Transplantation* 1981; 32:535

47. Cosimi AB, Colvin RB, Burton RC, et al: Use of monoclonal antibodies to T-cell subsets for immunologic monitoring and treatment in recipients of renal allografts. *N Engl J Med* 1981; 305:308

48. Reinherz EL, Meyer S, Gingras SP, et al: Antigen recognition by human T lymphocytes is linked to surface expression of the T3 molecular complex. *Cell* 1982; 30:735

49. Chang TW, Kung PC, Gingras SP, et al: Does OKT3 monoclonal antibody react with an antigen-recognition structure on human T cells? *Proc Nat Acad Sci USA* 1981; 78:1805

50. Landegren U, Ramstedt U, Axberg I, et al: Selective inhibition of human T cell cytotoxicity at levels of target recognition or initiation of lysis by monoclonal OKT3 and Leu-2a antibodies. *J Exp Med* 1982; 155:1579

51. Miller RA, Maloney DG, McKillop J, et al: In vivo effects of murine hybridoma monoclonal antibody in a patient with T-cell leukemia. *Blood* 1981; 58:78

52. Norman DJ, Barry JM, Funnell B, et al: OKT3 for treatment of acute and steroid- and ATG-resistent acute rejection in renal transplantation. *Transplant Proc* 1985; 17:2744

53. Ortho Multicenter Transplant Study Group: A randomized clinical trial of OKT3 monoclonal antibody for acute rejection of cadaveric renal transplants. *N Engl J Med* 1985; 313:337

54. Jaffers GJ, Fuller TC, Cosimi AB, et al: Monoclonal antibody therapy: Anti-idiotypic and non-anti-idiotypic antibodies to OKT3 arising despite intense immunosuppression. *Transplantation* 1986; 41:572

55. Goldstein G, Fuccello AJ, Norman DJ, et al: OKT3 monoclonal antibody plasma levels during therapy and the subsequent development of host antibodies to OKT3. *Transplantation* 1986; 42:507

56. Thistlethwaite JR, Gaber AO, Haag BW, et al: OKT3 treatment of steroid-resistant renal allograft rejection. *Transplantation* 1987; 43:176

57. Kirkman RL, Barrett LV, Gaulton GN, et al: Administration of an anti-interleukin 2 receptor monoclonal antibody prolongs cardiac allograft survival in mice. *J Exp Med* 1985; 162:358

58. Kupiec-Weglinski JW, Padberg W, Uhteg LC, et al: Anti-interleukin 2 receptor (IL-2R) antibody against rejection of organ grafts. *Transplant Proc* 1987; 19:591

59. Strober S: Transplantation: Approaches to graft rejection. *In:* Total Lymphoid Irradiation: Basic and Clinical Studies in Transplantation Immunity. Meryman HT (Ed). *Prog Clin Bio Res* 1986; 224:251

60. Najarian JS, Ferguson RM, Sutherland DER, et al: Fractionated total lymphoid irradiation as preparative immunosuppression in high risk renal transplantation: Clinical and immunological studies. *Ann Surg* 1982; 196:442

61. Waer M, Vanrenterghem Y, Kiam Ang K, et al: Comparison of the immunosuppressive effect of fractionated total lymphoid irradiation (TLI) versus conventional immunosuppression (CI) in renal cadaveric allotransplantation. *J Immunol* 1984; 132:1041

62. Levin B, Collins G, Hoppe RT, et al: Treatment of cadaveric renal transplant recipients with total lymphoid irradiation, antithymocyte globulin, and low-dose prednisone. *Lancet* 1985; ii:1321

63. Braun WE: Molecular, genetic and clinical aspects of the HLA system. *In:* Organ Transplantation and Replacement. Cerilli GJ (Ed). London, JB Lippincott Co, 1988, p 162

64. Cicciarelli J, Terasaki PI, Cecka M, et al: Is cyclosporine a match for tissue typing centers? Role of the zero HLA-A, B and DR mismatch effect. *Transplant Proc* 1987; 19:647

65. Mickey MR: HLA matching in transplants from cadaver donors. *In:* Clinical Kidney Transplants 1985. Terasaki PI (Ed). Los Angeles, UCLA Tissue Typing Laboratory, 1985, p 45

66. Opelz G, Mickey MR, Terasaki PI: HLA matching and cadaver kidney transplant survival in North America. Influence of center variation and presensitization. *Transplantation* 1977; 23:490

67. Krakauer H, Spees EK, Vaughn WK, et al: Assessment of prognostic factors and projection of outcomes in renal transplantation. *Transplantation* 1983; 36:372

68. Bashir HV, d'Apice A: Cadaver renal transplantation and HLA matching in Australia from 1971 to 1980. A report of the Australian and New Zealand combined dialysis and transplant registry. *Transplantation* 1982; 34:183

69. Cicciarelli J, Terasaki PI, Mickey MR: The effect of zero HLA Class I and II mismatching in cyclosporin-treated kidney transplant patients. *Transplantation* 1987; 43:636

70. Ting A, Morris PJ: Powerful effect of HLA-DR matching on survival of cadaveric renal allografts. *Lancet* 1980; ii:282

71. Goeken NE, Thompson JS, Corry RJ: A 2-year trial of prospective HLA-DR matching. Effects on renal allograft survival and rate of transplantation. *Transplantation* 1981; 32:522

72. Ting A: HLA and renal transplantation. *In:* Kidney Transplantation. Morris P (Ed). London, Grune & Stratton, 1984, p 159

73. Migliori RJ, Simmons RL, Fryd D, et al: HLA-DR tissue typing may be ignored for the first but not subsequent cadaver renal transplants. *Transplant Proc* 1987; 19:689

74. Gilks WR, Bradley BA, Gore SM, et al: Substantial benefits of tissue matching in renal transplantation. *Transplantation* 1987; 43:669

75. Cecka JM: The changing role of HLA matching. *In:* Clinical Transplants. Terasaki PI (Ed). Los Angeles, UCLA Tissue Typing Laboratory, 1986, p 14

76. Starzl TE, Marchioro TL, Holmes JH, et al: Renal homografts in patients with major donor-recipient blood group incompatibilities. *Surgery* 1964; 55:195

77. Gale RP, Feig S, Ho W, et al: ABO blood group system and bone marrow transplantation. *Blood* 1977; 50:185

78. Buckner CD, Clift RA, Sanders JE, et al: ABO-incompatible marrow transplants. *Transplantation* 1978; 26:233

79. Bensinger WI, Bucker CD, Thomas ED, et al: ABO-incompatible marrow transplants. *Transplantation* 1982; 33:427

80. Bensinger WI, Baker DA, Buckner CD, et al: Immunoabsorption for removal of A and B blood-group antibodies. *N Engl J Med* 1981; 304:160

81. Alexandre GPJ, Squifflet JP, De Bruyere M, et al: ABO-incompatible related and unrelated living donor renal allografts. *Transplant Proc* 1986; 18:452

82. Breimer ME, Brynger H, Rydberg L, et al: Transplantation of blood group A2 kidneys to O recipients. Biochemical and immunological studies of blood group A antigens in human kidneys. *Transplant Proc* 1985; 17:2640

83. Sommer BG, Henry ML, Ferguson RM: Sequential antilymphoblast globulin and cyclosporine for renal transplantation. *Transplant Proc* 1987; 19:1879

84. Sutherland DER, Ferguson RM, Aeder MI, et al: Total lymphoid irradiation and cyclosporine. *Transplant Proc* 1983; 15:2881

Self-Assessment Questions

Each of the following questions is followed by true or false answers based on information in the text. Any combination of answers may be correct. An explanation of the correct answers is given below.

1. Regarding the use of donor-specific transfusions:
   A. sensitization to donor antigens can be reduced by administering azathioprine during the period of transfusions

   B. patients receiving DST from an HLA-identical sibling donor should nevertheless be treated with maintenance cyclosporine following transplantation

   C. without exception, AZA-DST treatments preceding living-related donor renal transplantation is the treatment of choice for children with end stage renal disease

   D. evidence supports the use of AZA-DST for living-unrelated renal transplants

2. The use of cyclosporine in cadaver transplantation:
   A. has led to an improvement in 1-yr graft survival rates of more than 15% in all randomized clinical trials reported

   B. is primarily limited by infectious complications

   C. with multiple therapy regimens has reduced the incidence of CsA toxicity ten-fold

3. Which of the following OKT3 side-effects may be seen within 48 h after giving the first dose?
   A. pyrexia
   B. dyspnea
   C. chest pain
   D. nausea and vomiting

4. Characteristics of OKT3 administration include:
   A. an ineffective response when treating steroid or ALG-resistant acute graft rejection

   B. an anti-OKT3 antibody response which precludes repeated use of OKT3 in almost all patients

103

C. a high incidence (60%) of recurrent rejection after OKT3 therapy

D. an effect which results from blocking the generation of new functional effector T cells and inhibiting the activity of mature lymphocytes

5. Total lymphoid irradiation:

A. clearly superior to current immunosuppressive protocols for 12 month graft survivals

B. should optimally be administered using 1,200 rads

C. irradiation doses might be decreased with the use of CsA

D. as a primary therapeutic modality TLI should still be considered experimental

6. Human leukocyte antigen (HLA) matching:

A. uniformly accepted as beneficial in living-related, living-unrelated or cadaver donor kidney transplants

B. transplant centers with poor cadaver graft survival rates usually show a positive influence of HLA matching, whereas centers with good graft survival rates see little influence of HLA matching

C. in CsA-treated patients, little benefit is gained from HLA-A or HLA-B matching

D. HLA-DR matching may be of some benefit in second transplants or in highly sensitized patients

7. ABO-incompatible transplants:

A. two-year graft survival rates are significantly lower in ABO-incompatible than in ABO-compatible living donor transplants

B. require far more pretransplant preparation (i.e., donor specific platelet transfusion, plasmapheresis, splenectomy, injection of substance A or B blood group antigen, in addition to standard immunosuppression)

C. results from recent reports advocating the use of A2 kidneys transplanted into group O recipients have been substantiated by others

D. require the availability of immunoabsorbent columns to remove natural anti-A and anti-B isoagglutinins

Self-Assessment Answers

1. A. TRUE. Sensitization can be reduced from 30% to 15% with the use of azathioprine.
   B. FALSE. A majority of patients will have excellent long-term function without rejection and without the need for CsA.
   C. FALSE. In cases where it would be preferable to avoid the risk of sensitization that would then relegate the child to a cadaver transplant (i.e., only one living donor), AZA-DST may not be the treatment of choice.
   D. TRUE. Actuarial graft survival reported by the University of Wisconsin was 90% at 1 and 5 years.
2. A. TRUE. The European Multicenter Trial Group, the Canadian Multicenter Trial Group and the University of Minnesota have all shown significant improvement with the use of cyclosporine.

B. FALSE. Although other side-effects such as hypertension, hyperkalemia, and hyperuricemia have been reported, nephrotoxicity has clearly been the primary limiting factor.

C. TRUE. The incidence of CsA toxicity has dropped from 24% to 2% in the study reported from the University of Minnesota.

3. A. TRUE
   B. TRUE
   C. TRUE
   D. TRUE

4. A. FALSE. On the contrary, OKT3 has been highly effective in multiple studies comparing its efficacy in treating acute graft rejection to other standard therapies.

   B. FALSE. With concomitant administration of azathioprine or cytoxan, the incidence of anti-OKT3 response has been reduced to less than 40%.

   C. FALSE. In recent studies, the incidence of recurrent rejection has been reduced to approximately 20% by starting CsA 2 to 3 days prior to discontinuing OKT3.

   D. TRUE. OKT3 initiates these responses by binding directly to the T3 cell surface antigen on T-cells.

5. A. FALSE. When compared to results with current triple or quadruple therapy, TLI graft survival rates are not as good.

   B. FALSE. Optimum doses are in the range of 2,000 to 2,500 rads.

   C. TRUE. Current studies are evaluating low-dose TLI combined with low-dose CsA. Results are not yet available.

   D. TRUE. Widespread application of TLI should await further research.

6. A. FALSE. This is no longer true since the introduction of CsA and DST.

   B. TRUE. This is essentially the "center effect" discussed in the text.

   C. TRUE. This is probably also true for HLA-DR matching, with some exceptions.

   D. TRUE. These are two of the important exceptions.

7. A. FALSE. Although lower, 83% versus 92%, this was not statistically significant in Alexandre's study (81).

   B. TRUE. Most protocols have derived their basis from established bone marrow transplant protocols.

   C. FALSE. These results have not been readily repeated or accepted by others.

   D. TRUE. This is part of the pretransplant preparation.

Chapter 7

The Multiple Organ Failure Syndrome

Frank B. Cerra, MD

Outline

Educational Objectives

In this chapter the reader will learn:

1. about the multiple organ failure (MOF) syndrome, its clinical presentation, and its clinical course.

2. how MOF interacts with the adult respiratory distress syndrome (ARDS).

3. the basic characteristics of the physiology and metabolism of MOF.

4. the current concepts of MOF pathogenesis.

5. the current concepts of MOF management.

Hypermetabolism and the Multiple Organ Failure Syndrome

Background

The distinction between isolated or multiple organs failing postinjury and the syndrome of multiple organ failure (MOF) is a relatively new clinical differential (1-10). It was recognized that MOF was a cause of late mortality after trauma, typically after 14 to 21 days; it accounted for 7% to 10% of the overall mortality in polytrauma. In the setting of surgical sepsis, MOF continues to carry a high mortality risk, approaching 75% after septic shock.

This chapter will review the MOF syndrome as it is currently understood in its epidemiology, microbiology, physiology, metabolism, pathogenesis, and current treatment modalities.

Epidemiology of the Clinical Syndrome

The complex of injury, ARDS, and hypermetabolism followed by sequential organ failure is the classic form of the MOF syndrome The hypermetabolism characteristics have been statistically categorized into classes that indicate the degree of response which is present (Table 1). Several etiologies are now known and include: dead tissue, injured tissue, infection, perfusion insults, a failure to adequately restore perfusion, and a source of localized inflammation. Acute lung injury is usually present in some form within the spectrum of minimal lung injury to fulminant ARDS. Renal failure can precede the liver failure. In this setting, a cause of acute renal injury other than the metabolic alterations of MOF can usually be identified, with drug-induced and perfusion-induced renal injury being the most common. The metabolic alterations of MOF can still occur with the liver failure imposed on the renal insufficiency, usually resulting in renal failure requiring dialysis.

Table 1. Levels of metabolic response

Level	Urine Nitrogen (g/day)	Plasma[a] Lactate (mM/L)	Plasma[b] Glucose (mg%)	Insulin Resistance	$\dot{V}o_2$ (ml/min·m²)	Glucagon/ Insulin
low	<10	<1.5	<150	no	<140	1.5 - 3.0
mid	10 - 20	1.5 - 3.0	150 - 250	some	140 - 180	3.0 - 8
high	>20	>3	>250	yes	>180	>8

[a] With a lactate/pyruvate less than 20
[b] In the absence of diabetes mellitus, pancreatitis, and steroid therapy. The metabolic response to stress runs a spectrum, even within each clinical example. This variation is not predictable from clinical setting and necessitates the measurement of metabolism parameters, such as those listed in this table (6). A number of these parameters are laboratory-specific and values need to be adjusted into the measuring laboratory.

In most patients, control of the inciting source and supportive measures are associated with recovery of the patient over the next few days. In a smaller group of patients, a phase of persistent hypermetabolism, is entered (11). During this phase of stable hypermetabolism MOF is frequently not present. Once activated, even in the presence of control of the inciting source, it can persist for 14 to 21 days. Many patients require ventilatory support during this phase to meet the ventilatory demand. In those patients who recover, the hypermetabolism spontaneously abates. The mortality risk of this phase of persistent hypermetabolism seems to run in the 25% to 40% range.

Most MOF occurs in two forms relative to the initiating event (Fig. 1). In the first form, which is frequently seen after a primary pulmonary initiating event such as aspiration, the MOF is a terminal event, becoming manifest only within a few days of death (12, 13). In the second form, as in the case of septic shock with ARDS, the MOF is present nearly from the time of injury. There is a period of several days of relative stability and then progression over 7 to 14 days (11). A third clinical variety has recently been identified in a small number of cases. This form has progressive liver and renal failure in the absence of acute lung injury demonstrable by current methodology.

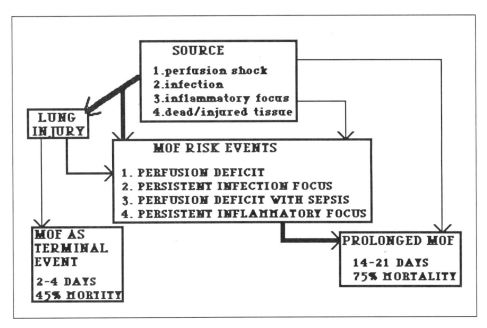

Fig. 1. The various clinical presentations and courses of the MOF syndrome are depicted in this flow diagram. The width of the connecting lines is meant to convey the relative frequency with which a particular pathway is observed (34).

Several clinical settings are associated with the transition from hypermetabolism to organ failure. These include: a persistent perfusion deficit; an unrecognized perfusion deficit; a persistent focus of infection; the combination of a perfusion deficit and a persistent or new septic focus, e.g., recurrent episodes of septic shock; and a persistent inflammatory focus in the absence of infection, such as acute fulminant pancreatitis. Because of the associated findings of progressive jaundice, biliary stasis, reduced hepatic amino acid extraction and reduced hepatic and total body protein synthesis, increased hepatic triglyceride production with reduced peripheral triglyceride clearance, increased ureagenesis even in the absence of protein loading, reduced hepatic redox potential as reflected in the betahydroxybutyrate/acetoacetate ratio, and, terminally, a failure of glucose release and hypoglycemia, the transition to clinical MOF seems to be the manifestation of clinical hepatic failure (14-21).

The transition to clinical MOF is a significant prognostic event. It heralds a change in mortality risk from the 25% to 40% range to the 40% to 60% range in the early stage, and to the 90% to 100% range in the late stages. The differentiation of early from late MOF is primarily a matter of the degree of liver and renal failure. Additional metabolic criteria are also used (Table 2).

Patients who survive hypermetabolism and MOF are in a markedly debilitated state, even with the use of aggressive nutritional support throughout the entire course. This debilitation seems to primarily be reflected in the skeletal muscle mass. The skeletal muscle mass disappears very rapidly during the phase of hypermetabolism, a phenomena referred to as autocannibalism (20). All muscle groups are affected. Consequently, weightbearing and exercise are major rehabilitation problems. Frequently, there is not sufficient muscle power

Table 2. Early and late organ failure

Criteria	Early	Late
Mentation	Light Coma	Deep Coma
ARDS	Present	Advanced
Muscle Mass	Some Wasting	Autocannibalism
Prerenal Azotemia	Some	A Lot
Bilirubin	<3 mg%	<8 mg%
Creatinine	<1.5	>2.5
Lactate [a]	<2	>3
BOHB/ACAC [b]	Normal	Increased
Phenylalanine	<100 UM/L	>100 UM/L
Triglyceride	<250	>250

[a] Beta hydroxybutyrate/acetoacetate ratio
[b] With normal lactate/pyruvate ratio

Most of the criteria for MOF and its severity relate to the onset of hepatic and renal dysfunction and then failure. The bilirubin value is in the absence of other causes such as resolving hematoma, biliary tract obstruction, hemolysis, or drug-induced cholecystosis. ARDS is present during hypermetabolism when organ failure is neither clinically present nor necessarily predictable from the existing clinical setting.

to support ventilation, even at low minute ventilation ($\dot{V}E$) requirements, necessitating prolonged periods of ventilatory support. Rehabilitation becomes a long, slow process of rebuilding skeletal muscle mass, joint stability, and bone strength. A form of peripheral neuropathy has recently been identified as a sequelae of hypermetabolism and MOF (22). The problem is characterized by a motor and sensory peripheral neuropathy together with evidence of skeletal muscle denervation. The cause is unknown; the treatment is supportive and "tincture of time."

Physiology of Multiple Organ Failure

The pulmonary involvement in the MOF syndrome occurs on at least three levels: primary lung involvement, secondary lung involvement, and the mechanics of meeting the ventilatory demands of the systemic hypermetabolism. Primary lung pathology is usually in the form of microbial pneumonitis. This infection can be the inciting source for the hypermetabolism/MOF response, and can be the vent that triggers ARDS. Primary pneumonitis is also a secondary infection occurring during the course of hypermetabolism/MOF. Secondary lung involvement occurs in ARDS induced by a variety of nonlung events including bleeding shock, septic shock, severe sepsis, local inflammatory events such as pancreatitis, acute intracranial events, and polytrauma. In the former case, the MOF tends to occur over a few days as a preterminal event (12, 13). In the latter case, the MOF is present early, tends to be stable for 7 to 10 days, and then progressively worsens (8, 11, 23). In both cases, the ventilatory demand of the hypermetabolism is significantly increased. Typically, 15 to 20 L of $\dot{V}E$ is necessary. The combination of the ventilatory demand and the intrinsic lung pathology usually necessitate mechanical ventilation.

Control of the inciting source is an important component of therapy. That is not to say, however, that the ARDS will immediately resolve. Rather, once triggered, the ARDS tends to run its course and proceed from the acute inflammatory phase into the healing phase, with return of lung function requiring several months (if at all) (24-26). The acute ICU course is usually 14 to 21 days for ARDS. This course almost always has associated hypermetabolism. Undoubtedly, lesser forms of acute lung injury occur that resolve at a much faster rate, particularly with source control. When MOF occurs coincident with the ARDS, as in severe sepsis or septic shock, the prognosis is much worse, with at least a 75% mortality rate even though death may not occur for 21 to 28 days (27).

The primary event in the systemic response seems to be an increase in O_2 consumption ($\dot{V}O_2$) demand. This demand must be met by an increase in supply if survival is to occur. This increase in supply necessitates an increase in cardiac output and an increase in $\dot{V}E$ to maintain oxygenation and facilitate CO_2 removal. The primary physiologic response that induces flow appears to be a fall in systemic vascular resistance (SVR), the auto-unloading phenomenon. In the presence of increased vasoactive amines and autonomic outflow with increased venous return, the high cardiac output state is induced. The absence of this response is associated with an increased mortality risk, and usually occurs for one of three reasons: inadequate preload, pre-existing cardiac disease, or acquired cardiac dysfunction (23, 28, 29).

The precise origin of this response is not clear. The decrease in SVR is independent of flow and presumably is a response to the primary increase in $\dot{V}O_2$ demand (29, 30). In the adequately resuscitated state, major percentages of the flow are going to the skeletal muscle and visceral compartments. How much of this flow is nutrient and how much is for metabolic transport is unknown. It is clear that the skeletal muscle compartment is a primary source for metabolites such as amino acids. This increase in visceral compartment blood flow and $\dot{V}O_2$ seems necessary for optimum survival potential (30). The putative origin of this increased visceral perfusion resides in the synthetic activity present in this compartment, particularly hepatic amino acid clearance and protein synthesis. A failure of central amino acid clearance and hepatic protein synthesis both seem to be major determinants of mortality (11, 21, 31).

Metabolism of Multiple Organ Failure

Energy expenditure is increased during hypermetabolism and MOF. This augmented use is reflected in the increased $\dot{V}O_2$ and CO_2 production. The endogenous RQ appears to run 0.78 to 0.82, reflecting a mixed fuel source, i.e., the carbon source for oxidative production of ATP is not pure glucose, but rather a mixture of carbohydrate, fat, and amino acid. In the higher levels of hypermetabolism, relative to starvation, there is a significant reduction in the fractional calories derived from glucose and fat, and an increase in those derived from amino acids. Because of the increase in total energy expenditure to 1.5 to 2.0 times basal energy expenditure, however, there is an absolute increase in the amount of glucose and fat oxidized relative to a comparable period of starvation. The fats oxidized are primarily medium-chain and short-chain fatty acids, but with a significant contribution of the long-chain fatty acids. The carbohydrate carbon sources include glucose, glycerol, and lactate. The principle user of lactate appears to be cardiac muscle. The amino acids primarily oxidized for energy production appear to be predominantly the branched-chain amino acids, leucine, isoleucine, and valine, and primarily in skeletal muscle. The nitrogen released is used in urea production. The production of ATP appears to be efficiently maintained as long as appropriate resuscitation has occurred. A true failure of energy production seems to only occur during perfusion shock episodes and as a terminal event in MOF (11).

An excess of total calories or an excess of glucose calories has been shown to have a number of detrimental effects on metabolism and organ structure and function. These effects include: fatty liver syndrome, hyperosmolar states, excess CO_2 production and $\dot{V}O_2$, stimulation of catecholamine release, increased lactate formation, a failure to suppress gluconeogenesis, a failure to alter catabolic or synthetic rates, and increased gas production and bowel distension when used enterally. Not exceeding the total caloric requirement and the substitution of fat calories for glucose calories can alleviate the adverse effects of excess glucose administration (11, 32-34).

Hepatic glucose release is increased. This derives in part from increased gluconeogenesis and in part from increased glycogenolysis. The gluconeogenic substrates include: lactate, alanine, glutamine, glycine, serine and glycerol. The alanine and glutamine are nitrogen carriers from the peripheral tissue and represent transamination products from amino acids. A major source of this nitrogen is from amino acids whose carbon skeletons are entering the Krebs cycle for ATP production and, thus, give us their amino nitrogens. These nitrogens and those from the other gluconeogenic amino acids entering into glucose production provide nitrogen for urea production. The gluconeogenesis appears to be driven by a number of mechanisms including the amount of substrate presented, the existing hormone milieu, particularly a high glucagon/insulin ratio, and inflammatory mediators. Some studies also indicate that a significant source of the released glucose is from glycogen breakdown (11, 35-37).

The glucose space is increased; the mass flow of glucose to the periphery is increased; the peripheral uptake of glucose is increased; and the fractional oxidation of glucose as a percent of total calories oxidized is reduced. The addition of insulin into a setting where the levels of insulin are already high serves to increase the peripheral uptake of glucose, but does not appear to significantly change its oxidative use. In the absence of a perfusion deficit, there is an increased conversion of pyruvate to lactate in a stoichiometric relationship such that there is no excess lactate production. These phenomena have been interpreted as a reduction in the oxidation of pyruvate, presumably through a reduced activity of pyruvate dehydrogenase. Indeed, a relative reduction in enzyme activity has been demonstrated in experimental models. Stimulation of PDH with dichloroacetate has increased the oxidation of pyruvate and decreased that of lactate. In a controlled trial, however, this effect was no greater in the hypermetabolism of burns than it was in the nonhypermetabolic control group (38). Thus, the increased proportionate production of lactate and pyruvate may reflect hypermetabolism with an increased rate of glycolysis. As the progression into MOF occurs, lactate and pyruvate productions progressively increase but without excess lactate production until the cardiac output falls. Ultimately, glucose release fails and hypoglycemia occurs as a terminal event (11).

112

Early on, alpha and beta-regulated lipolysis are reduced. After a few days, lipolysis is increased with a marked increase in beta stimulation. Plasma ketones are very low, even in the absence of any glucose or other substrate administration. A picture of long-chain fatty acid deficiency develops in the plasma immediately following injury. The increase in oleic acid can be suppressed by the administration of current fat emulsions, but the reductions in linoleic and arachidonic acid are not. It also appears that exogenous lipid can increase the metabolism of arachidonic acid with an increased production of its metabolites (39, 40).

As MOF progresses, the endogenous RQ exceeds 1.0, indicating net lipogenesis. The site of this increased lipogenesis appears to be primarily liver. In addition, the peripheral clearance of triglyceride is reduced. In part, this latter phenomenon reflects a reduced lipoprotein lipase activity in skeletal muscle and adipose tissue. The plasma polyunsaturated fatty acid profile comes to resemble that reported for hepatic failure (11).

Total body protein catabolism is markedly increased. Total body protein synthesis is increased relative to starvation but is significantly less than the rate of catabolism. Thus, the rate of net catabolism is markedly increased (15, 16, 41-43). The lean body mass can become significantly depleted in 7 to 10 days. The clinical correlates of these phenomena are the rapid loss of skeletal muscle mass and high urine nitrogen excretions, frequently exceeding 20 g/day. Inherent in this is the meaning of the term "autocannibalism" (20). The primary sites of this amino acid efflux are from the mobile amino acid pools in skeletal muscle, connective tissue, and unstimulated gut. It is also reflected in the plasma amino acid profile with low levels of branched-chain amino acids relative to starvation and increased levels of aromatic amino acids, methionine, threonine, alanine, glutamine, and gluconeogenic amino acids (3, 14, 44). The uptake of amino acids by skeletal muscle is suppressed, further potentiating the net catabolism (45-47).

The hepatic uptake of amino acids is increased, as is hepatic protein synthesis. This increase in hepatic protein synthesis, however, is not uniform. Rather, certain proteins such as albumin and transferrin have selectively decreased synthesis, while others such as the acute-phase reactant proteins are increased. Other places where there seems to be an increase in amino acid use are active sites of inflammation, wounds, and in mononuclear cells producing cytokines. One of the manifestations of this increased flux and turnover of amino acids is an increase in urea production and the clinical manifestation of prerenal azotemia that becomes aggravated as the glomerular filtration falls. Thus, the lean body mass becomes redistributed from the stores to the sites of active protein synthesis, oxidation, and conversion to other substrates such as glucose.

The catabolism is not very responsive to exogenous amino acids. The total body synthetic rate, however, is. As the load of exogenous amino acids is increased, the synthetic rate is increased (47). This process can occur until the synthetic rate equals the catabolic rate. At that point, nitrogen equilibrium is achieved and the rate of net catabolism is minimized by increasing the rate of synthesis and not by decreasing the rate of catabolism. With malnutrition, which can develop rapidly, hepatic protein synthesis can fail and is reflected by a further fall in transferrin and a fall in acute phase reactants. Exogenous amino acids can restore this reduction in synthesis. In patients who are going to survive, this stimulation of protein synthesis rates in response to exogenous amino acids is characteristic. Patients in whom this phenomenon does not occur have a much higher mortality risk (3, 5, 6, 20).

As MOF progresses, total body and hepatic protein synthesis rates fall, and the rates of absolute and relative catabolism increase. A reflection of this is in the increased rate of ureagenesis and the magnitude of the observed pre-renal azotemia. The plasma amino acid profile also reflects this hepatic insufficiency as the levels of all amino acids including the branched-chain amino acids, begin to rise and total amino acid clearance is reduced. With hepatic necrosis, marked elevations are observed in all the plasma amino acids. In this latter phase, exogenous amino acid support is of little therapeutic benefit (11) (Fig. 2).

Pathogenesis of Multiple Organ Failure

There are at least three mediator systems that can translate the injury into a recognizable response: the CNS, the classic endocrine system, and the cell-cell system (48-51). It is apparent that: a) these systems interact with each other at multiple interfaces; b) a full blown response requires all three systems; c) deficiencies in one system can be compensated for by the others; and d) different pathways may predominate in response to different initiating agents.

Most inciting events start with a local injury from trauma, infection or lack of perfusion. A local inflammatory response occurs, presumably from the products of platelet activation, endothelial injury and tissue factor release with activation of complement, coagulation, and the kallekrine system. The local "soup" that develops can then initiate a systemic response. With microbes, local and systemic responses can also be induced by direct action of the microbial toxins or components of the microorganism. In addition, the antigen processing mechanisms are initiated and the "joining" of the immune and inflammatory response occurs. The result is the systemic inflammatory response called hypermetabolism or sepsis syndrome. The cell-cell system seems to be important in the mediation of local responses and in translating the local into the systemic reaction. The neuroendocrine system seems to modulate more global responses, either being directly activated by the injury itself or indirectly through the cell-cell system.

The interleukin group of mediators are all metabolically active and have the capacity to act directly at the cell level, or indirectly through the CNS. They can induce many of the observed responses: fever, leukocytosis, increased gluconeogenesis, and proteolysis. IL1 can directly stimulate the adrenal cortex. In inflammatory wounds, muscle purine metabolism is strongly influenced by a high-energy phosphate-promoting factor released by inflammatory macrophages (52). Local wound factors can also affect metabolic processes in organs removed from the localized inflammatory site (51). A product of the endotoxin-activated macrophage can inhibit skeletal muscle amino acid uptake (53).

Tumor necrosis factor is another cytokine released by activated macrophages. An intact adrenal cortex is necessary to experimentally reproduce the metabolic effects of endotoxin-stimulated TNF (54, 55). These effects can also be largely reversed by insulin administration (56). Numerous metabolically active peptides continue to be identified. These peptides can modulate skeletal muscle

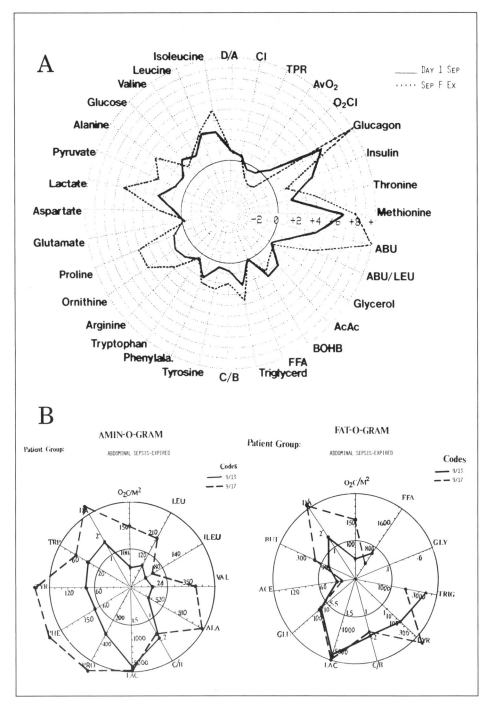

Fig. 2. The plasma amino acids undergo characteristic changes as the MOF metabolism progresses. In A, data from a longitudinal study in septic patients is presented in statistical circles. The innermost circle represents the mean values from the control group. Each circle going outward represents one standard deviation from that mean (14). The mean values from early hypermetabolism and late MOF are plotted. In B, the plasma amino acid profile from hepatic necrosis is presented. A clearance failure for all amino acids has occurred.

115

amino acid uptake (47) and release, and can modulate the alpha and beta-receptor-sensitive lipase system (57).

The hypermetabolic state can be experimentally reproduced by repeated small doses of endotoxin (58). Intestinal translocation of bacteria and toxins can be induced by endotoxins as well as being a source for endotoxin (59). Endotoxin-induced liver damage appears to be, in part, mediated by lipid peroxidation (60). PMN activation by endotoxin can also occur in the absence of activated complement. Endotoxin can induce macrophage-mediated microthrombosis (61); this effect on procoagulant production may be independent of prostaglandin synthesis (62).

A trade-off for this type of regulatory system is a progressive insensitivity to outside intervention as the degree of metabolic control increases. Thus, the administration of glucose does not readily affect the rate of lipolysis (63) or gluconeogenesis (64), and betahydroxybutyrate ineffectively modulates lipolysis (11). The counterregulatory hormones override the insulin effects on hormone-sensitive lipase in adipose tissue, but not the effects on fatty acid esterases and ketosis. The close interaction of pathways may also help to explain the inability of single-agent mediator-blocking regimens to achieve a consistent and reasonable degree of clinical or experimental results.

The mechanisms of cell injury that lead to MOF appear to be multiple and include microcirculatory hypoxia, and mediator and microbial toxin-induced injury. When there is inadequate systemic resuscitation, tissue hypoxia exists. When flow-dependent $\dot{V}O_2$ and excess lactate production are controlled, as determined by systemic sampling, it is not clear that all organ beds have an adequate matching of microcirculatory flow and cell demand for O_2.

Mediator-induced injury also seems to occur. Complement-mediated endothelial damage in acute lung injury is a well described phenomenon in acute lung injury. Oxygen radical generation with injury is an increasingly recognized potential mechanism for reperfusion injury to intracellular organelles and membrane transduction mechanisms. Excessive PGE_2 production is immunosuppressive and may potentiate infectious complications (65, 66). Leukotriene can cause profound cardiac contractility depression. Microbial toxins or components can cause cell injury. Endotoxin can directly inhibit intracellular glycolytic enzymes and can directly alter hepatocyte protein synthesis. It can also produce indirect effects by stimulating the macrophage, which then can alter a target cell function (67).

Another mechanism of injury is best categorized as metabolic dysregulation. In this model, products of metabolism in one area adversely alter metabolism in another area. As an example, plasma proteases may hydrolyze peptide mediators into smaller peptides that are also metabolically active. PIF is being increasingly recognized as a peptide derived from IL1 (68). SAP is hypothesized to be a peptide derived from fibronectin. Octopamine is a vasoactive amine derived from the nonoxidative metabolism of phenylalanine that can induce the low SVR and high cardiac output state.

As has been illustrated in the section on hypermetabolism, the macrophage appears to play a central role in modulating the activity of anatomically associated target cells. The potential exists for the activated macrophage to dysregulate or injure the target cells. Definitive evidence for this phenomenon, however,

116

is yet to be produced. Signal transduction failure may occur and be manifest as altered cell metabolism. Intensive research is proceeding in these areas.

Current Therapy and Future Directions

Current MOF therapy is aimed at prevention and supportive care (Fig. 3). Three general areas are emphasized: source control, restoration, and maintenance of O_2 transport and metabolic support. Source control is a major emphasis, as persistence of a source guarantees a high MOF mortality risk. Whenever possible, excision or removal of the inciting cause is desirable. In many cases, however, this is not possible; as in primary pneumonias, pancreatitis, fractures and soft tissue injury, and hematoma. Appropriate antimicrobial agents are particularly important where the septic focus cannot be removed; these agents are usually effective in eradicating these foci. Fracture stabilization and early burn excision and grafting are other examples of the application of this principle.

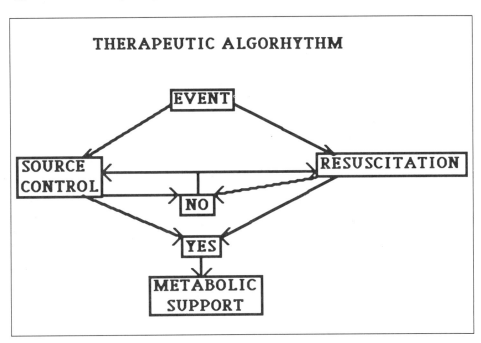

Fig. 3. A current treatment algorithm is presented. The approach emphasizes the simultaneous actions of resuscitation and source control followed by nutrition/metabolism support.

With the recognition of subclinical flow-dependent $\dot{V}O_2$ in settings of pancreatitis, ARDS, and septic and volume shock, i.e., that the clinical criteria of perfusion have a significantly decreased sensitivity and specificity in these settings, increased emphasis is being placed on invasive techniques of resuscitation using $\dot{V}O_2$ criteria. Flow-dependent $\dot{V}O_2$ is treated with increased O_2 content and increased flow until it is no longer present and excess lactate production has ceased. Pre- and postoperative studies continue to indicate a decrease in mortality, infectious complications, and MOF when these principles are used (29, 68-70).

Malnutrition is a primary manifestation of MOF. It seems increasingly clear from the studies that nutritional support per se does not alter the course of the disease process, but can effectively control the visceral malnutrition and limit the lean body mass loss as a covariable in mortality. To effectively achieve this end, several principles have evolved (11):

1. Avoid excess total calories and excess glucose. As guidelines, 30 to 35, non-protein cal/kg·day with 0.5 to 1.0 g/kg·day from current fat emulsions are useful starting points (11).

2. Achieve nitrogen equilibrium by titrating the dose of amino acids (71-76). 1.5 to 2.0 g/kg·day is the usual starting dose. Because of the methodology of doing bedside nitrogen balance, achieving a calculated 2 to 4 g/day of positive balance is usually necessary. A second guideline is to maintain the BUN proportionate to the creatinine or under 110 mg%. Current clinical studies indicate that the modified amino acids are a more efficient protein source at achieving nitrogen retention with a higher rate of protein synthesis than are the standard amino acid formulas (71, 77, 78).

3. Achieve a rising or normal range of hepatic protein synthesis as reflected in the plasma transferrin or prealbumin. The modified amino acid formulas appear to be more efficient at attaining this end-point. When this end-point occurs, an improved survival potential also seems to be present (1-6, 20, 71, 72, 78).

When this algorithm is applied in clinical practice by knowledgeable practitioners, a reduction in overall mortality, the incidence of MOF, and the mortality of MOF are significantly reduced. The incidence and mortality risk of ARDS, however, seems to go on unchanged (27) (Table 3).

Table 3. Effect of aggressive critical care on MOF

Year	Number	% Die	% MOF	% Die MOF	% ALI	% Die ALI
1976-80	432	19 ± 4	7.2 ± 1.9	39 ± 13	43 ± 4	39 ± 8
1981-85	409	11 ± 3*	2.7 ± 1.7*	22 ± 14*	46 ± 7	54 ± 27

* $p < .01$
Values: Mean ± SD
ALI = acute lung injury

The results of a 10-yr epidemiologic study are summarized. The two 5-yr periods represent the time before and after instituting a program of aggressive source control, O_2 transport manipulation, and nutritional/metabolic support (started in 1981) (34).

Based on experimental databases, a number of new support and therapeutic regimens are currently undergoing clinical testing. Monoclonal antibodies and FAB fragments directed against various components of lipolysaccharide are being tested as an alternate of adjuvant means of controlling septic sources. It has been hypothesized that intestinal overgrowth with colonic flora, especially in the presence of gastric alkalinization, may potentiate the incidence of pneumonia by enteric organisms. Intestinal translocation of enteric bacteria, especially in the presence of reduced gut perfusion and/or malnutrition, has been hypothesized to be a primary variable in septicemia and liver failure. Several approaches are being taken to try and control these phenomena (73-75): a) using mucosal barrier or mucosal cytoprotection to control stress ulceration instead of pH control with antacids and/or H2 receptor antagonists; b) controlling the enteric flora and their migration and translocation by various gut decontamination regimens; and c) early, aggressive use of enteral nutrition. All these modalities are in various stages of clinical testing and definitive data are not yet available.

It is understood that the mediator systems are controlling the carbon flow for energy production. Energy production per se does not seem to be the major clinical problem, except as a preterminal event. It also appears as if achieving energy (caloric) equilibrium does not improve the statistical likelihood of survival, as seems to be the case with achieving nitrogen equilibrium (11, 68-76). The efficacy of the newer energy-producing substrates remains to be demonstrated in clinical practice.

One of the major endpoints of metabolic support is focusing on the preservation of organ structure and function and the promotion of repair in organ structure and function after injury has occurred. The polyunsaturated fatty acids are beginning to play a pivotal role in this process. In an animal model of the respiratory distress syndrome, the addition of intravenous lipid emulsion to the parenteral nutrition regimen improved lecithin production and the return of more normal compliance (65, 66).

Clinical trials of single agent chemotherapy such as insulin, steroids, and PgE_1 have shown no significant improvement in survival or the occurrence of MOF. In some cases, outcome was worsened. Experimental studies with other single-agent chemotherapies are continuing to produce conflicting results. It is beginning to appear as if there is no "magic bullet." Some encouraging results with experimental combination chemotherapy are beginning to occur where multiple mediator pathways are being influenced. Hormone manipulation by hormone administration, e.g., growth hormone, is being attempted.

Hopefully, some of these newer approaches will provide improved therapeutic or support regimens.

References

1. Border JH, Chenier R, McMenamy RH: Multiple systems organ failure: Muscle fuel deficit with visceral protein malnutrition. *Surg Clin North Am* 1976; 56:1147

2. Clowes GHA, O'Donnell TF, Blackburn G: Energy metabolism and proteolysis in traumatized and septic man. *Surg Clin North Am* 1976; 56:1169

3. Moyer F, Border JR, McMenamy R, et al: Multiple systems organ failure V: Alterations in plasma protein profile in septic-trauma effect of intravenous amino acids. *J Trauma* 1981; 21:645

4. McMenamy R, Birkhan R, Oswald R, et al: Multiple systems organ failure II: The effect of infusion of amino acids and glucose. *J Trauma* 1981; 21:228

5. Moyer ED, McManemy R, Cerra FB, et al: Multiple systems organ failure III. Contrasts in plasma amino acid profiles in septic trauma patients who subsequently survive and do not survive effects of intravenous amino acids. *J Trauma* 1981; 21:263

6. Moyer G, Border JR, Cerra FB, et al: Systems organ failure IV: Imbalances in plasma amino acids associated with exogenous albumin in the trauma-septic patient. *J Trauma* 1981; 21:543

7. Tilney N, Bailey G, Morgan A: Sequential system failure after rupture of abdominal aortic aneurysms. *Ann Surg* 1973; 118:117

8. Deutschman C, Simmons RL, Cerra FB: The systemic response to cytomegalovirus: Further evidence for a host dependent response. *Arch Surg* (In Press)

9. Carrico CJ, Meakins J, Marshall J, et al: Multiple organ failure syndrome. *Arch Surg* 1986; 121:196

10. Pine RW, Wertz MJ, Lennard ES, et al: Determinants of organ malfunction or death in patients with intraabdominal sepsis. *Arch Surg* 1983; 118:242

11. Cerra FB: Hypermetabolism, organ failure, and metabolic support. *Surgery* 1987; 191:1

12. Fowler AA, Hammon RF: ARDS: Prognosis after onset. *Am Rev Respir Dis* 1985; 132:472

13. Montgomery AB, Stager MA: Causes of mortality in patients with ARDS. *Am Rev Respir Dis* 1985; 132:485

14. Cerra FB, Siegel JH, Border J, et al: The hepatic failure of sepsis: Cellular vs substrate. *Surgery* 1979; 86:409

15. Long CL, Jeevanaudan M, Kinney JM: Whole body protein synthesis and catabolism in septic man. *Am J Clin Nutr* 1977; 30:1340

16. Cerra FB, Caprioli J, Siegel J, et al: Proline metabolism in sepsis, cirrhosis, and general surgery: The peripheral energy deficit. *Ann Surg* 1979; 190:577

17. Giovannini I, Boldrini G, Castagnato M, et al: Respiratory quotient and patterns of substrate utilization in human sepsis and trauma. *JPEN* 1983; 7:226

18. Imamura M, Clowes GH, Blackburn G: Liver metabolism and gluconeogenesis in trauma and sepsis. *Surgery* 1975; 77:868

19. Robin AP, Askanazi J, Greenwood M, et al: Lipoproteinlipase activity in surgical patients: Effects of trauma and sepsis. *Surgery* 1981; 90:401

20. Cerra FB, Siegel JH, Colman B, et al: Autocannibalism, a failure of exogenous nutritional support. *Ann Surg* 1980; 192:570

21. Pearl RH, Clowes GHA, Hirsch EF, et al: Prognosis and survival as determined by visceral amino acid clearance in severe trauma. *J Trauma* 1985; 25:777

22. Bolton C, Young G: Sepsis and septic shock: Central and peripheral nervous systems. *In:* Prospectives in Sepsis and Septic Shock. Sibbald W, Sprung C (Eds). Society of Critical Care Medicine, Fullerton, CA, 1985, pp 157-171

23. Siegel JH, Cerra FB: Physiological and metabolic correlations in human sepsis. *Surgery* 1979; 86:163

24. Rinaldo JE, Rogers RM: ARDS: Changing concepts of lung injury and repair. *N Engl J Med* 1982; 306:900

25. Bell RC, Priboda TJ, Andrews CP: Long term pulmonary function in survivors of ARDS. *Chest* 1983; 94:343A

26. Alberts WM, Priest GR, Moser KM: The outlook for survivors of ARDS. *Chest* 1983; 84:272

27. Cerra FB, Eyer S, Perry JP: Acute lung injury and MOFS. *Crit Care Med* (Submitted)

28. McLean L, Mulligan W, McLean A: Patterns of septic shock in man. *Ann Surg* 1967; 166:543

29. Shoemaker W: Hemodynamic and oxygen transport patterns in septic shock: Physiologic mechanisms and therapeutic implications. *In:* Prospectives in Sepsis and Septic Shock. Sibbald W, Sprung C (Eds). Society of Critical Care Medicine, Fullerton, CA, 1985, pp 203-234

30. Groenveld ABJ, Bronsveld W, Thijs LG: Hemodynamic determinants of mortality in human septic shock. *Surgery* 1986; 99:140

31. Clowes GHA, Hirsch E, George BC, et al: Survival from sepsis. The significance of altered protein metabolism regulated by proteolysis inducing factor, the circulating cleavage product of interleukin-1. *Ann Surg* 1985; 202:446

32. Shaw JHF, Wolfe RR: Glucose and urea kinetics in patients with early and advanced gastrointestinal cancer: The response to glucose infusion, parenteral feeding, and surgical resection. *Surgery* 1987; 101:181

33. Keim NL: Nutritional effectors of hepatic steatosis induced by parenteral nutrition in the rat. *JPEN* 1987; 11:18

34. Sax HC, Talamini MA, Brackett K, et al: Hepatic steatosis in total parenteral nutrition: Failure of fatty infiltration to correlate with abnormal serum hepatic enzyme levels. *Surgery* 1986; 100:697

35. Elwyn DH, Kinney JM, Juvanandum M: Influence of increasing carbohydrate intake on glucose kinetics in injured patients. *Ann Surg* 1979; 190:117

36. Carpentier Y, Askanazi J, Elwyn D, et al: The effect of carbohydrate intake on lipolysis rate in depleted patients. *Metabolism* 1980; 29:974

37. Wolfe R, Allsop J, Burke J: Glucose metabolism in man: Responses to intravenous glucose infusion. *Metabolism* 1979; 28:210

38. Miyoshi H, Jahoor R, Herndon DN, et al: Stimulation of pyruvate dehydrogenase activity increases pyruvate oxidation and decreases lactate production in severely burned patients. *Surg Forum* 1987; 38:26

39. Alden PB, Svingen BA, Holman R, et al: Essential fatty acid states in isolated closed head injury. *J Trauma* 1987; 27:1039

40. Alden PB, Svingen BA, Holman R, et al: Partial correction of exogenous lipid of abnormal patterns of PUFA in stressed and septic patients. *Surgery* 1986; 100:671

41. Birkhan R, Long C, Fitkin DL, et al: A comparison of the effects of skeletal trauma and surgery on the ketosis of starvation in man. *J Trauma* 1981; 21:513

42. Waterlow JC, Golden M, Picou D: Measurement of rates of protein turnover synthesis and breakdown in man and effects of nutritional status and surgical injury. *Am J Clin Nutr* 1977; 30:1333

43. Powell-Tuck J, Fern E, Garlich P, et al: The effect of surgical trauma and insulin on whole body protein turnover in parenterally-fed undernourished patients. *Human Nutr Clin Nutr* 1984; 38:11

44. Cerra FB, Siegel JH, Border J, et al: Correlations between metabolic and cardiopulmonary measurement in patients after trauma, general surgery and sepsis. *J Trauma* 1979; 19:621

45. Hasselgren PO, Talamini M, James JH, et al: Protein metabolism in different types of skeletal muscle during early and late sepsis in rats. *Arch Surg* 1986; 121:918

46. Hasselgren PO, James JH, Fischer JE: Inhibited muscle amino acid uptake in sepsis. *Ann Surg* 1986; 203:360

47. Hasselgren PO, James JH, Warner BW, et al: Reduced muscle amino acid uptake in sepsis and the effects in vitro of septic plasma and interleukin-1. *Surgery* 1986; 100:222

48. Bessey PQ, Watters JM, Aoki TT, et al: Combined hormonal infusion stimulates the metabolic response to injury. *Ann Surg* 1984; 200:264

49. Watters JM, Bessey PQ, Dinarello CA, et al: Both inflammatory and endocrine mediators stimulate host response to sepsis. *Arch Surg* 1986; 121:179

50. Wilmore DW, Orlick L: Systemic response to injury and the healing wound. *JPEN* 1980; 4:147

51. Amaral JF, Shearer JD, Caldwell MD: Examination of lactate metabolism in the cellular infiltrate of wounded tissue. *Surg Forum* 1987; 38:31

52. Morris AS, Shearer JD, Forster J, et al: The relationship of purine metabolism to the macrophage-mediated increase of high energy phosphates in skeletal muscle. *J Surg Res* 1986; 41:339

53. Hummel RP III, Warner BW, Pedersen P, et al: In vitro effects of the TNF. IL-1 and other monokines on skeletal muscle amino acid uptake and protein degradation. *Surg Forum* 1987; 38:13

54. Michie HR, Spriggs DR, Rounds J, et al: Does cachectin cause cachexia? *Surg Forum* 1987; 38:38

55. Starnes HF, Warren RS, Conti PS, et al: Redistribution of amino acids in rat liver and muscle induced by tumor necrosis factor requires the adrenal response. *Surg Forum* 1987; 38:41

56. Fraker DL, Norton JA: Reversal of the toxic effects of cachectin by insulin. *Surg Forum* 1987; 38:18

57. St.Vil D, Gagner M, Forse RA: Control of human adipocyte lipolysis by septic plasma mediators. *Surg Forum* 1987; 38:15

58. Demling RH, Lalonde CC, Jin LJ, et al: The pulmonary and systemic response to recurrent endotoxemia in the adult sheep. *Surgery* 1986; 100:876

59. Deitch EA, Berg R, Specian R: Endotoxin promotes the translocation of bacteria from the gut. *Arch Surg* 1987; 122:185

60. Sugino K, Dohi K, Yamada K, et al: The role of lipid peroxidation in endotoxin-induced hepatic damage and the protective effect of antioxidants. *Surgery* 1987; 101:746

61. Moore FD, Moss NA, Revhaug A, et al: A single dose of endotoxin activates neutrophils without activating complement. *Surgery* 1987; 102:200

62. Maier RV, Hahnel GB: Is macrophage-induced microthrombosis during endotoxemia dependent on prostaglandin synthesis? *J Surg Res* 1986; 40:238

63. Shaw JHF, Wolfe RR: Fatty acid and glycerol kinetics in septic patients and in patients with gastrointestinal cancer. The response to glucose infusion and parenteral feeding. *Ann Surg* 1987; 205:368

64. Long C, Kinney J, Geiger J: Nonsuppressability of gluconeogenesis in septic patients. *Metabolism* 1976; 25:193

65. Alexander JW, Saito H, Trocki O, et al: The importance of lipid type in the diet after burn injury. *Ann Surg* 1986; 204:1

66. Billiar T, Svingen B, West M, et al: Diet high in fish oil suppressed Kupffer cell prostanoid production while preserving Il-1 response to endotoxin. *Surgery* 1987 (In Press)

67. West MA, Keller G, Hyland B, et al: Hepatocyte function in sepsis: Kupffer cells mediate a biphasic protein synthesis response in hepatocytes after endotoxin and killed *E. coli. Surgery* 1985; 98:388

68. Clowes G, George B, Villes J: Muscle proteolysis induced by a circulating peptide in patients with sepsis and trauma. *N Engl J Med* 1983; 308:545

69. Eyer S, Cerra FB: Cost-effective use of the surgical intensive care unit. *World J Surg* 1987; 11:241

70. Jensen JA, Riggs K, Vasconez LO, et al: Clinical assessment of postoperative peripheral perfusion. *Surg Forum* 1987; 38:66

71. Bower RH, Muggin-Sullam M, Vallgren S, et al: Branched chain amino acid-enriched solutions in the septic patient: A randomized, prospective trial. *Ann Surg* 1986; 203:13

72. Cerra FB, Mazuski J, Chute E, et al: Branched chain metabolic support. *Ann Surg* 1984; 199:286

73. Deitch EA, Winterton J, Berg R: The gut as a portal of entry for bacteremia. Role of protein malnutrition. *Ann Surg* 1987; 205:682

74. Baker JW, Deitch EA, Berg R, et al: Hemorrhagic shock impairs the mucosal barrier, resulting in bacterial translocation from the gut and sepsis. *Surg Forum* 1987; 38:73

75. Guzman-Stein G, Bonsack M, Liberty J, et al: Intestinal handling facilitates enteric bacterial translocation. *Surg Forum* 1987; 38:75

76. Cerra FB, Chung NK, Fischer JE, et al: Disease-specific amino acid infusion (FO80) in hepatic encephalopathy: A prospective, randomized, double-blind controlled trial. *JPEN* 1985; 9:288

77. Cerra F, Blackburn G, Hirsch J, et al: The effect of stress level, amino acid formula, and nitrogen dose on nitrogen retention in traumatic and septic stress. *Ann Surg* 1987; 205:282

78. Cerra FB, Upson D, Angelico R, et al: Branched chains support postoperative protein synthesis. *Surgery* 1982; 92:192

Self-Assessment Questions

1. The MOF syndrome refers to:
   A. adult respiratory distress syndrome
   B. liver failure
   C. the sequential failure of lung, liver and kidney
   D. renal failure
   E. encephalopathy

2. Risk factors for developing MOF include all of the following except:
   A. recurrent episodes of shock
   B. an uncontrolled septic focus
   C. a persistent inflammatory focus
   D. enteral nutrition
   E. pelvic fractures with large retroperitoneal hematoma and muscle injury

3. The physiologic hallmarks of MOF include all of the following except:
   A. increased $\dot{V}o_2$
   B. increased CO_2 production
   C. increased cardiac output
   D. increased SVR
   E. increased splanchnic perfusion

4. Muscle metabolism in MOF is characterized by:
   A. increased amino acid release
   B. decreased oxidation of branched-chain amino acids
   C. increased amino acid uptake
   D. increased protein synthesis
   E. decreased protein catabolism

5. Total calories and glucose calories in excess of demand are associated with all of the following except:
   A. fatty liver syndrome
   B. increased CO_2 production
   C. decreased $\dot{V}O_2$
   D. RQ > 1.0
   E. increased catecholamine output

6. Metabolic support principles in MOF include all of the following except:
   A. 30 to 35 nonprotein cal/kg·day
   B. 1.5 to 2.0 g/kg·day of amino acids
   C. 0.5 to 1.0 g/kg·day of lipid emulsion
   D. increasing the calorie loads until RQ > 1
   E. giving multivitamins, Mg, Zn, and trace elements

7. Therapeutic end-points in the therapeutic algorithm of MOF include all of the following except:
   A. control of the inciting source
   B. nutritional/metabolic support
   C. achieving positive nitrogen balance
   D. the presence of flow-dependent $\dot{V}O_2$
   E. a falling serum creatinine

8. Preventive measures for MOF include all of the following except:
   A. fracture stabilization
   B. burn excision
   C. antibiotics appropriate to an infection
   D. malnutrition
   E. surgical control of a septic focus

9. The systemic response as observed in the clinical presentation, physiology, and metabolism can be the same for all of the following except:
   A. anaerobic sepsis
   B. Candida sepsis
   C. CMV sepsis
   D. Gram-positive or negative sepsis
   E. narcotic overdose

10. Hypermetabolism can be seen after each of the following except:
    A. septic shock
    B. pancreatitis
    C. severe polytrauma
    D. aspiration pneumonia
    E. simple congestive heart failure

Self-Assessment Answers

1. C	6. D
2. D	7. D
3. D	8. D
4. A	9. E
5. C	10. E

Case Studies

Case One

A 27-yr-old male was injured in a car accident in which he sustained a right midshaft femur fracture, closed-head injury, right-sided pulmonary contusion, and a ruptured spleen. He is resuscitated and undergoes an uneventful splenectomy.

Three days postinjury he is confused, tachypneic, tachycardic, and has diffuse, bilaterally symmetric infiltrates on his chest x-ray. His Pao_2 is 45 torr on room air; rectal temperature is 101°F and the WBC is 15,000.

The most likely diagnosis is [Decision 1]:

A. ARDS post-trauma

B. pulmonary emboli

C. primary pneumonia

D. drug reaction

He is intubated, begun on positive pressure ventilation with continuous distending pressure. He is also resuscitated and his measurements include: cardiac output 12 L/min; $\dot{V}o_2$ 200 ml/min·m²; SVR 500 dyne/cm; plasma lactate 2.0 mg%; plasma glucose 200 mg%; urinary urea nitrogen of 18 g/day; serum bilirubin 1.0 mg; creatinine 1.0 mg%.

The patient also has [Decision 2]:

A. hypermetabolism

B. a hyperdynamic state

C. MOF

D. a hyperdynamic state with hypermetabolism

He persists in a hemodynamically stable state for the next 10 days. An episode of line sepsis and a urinary tract infection occur. On day 21 postinjury, the hyperdynamic-hypermetabolic state abates; the ARDS improves, and the patient is extubated and does well.

Decisions - Case One

[1]. A

[2]. D

Case Two

A 67-yr-old female enters with a free-ruptured diverticulum of the sigmoid colon with associated peritonitis and septic shock. She undergoes fluid resuscitation and antibiotics but remains relatively hypotensive and unstable. Her cardiac output was 5 L/min, SVR 2350 dyne/cm, and lactate 4.5 mg%. She is treated with dobutamine, with an improvement in flow and lactate, and taken to the operating theater where she undergoes an exteriorization resection of her sigmoid colon followed by feces removal from her abdomen and antibiotic ingestion.

In the postoperative period her $\dot{V}O_2$ is 140 ml/min·m²; lactate 2.5 mg%; cardiac output 8 L/min; SVR 1600 dyne/cm; and pulmonary wedge pressure 18 cm H_2O.

She is treated with nipride and dopamine is added. Her repeat studies show:

$\dot{V}O_2$ 200 ml/min·m²; lactate 2.0%; cardiac output 10 L/min; SVR 700 dyne/cm; serum bilirubin 2.0 mg%; and creatinine 1.5 mg% with PaO_2/FIO_2 of 260 on an FIO_2 of .50 and PEEP 15 cm H_2O. The patient has [Decision 1]:

A. acute lung injury

B. hypermetabolism

C. MOF

D. 1 and 2 above

E. 1, 2 and 3 above

She is begun on metabolic support. She remains on antibiotics; the surgical cultures grow multiple enteric organisms and Candida. She is stable for 8 days and then develops hemodynamic instability, fever, serum bilirubin 3.0 mg%, creatinine 1.5 mg%, and grows Candida from her sputum and blood; amphotericin B is started. All lines are changed; sinus x-rays and CT scan of chest and abdomen are negative.

She clears the fungus infection but $\dot{V}O_2$ remains 200 ml/min·m² plasma lactate 2.5 mg%, $\dot{V}E$ of 18 L/min, and a PaO_2/FIO_2 200 on an FIO_2 of .60 and 15 cm H_2O PEEP.

She now grows Gram-negative bacteria from her tracheal aspirate with an associated increase in secretions, and cultures grow herpes simplex from her tracheal aspirate and blood. She is begun on appropriate antimicrobials and her cultures clear. A sinusitis is diagnosed on x-ray and a tracheostomy is done with resolution of the sinusitis.

She persists with $\dot{V}O_2$ 200 ml/min·m²; lactate 2.2 mg%; cardiac output 11 L/min; nitrogen balance 4 mg/day; SVR 600 dyne/cm; transferrin 130 mg%, bilirubin 5 mg%; creatinine 2.0 mg%; PaO_2/FIO_2 150 on and FIO_2 of .60; and 15 cm H_2O PEEP.

The patient has progressed to [Decision 2]:

A. early MOF

B. late MOF

C. persistent hypermetabolism

D. sepsis syndrome

E. late ARDS

On day 18 postinjury a CT scan was done which revealed a walled left upper quadrant abscess. A percutaneous catheter was placed; pus was removed and the cavity was well-drained. The patient persisted with nearly the same data as above until day 28 postinjury. At that time, she began to improve; she was discharged from the ICU on day 40 postinjury. She remained in the hospital for an additional 30 days of rehabilitation and returned to work 10 months postinjury.

Decisions - Case Two

[1]. D

[2]. A

Chapter 8

Intestinal Transplantation

Marc I. Rowe, MD and Samuel D. Smith, MD

Outline

I. INTRODUCTION

II. REJECTION

III. GRAFT VS. HOST DISEASE (GVH)

IV. BOWEL PRESERVATION

V. SURGICAL TECHNIQUE

VI. HUMAN INTESTINAL TRANSPLANTATIONS
The Current Approach

Educational Objectives

In this chapter the reader will:

1. learn the major problems associated with bowel transplantation.

2. review the known clinical cases of bowel and multivisceral transplantation.

3. learn the author's current clinical approach that offers the greatest chance for successful intestinal transplantation.

Introduction

A large number of pediatric and adult patients are now surviving despite insufficient intestinal function to sustain life. Most have short lengths of intestine as a result of congenital anomalies, inflammatory bowel disease, or trauma. Others suffer from intestinal motility problems or secretory diarrhea. The key factor in their survival has been the development of total parenteral nutrition (TPN) by Wilmore and Dudrick in 1968 (1). TPN provides sufficient nutrients intravenously to achieve growth and development for long periods. Recently, this technique has become more practical and less expensive as a result of the organization of home TPN programs (2). However, it is apparent that aside from the expense and impact on the quality of life, this technique has formidable limitations and complications. Chief among the limiting factors is the eventual loss of access to the central venous system. As more and more veins thrombose, catheter insertion into the central system becomes increasingly difficult and finally impossible. The patient has then lost his only means of obtaining nutrition. The most common serious complication of TPN is infection. Recurrent bouts of septicemia often necessitate removal of the intravenous line with possible loss of the access site. Serious infection, particularly by fungi and Gram-negative organisms, may lead to death. Progressive liver disease leading to hepatic fibrosis and liver failure is at present an intractable complication that results in death.

An obvious solution to the problem of short bowel syndrome is the transplantation of a sufficient length of functioning intestine before all venous access has been lost or before liver failure develops. Twenty-nine years ago, Lillehei et al. (3) clearly demonstrated that transplantation of the entire small bowel was technically feasible. He achieved long-term survival following autotransplantation of the intestine in the dog. Intestinal allografts, however, survived for only 5 days before rejection occurred. It was apparent to investigators at that time that successful allografts would require control of the rejection process. In the ensuing years, steady advances were made in the understanding of transplantation immunology, and with the use of immunosuppressive agents successful transplantation of the kidney in particular was achieved. Over the past 12 yr, the success rate of kidney, liver, heart, and lung transplantation has markedly accelerated, fueled by the introduction of cyclosporine and the more effective utilization of other immunosuppressive agents. Paradoxically, there has been no parallel success in intestinal transplantation. A long-term functional survival of an intestinal transplant in a human patient has not been reported. The purpose of this review is to discuss the major problems associated with bowel transplantation: a) rejection of the graft, b) graft vs. host (GVH) disease, c) preservation of the graft, and d) surgical technique. The known clinical cases of transplantation and multivisceral transplantation will be reviewed, and will include a brief description of a current multivisceral transplant patient surviving for over 90 days with functional intestine. The final section will discuss what the authors believe is the current clinical approach that offers the greatest chance for successful intestinal transplantation and will indicate the areas in which progress is being made and new approaches may soon be used. Important subjects such as control of infection, postoperative metabolic care, and pre and postoperative nutritional management will not be covered or only briefly mentioned because of space limitations.

Rejection

Bowel transplantation utilizing microvascular techniques in inbred strains of rat (4) is the principal tool used to probe the mechanisms of rejection of intestinal allografts. The use of inbred strains allows the isolated study of rejection without associated GVH disease. The transplantation of a brown Norway-Lewis hybrid donor into a brown Norway recipient allows isolated allograft rejection without GVH disease, since only the recipient recognizes the donor graft as foreign. Liedgens' group (5), using this model, demonstrated the central role of T-cells in rejection. Maximum signs of rejection were observed by day 10. There was progressive damage to the mucosa in the villi with infiltration of mononuclear cells in the intestinal wall. Monoclonal antibodies demonstrated that most of these cells were T-helper cells.

Since cyclosporine is effective in controlling T-cells with little myelotoxicity, its development and implementation were anticipated as major breakthrough for small bowel transplantation. Initial use in the rat model was encouraging. Utilizing cyclosporine as the sole immunosuppressive agent, Schraut's group (6) reported long-term survival of small bowel allografts. Without immunosuppressive therapy, all animals died of acute rejection after an average of 9 days. All recipients who received intramuscular cyclosporine therapy until postoperative day 28 remained healthy and free of signs of graft rejection for 17 months.

The results in larger animals were variable. Ricour et al. (7), Graddock et al. (8), Diliz-Perez et al. (9), and Pritchard et al. (10) prevented acute rejection in the pig and dog with parenteral cyclosporine. However, the number of long-term survivors was a small percentage of the total number of animals transplanted. The majority of the failures were attributed to technical problems and infection. Parenteral administration of cyclosporine was significantly more effective than the oral route. Rejection in some cases was found to be the result of ineffective absorption of oral cyclosporine from the grafted intestinal tract.

The ideal dosing interval and duration of cyclosporine administration are still not settled. When two patients received the dose of cyclosporine (11, 12), commonly used for solid organ transplantation (such as kidney or liver), they developed late and chronic rejection of their intestinal graft. This suggests that higher blood levels of cyclosporine may be necessary to prevent rejection of the intestine compared to other organs. Our own experience with high-dose cyclosporine in a current case of multivisceral transplantation, including the small intestine, supports this contention.

As the blood level of cyclosporine increases, the risk of renal, neurologic, and septic complications becomes a limiting factor. New, more effective, and less-toxic immunosuppressive agents are being introduced. FK506 was developed in Japan and acts in a manner similar to cyclosporine but is many times more potent with less renal and neurologic toxicity. A recent report (13) demonstrated the synergistic effectiveness of low-dose FK506 and cyclosporine combination therapy for cardiac transplantation in rats. This drug alone or in combination with cyclosporine may be more effective for bowel transplantation than cyclosporine alone.

The standard approach to control rejection is altering the recipient's responses to the foreign graft. A different and promising approach is to alter the graft itself — immunomodulation of the donor organ to decrease its immunogenicity. Dendritic cells (antigen-presenting cells or passenger leukocytes) appear to play a major role in the activation of recipient T-cells and the initiation of the rejection process. A number of methods have been developed to pretreat the donor or the donor's organ to alter its immunogenicity, including antilymphocytic serum, ultraviolet radiation, x-ray, and monoclonal antibodies. Experimentally (14, 15), rejection is best controlled if these treatments are administered 4 or 5 days prior to transplantation. At present, this delay would be a serious limiting factor. There is also evidence that the treatments currently available to achieve immunologic modulation only temporarily inactivate or eliminate the dendritic cells or passenger leukocytes.

The combination of administering immunosuppressive agents and monitoring to detect early signs of rejection is currently the most practical approach to control rejection before irreversible damage takes place. Monitoring must be sensitive enough to allow possible rescue of the graft by increasing doses of cyclosporine, bolus steroid therapy, or monoclonal antibody therapy. However, small bowel rejection may be more serious and life-threatening than rejection of other organs because there is loss of mucosal integrity that allows bacterial invasion of the graft (16). This may lead to bowel necrosis, systemic sepsis, or progressive graft fibrosis with loss of function.

The most direct method for detecting rejection is microscopic examination of the intestinal graft. This is accomplished by mucosal biopsy through the distal stoma of an intestinal graft that is in proximal continuity, through either the proximal or distal stoma of an isolated intestinal loop of the grafted intestine, or endoscopically either perorally or rectally of an intestinal graft that is in complete continuity. Stauffer (17) has demonstrated that microscopic changes in mucosal suction biopsies precede gross evidence of rejection by 24 to 36 h. Further precision was added by a quantitative morpho-metric analysis of the mucosa. Rejection was then identified 3 or 4 days before macroscopic signs. Because of the technical difficulties in obtaining biopsies, and the variability in distribution and intensity of histologic changes, functional tests have been recommended to detect rejection. Maltose absorption was compared to serial biopsies and found to be a sensitive method for determining functional integrity of the small bowel allograft (18). Maltose is a disaccharide and must be split into glucose by the brush border enzyme maltase. The glucose is then actively absorbed and can be measured in the blood. The test is performed by administering maltose into the GI tract and measuring serial blood glucose levels. Other absorption tests that appeared to detect rejection include D-xylose (19), glucose-14C, and cyclosporine uptake (20).

Graft vs. Host Disease

GVH disease is frequently seen in bone marrow transplantation. The classic clinical picture includes an erythematous macular papular rash, liver dysfunction, secretory diarrhea, and pancytopenia. The disease can be crippling or fatal. Many investigators believe that GVH disease may also be a serious problem in bowel transplantation due to the presence of large numbers of lymphocytes in the mucosa, peyers patches, and mesenteric lymph nodes. The rat has served as the major model by which to study GVH disease. Isolated GVH disease can be created by using a Lewis rat as the intestinal donor and a Brown-Norway Lewis F1 hybrid animal as recipient. Since only the Lewis donor lymphocytes can recognize the Brown-Norway antigens of the recipient as foreign, isolated GVH reaction occurs without rejection. Using this model, allograft survival has been approximately 15 days without treatment. To help distinguish GVH disease from rejection, these two immunologic responses were compared (21). Rejection usually occurs by day 7, and the first signs of GVH disease appeared between days 8 and 11. GVH disease in the rat presented with redness and swelling of the ears, nose, feet, and periocular region, progressing to scaling and hair loss. There was diarrhea, marked enlargement of all lymphoid tissue, splenomegaly, and enteritis of the native bowel. A key point was that the transplanted bowel itself appeared normal. Skin changes occurred late in the course of GVH disease in these animals in comparison to the early skin changes seen in GVH disease in bone marrow transplant patients. The clinical diagnosis of GVH disease may be difficult. Clinical findings include maculopapular rash, liver enzyme changes, and pancytopenia, all nonspecific. To differentiate GVH disease from rejection, biopsy of the allograft and a recipient lymph node, as well as performing a bowel functional test such as maltose absorption, can be helpful. Abnormalities in maltose absorption and allograft biopsy changes suggest rejection, while histologic changes in the recipient lymph node suggest GVH disease.

The use of prolonged cyclosporine or antilymphocyte serum (16) to control GVH disease has been utilized in clinical bone marrow transplantation. There are also several experimental approaches to treating GVH disease currently being tested, including the administration of thalidomide (22). Since the treatments of established GVH disease have met with variable success, most investigators have focused on prevention. Kirkman et al. (23) demonstrated that donor T-cells are necessary to cause GVH disease in the recipient; T-cell depletion of the donor successfully prevented GVH disease. He then found that subsequent bone marrow reconstitution of the donor utilizing T-cells reinstituted GVH disease once the donor bowel was transplanted. He also found that cyclosporine can prevent GVH disease but continuous administration is required. The best approach to GVH disease in small bowel transplantation appears to be prevention by rendering the graft lymphocytes inactive. The in vitro irradiation of the donor bowel with 1,000 rads after harvesting prevented GVH disease in the rat model (24), and did not lead to injury or malfunction of the allograft.

The question has been raised whether GVH disease in gut transplantation is in fact a serious clinical problem or simply a finding in experimental models. Although it is easily produced in the rat, studies of GVH disease in the dog are less clear-cut. It was found by Cohen et al. (25) and Lillehei et al. (26), but not by Resnick et al. (27). Fujiwara et al. (28) noted simultaneous GVH disease and rejection in the dog model with a decrease in functional mucosa, mass splenic changes, and mesenteric node changes. They felt that the weakening of these immune structures of the recipient and graft predispose to catastrophic enterogenous infections, perhaps explaining the large number of animals that die without overt signs of rejection. GVH disease may have contributed to the intestinal transplant failure and death of two patients (11, 12). There has been a recent report of what appears to be GVH disease in liver transplantation patients (29). We have not encountered any evidence of GVH disease in our current multivisceral transplant patient.

Bowel Preservation

Effective preservation of the intestine during the time between harvesting and implantation is an obvious prerequisite to a successful outcome. Small bowel mucosa is extremely sensitive to ischemia and reperfusion. Damage to the mucosa is thought to result from the generation of O_2 free radicals, liberation of endotoxin from the indigenous bacterial flora, and massive fluid loss from intestinal secretion following reperfusion. There are currently two major methods of organ preservation: simple cold storage and cold storage with pulsatile perfusion. The most common preservation method includes intravascularly and intraluminally flushing with cold (4°C) crystalloid solution. The organ is then placed in a sterile plastic bag and stored in ice. The duration of successful cold storage preservation varies according to the organ; kidneys tolerate up to 40 h, the liver 10 h, and the heart 4 to 5 h (30). Bowel has been preserved from 6 to 20 h in animals (31, 32). Successful preservation was increased to 12-24 h by adding fructose to the perfusate (33). Allopurinol (34) and lidoflazine (calcium channelblocker) (35) have been added to the perfusate and appear to decrease mucosal injury by decreasing the generation of O_2 free radicals.

A solution recently developed at the University of Wisconsin has allowed successful preservation of human livers for over 30 h (36). It contains nonbiodegradable colloid-dialyzed hydroxyethyl starch, raffinose, potassium lactobionate, and allopurinol. It is logical to assume that the preservation of intestinal grafts will similarly be prolonged by its use.

While simple cold storage is the most frequently employed technique, cold storage with pulsatile perfusion has been reported to allow successful bowel preservation in dogs for as long as 24 h (37). In these experiments, a solution of fresh frozen plasma, $MgSO_4$, ampicillin, kanamycin, methylprednisolone, chlorpromazine, and O_2 were perfused via a pulsatile pump into the arterial side of the intestinal graft at 7°C. Similar methods have been used clinically for renal storage. This method is complex and requires maintenance of continuous perfusion during transportation and storage. Since comparable results are achieved with technically simpler cold storage, the pulsatile method is not widely used.

Surgical Technique

The route of venous outflow from the graft is the major technical decision in bowel transplantation. Drainage may be directed into the systemic venous system by placement of the donor portal vein into the recipient inferior vena cava, creating a portosystemic shunt and bypassing the liver. A more "normal" route is accomplished by placement of the donor portal vein end-to-side to the recipient portal vein so that blood passes directly into the liver. The advantages of portosystemic drainage over the porto-porto anastomosis include the ease of performing the anastomosis and removing the graft if necessary. Venous thrombosis does not carry as high a risk with a portosystemic compared to a porto-porto anastomosis. If venous thrombosis occurs in a porto-porto anastomosis, the clot may extend into the recipient portal vein, creating portal hypertension. The metabolic consequence of bypassing the liver in portosystemic drainage also must be considered. Portal venous drainage was compared to systemic venous drainage in the rat (37, 38). Portal drainage moderately extended the survival of allografts but resulted in altered plasma amino acid levels similar to those in hepatic encephalopathy. Despite the possible drawbacks, the majority of investigators use the portosystemic route because of its safety and technical ease.

The length of the bowel to be transplanted, and whether ileum or jejunum is the most important segment to include, are questions that have not as yet been definitely answered. In children with a contracted peritoneal cavity, the intestine mass becomes particularly critical. The larger the intestine mass the greater the immunologic burden on the host, but the greater the digestive function and absorptive surface. Kimura et al. (39) demonstrated in rats that the longer the length of bowel transplanted the greater the risk of dying from either graft rejection or GVH disease. In the adult patients, at least 100 cm of bowel has been transplanted but no long-term functional information is available. We believe that the ideal choice is to use the entire small intestine from a donor who is significantly smaller than the recipient.

There are several methods of dealing with the proximal and distal ends of the bowel graft once vascular continuity has been established. In the majority of animal and human transplantations, both ends of the bowel were exteriorized as stomas, creating a defunctionalized or a Thiry-Vella loop. There are several advantages to a Thiry-Vella loop; there are no anastomoses, thus eliminating the risk of suture line leak. Since the bowel is defunctionalized, if vascular thrombosis or rejection occurs the resulting necrosis does not lead to escape of intestinal contents and peritonitis. The two stomas allow access for mucosal biopsies.

Other methods of handling the bowel ends include: a) establishing continuity with the native bowel proximally and distally, or b) establishing proximal continuity and constructing a distal stoma. Experimental studies (40) suggest that exposing the mucosa to intestinal secretions and nutrients is important to maintain small intestinal mass, normal disaccharidase activity, and the normal proximal-to-distal gradient of intestinal mucosa mass. There might, therefore, be a potential advantage to keeping the transplanted bowel in continuity. A stoma is still available for mucosal biopsy. We chose this arrangement in our present case.

Human Intestinal Transplantations

At least 14 human small bowel transplants have been performed (Table 1). Not all have been formally reported in the medical literature. For this reason, the case summaries by necessity are brief and not all the facts can be verified. Deterling in 1964 performed two separate transplants in children (41). One child received an ileal segment from his mother and died after 12 h. The second patient had a cadaver graft that was removed in 2 days due to graft necrosis. In 1967, Lillehei et al. (26) performed a cadaver transplant in a 46-yr-old woman who died with 12 h from multiple pulmonary infarcts. In 1968, Okumura et al. (42) transplanted intestine from a cadaver undergoing cardiac massage. The graft suffered necrosis and the patient expired after 12 days. In 1969, Olivier et al. (43) transplanted small bowel and colon in a 35-yr-old male with Gardner's syndrome. Despite immunosuppression with azathioprine, cortisone, and antilymphocyte globulin, the patient died on the 26th post-transplant day of irreversible rejection. Alican et al. (44) in the same year, transplanted 1 m of ileum from a living related maternal donor into a 10-yr-old boy who had lost his intestine secondary to strangulation by a mesenteric band. On the 7th postoperative day, the graft was removed for necrosis without clear-cut evidence of rejection. The patient subsequently died of sepsis. In 1970, Fortner et al. (11) transplanted 170 cm of lower jejunum and upper ileum from a HLA-identical sister into a 37-yr-old female with Garnder's syndrome. An auxiliary donor intestinal pouch was created for serial biopsy. Immunosuppression was initially azathioprine and antilymphocyte globulin (ALG) but steroids were added when rejection was identified on day 17. Damage appeared to be confined to the mucosa. Progressive weakness developed with muscle atrophy and liver dysfunction. The patient subsequently died of *E. coli* sepsis on the 76th postoperative day. In 1984 Starzl et al. (45) reported two cases of pancreatic duodenal transplantation which included long segments of jejunum. Both patients required jejunal graft removal due to severe protein-losing enteropathy from loss of jejunal mucosa.

In 1985 Cohen et al. (12) transplanted the entire small bowel from a 10-yr-old blood group O to a 26-yr-old blood group A woman with short gut secondary to Gardner's syndrome. Immunosuppression was with cyclosporine and cortisone. A hemolytic reaction developed on the 6th postoperative day secondary to anti-A antibodies from lymphocytes originating in the intestinal graft. On the 9th postoperative day, the patient collapsed and became comatose. The following day she suffered cardiac arrest but was resuscitated. The graft was subsequently removed but the patient died 17 days after transplantation. Pathologic examination of the graft demonstrated moderate rejection. The liver and spleen were enlarged and there was cholestatic changes and microinfarcts in the liver. Review of the serial transplant bowel biopsies were consistent with rejection by day 9. The cause of death was not clear. In future cases, Cohen recommend matching the donor and recipient for ABO compatibility or possible irradiation

Table 1. Summary of human small bowel transplantation

Team	Year	Immunosuppression	Venous Drainage	Intestinal Drainage	Complication	Outcome
Small Bowel Transplants						
1. Detering et al (41)	1964	—	?	?	?	Died after 12 h
2. Detering et al (41)	1964	—	?	?	Graft necrosis	Died after 48 h
3. Lillehei et al (23)	1967	—	Inferior vena cava	Thiry-Vella	Massive pulmonary infarct	Died after 12 h
4. Okumura et al (42)	1968	—	Left iliac vein	Thiry-Vella	Graft necrosis	Died after 12 h
5. Oliver et al (43)	1969	Azathioprine, steroids, antilymphocyte globulin	Portal vein	Proximal anastomosis, distal stoma	Irreversible rejection	Died on day 26
6. Alican et al (44)	1969	Azathioprine, steroids, antilymphocyte globulin	Left renal vein	Thiry-Vella	Graft necrosis, sepsis	Graft removed 7 days later, died after 30 days
7. Fortner et al (11)	1970	Azathioprine, steroids, antilymphocyte globulin	Right iliac vein	Proximal and distal anastomosis with isolated pouch	Rejection, sepsis, liver dysfunction	Died on day 76
8. Cohen et al (12)	1985	Steroids, cyclosporine	Inferior vena cava	Thiry-Vella	Hemolytic reaction day 6, coma day 9, cardiac arrest day 10	Graft removed 11 days later, died after 12 days
9. Ricour et al (46)	1987	Steroids, cyclosporine	?	Thiry-Vella	Rejection day 13, liver dysfunction	Graft removed after 6½ mo, died 6 days later
Pancreatic duodenal jejunal transplants						
10. Starzl et al (47) 11. (Two patients)	1983	Steroids, cyclosporine	Common iliac	Roux en y, jejunal limb	Protein losing enteropathy	Resection, transplant bowel; pts alive
Multivisceral transplants						
12. Starzl et al	1984	Steroids, cyclosporine	Total viscera transplantation, caval sleeve	Primary anastomosis	OR hemorrhage, irreversible shock	Died in OR
13. Williams et al	1987	?	?	?	Early postop bleeding	Died 2 days later
14. Starzl et al	1987	Steroids, cyclosporine	Hepatic veins to vena cava	Primary anastomosis	Anastomotic leak, sepsis, liver dysfunction	Alive >120 days

of the graft. Ricour's group (46) has recently reported the case of a 9-yr-old girl who received 120 cm of small intestine from an iso-blood group A donor. Both the graft and native bowel were exteriorized as stomas. Immunosuppression included methylprednisolone sodium succinate 2 mg/kg·day (Solu-medrol) and 10 mg/kg·day cyclosporine. Graft rejection treated with steroids and ALG developed on day 13. She developed progressive liver and renal failure with coagulopathy. Because of the severe liver dysfunction, the cyclosporine was stopped and the graft removed 6-1/2 months after transplant. She died 6 days later of progressive liver failure. The cause of the liver failure was felt to be secondary to cyclosporin toxicity or long-term TPN.

Multivisceral transplantation or transplantation of the liver, stomach, small bowel, pancreas, and large bowel en block has been performed in three cases. These patients had inadequate intestinal function due to short bowel syndrome, and liver failure as a result of long-term TPN. Since neither an isolated intestinal or liver transplantation would solve their separate problems, a single block of organs was transplanted by anastomosing from the graft vena cava to the donor vena cava and the graft aorta to the recipient aorta. This procedure was first described by Starzl et al. (47) in 1968. The first case was performed in Pittsburgh on a 13-yr-old girl with short bowel and liver failure. Her condition was moribund preoperatively and she died at the completion of the operation. A multivisceral transplant performed in Chicago resulted in death soon after operation. The details are yet to be reported. The second multivisceral transplant in Pittsburgh was performed in a 3-yr-old girl 4 months prior to preparation of this manuscript. There has been no evidence of rejection or GVH disease. Immunosuppression has been high-dose cyclosporine and steroids. This patient is clinically well and has satisfactory intestinal and liver function.

The Current Approach

Below is our concept of the current state of the art approach to bowel transplantation based on animal studies, clinical reports, and data obtained from our current patient. Prime candidates for intestinal transplantation are patients with short bowel syndrome confirmed by measurement at operation, and radiologic follow-up. These patients should be unable to absorb sufficient nutrients through the GI tract to sustain life. At present, bowel transplantation must be considered experimental and only done when there are no other alternatives. This situation occurs when progressive liver failure develops as a result of TPN or if the patient is no longer able to be maintained on TPN because of a loss of venous access.

Bowel transplantation should not be done across ABO groups. The donor should be smaller than the recipient. The most practical method of intestinal preservation currently is simple cold storage. The use of the University of Wisconsin solution will likely extend preservation time significantly. The addition of other agents, such as superoxide radical scavengers, may further increase this time. Efforts should be made to reduce storage time to the minimum, preferably by harvesting the organ and performing the transplantation in the same institution.

Some method of graft pretreatment may reduce immunogenicity and the later danger of GVH disease. The most promising approach appears to be irradiation of the graft and infusion of T-cell monoclonal antibodies into the graft.

The best functional results, despite the increased antigenic load, can be achieved if the jejunum and ileum are transplanted. Venous outflow is most simply established by portosystemic drainage into the inferior vena cava. We favor anastomosis of the upper intestine of the recipient to the proximal end of the graft. The distal transplanted bowel is brought out as a stoma. A gastrostomy tube is placed for decompression and early feeding.

Cyclosporine with steroids presently offers the greatest chance for prevention of graft rejection and GVH disease. The dose of cyclosporine reflected by blood levels should be higher than is commonly used in solid organ transplantation. In our present patient, the combination of high-dose cyclosporine and steroids has resulted in no evidence of GVH disease or rejection for over 3 months. To detect early signs of rejection, serial intestinal biopsies and a functional bowel study such as maltose absorption should be considered.

The use of high-dose cyclosporine complicates the postoperative care. Hypertension and reduced renal function occur early. Precise management of fluid, electrolyte, and protein intake is necessary. Bacterial, fungal, and viral infections are common complications of all immunosuppressed patients, but the intestinal transplantation patient may present added risk because of intestinal flora. Judicious use of antibiotics and a system of surveillance cultures are important. Meticulous care of the intravascular lines and their removal at the first signs of infection are mandatory. Control of the bowel bacterial flora may be an important adjunct to therapy.

In order to maintain healthy mucosa, it may be helpful to immediately expose the transplanted intestine to digestive secretions and nutrients. Small volumes of iso-osmolar electrolytes, amino acids, carbohydrates, and possibly short-chain fatty acids can be infused into the transplanted GI tract.

The method of feeding and the choice of feeds after bowel transplantation have not been studied. From our limited experience, it appears that feedings are best delivered through a gastrostomy. Early continuous infusions of an iso-osmolar elemental diet should be used initially. As intestinal function improves, the volume and concentration of the formula can be progressively increased. This allows a rapid reduction of TPN to minimize TPN liver damage. The time of introduction of more complex nutrients has not been determined.

References

1. Wilmore DW, Durick SJ: Growth and development of an infant receiving all nutrients exclusively by vein. *JAMA* 1968; 203:860

2. Jeejeebhoy DN, Langer B, Tsallas G, et al: Total parenteral nutrition at home: Studies in patients surviving 4 months to 5 years. *Gastroenterology* 1976; 71:943

3. Lillehei RC, Goott B, Miller FA: The physiological response of the small bowel of the dog to ischemia including prolonged in vitro preservation of the bowel with successful replacement and survival. *Ann Surg* 1959; 150:543

4. Monchik GJ, Russell PS: Transplantation of small bowel in the rat: Technical and immunologic considerations. *Surgery* 1971; 70:693

5. Liedgens P, Muller-Hermelink HK, Deltz E: Rejection in heterotopic small-bowel transplantation. *In*: Small Bowel Transplantation. Deltz E, Thiede A, Hamelmann H (Eds). New York, Springer Verlag, 1986, pp 116-120

6. Schraut WH, Lee KKW: Long-term survival of orthotopic small-bowel allografts using cyclosporine A. *In*: Small Bowel Transplantation. Deltz E, Thiede A, Hamelmann H (Eds). New York, Springer Verlag, 1986, pp 156-165

7. Ricour C, Revillon Y, Arnand-Battandier F, et al: Successful small bowel allotransplantation in piglets using cyclosporine. *Transplant Proc* 1983; 15:3019

8. Graddock GN, Nordgren SR, Reznick RK, et al: Small bowel transplantation in the dog using cyclosporin. *Transplantation* 1983; 35:284

9. Diliz-Perez HS, McClure J, Bedetti C, et al: Successful small bowel allotransplantation in dogs with cyclosporine and prednisone transplantation. *Transplantation* 1984; 37:126

10. Pritchard TJ, Madara JL, Tapper D, et al: Failure of cyclosporine to prevent small bowel allograft rejection in pigs. *J Surg Res* 1985; 38:553

11. Fortner JG, Sichuk G, Litwin SD, et al: Immunological responses to an intestinal allograft with HL-A-identical donor-recipient. *Transplantation* 1972; 14:531

12. Cohen Z, Silverman RE, Wassef R, et al: Small intestinal transplantation using cyclosporine. *Transplantation* 1986; 42:613

13. Murase N, Todo S, Lee PH, et al: Heterotopic heart transplantation in the rat receiving FK-506 alone or with cyclosporine. *Transplant Proc* 1987; 19:71

14. Gullman RE, Lindquist RR: Renal transplantation in the inbred rat. Reduction of allograft immunogenicity by cytoxic drug pretreatment of donors. *Transplantation* 1969; 8:490

15. Steinmuller D, Warden G, Coleman M, et al: Prolonged survival of rat heart and kidney allografts irradiated in vitro. *Transplantation* 1971; 12:153

16. Schraut WH: Current status of small-bowel transplantation. *Gastroenterology* 1988; 94:525

17. Stauffer VG: Monitoring of small-bowel grafts by mucosal suction biopsies. *In*: Small Bowel Transplantation. Deltz E, Thiede A, Hamelmann H (Eds). New York, Springer Verlag, 1986, pp 234-240

18. Billiar TR, Garberoglis C, Schraut WH: Maltose absorption as an indicator of small intestinal allograft rejection. *J Surg Res* 1984; 37:75

19. Ruiz JO, Uchidu H, Schultz LS, et al: Problems in absorption and immunosuppression after entire intestinal allotransplantation. *Am J Surg* 1972; 123:297

20. Nordgren S, Cohen Z, Mackenzie R, et al: Functional monitors of rejection in small intestinal transplants. *Am J Surg* 1984; 147:152

21. Schraut WH, Lee KKW: Clinicopathologic differentiation of rejection and graft-vs-host disease following small bowel transplantation. *In*: Small Bowel Transplantation. Deltz E, Thiede A, Hamelmann H (Eds). New York, Springer Verlag, 1986, pp 98-108

22. Vogelsang GV, Hess AD, Gordon G, et al: Treatment and prevention of acute graft versus host disease with thalidomide in a rat model. *Transplantation* 1986; 41:641

23. Kirkman RL, Lear PA, Madara JL, et al: Small intestine transplantation in the rat — Immunology and function. *Surgery* 1984; 96:280

24. Lee KKW, Schraut WH: In vitro allograft irradiation prevents graft-versus-host disease in small bowel transplantation. *J Surg Res* 1985; 38:364

25. Cohen Z, Macgregor AB, Moore KTH, et al: Canine small-bowel transplantation: A study of immunologic responses. *Arch Surg* 1976; 111:248

26. Lillehei RC, Idezuki Y, Feemster JA, et al: Transplantation of stomach, intestine, and pancreas: Experimental and clinical observation. *Surgery* 1967; 62:721

27. Reznick RK, Craddock GN, Langer B, et al: Structure and function of small-bowel allografts in the dog: Immunosuppression with cyclosporin A. *Can J Surg* 1982; 25:51

28. Fujiwara H, Raju S, Grogan JB, et al: Total orthotopic small bowel allotransplantation in the dog. *Transplantation* 1987; 44:747

29. Badosa F, DeOca J, Figueras J, et al: Is there a (graft-versus-host) reaction in liver transplantation? *Transplant Proc* 1987; 19:3822

30. Diethelm AG, Barger BO, Whelchel JD, et al: Organ Transplantation. *In*: Clinical Surgery. Davis JH, Dracker WR, Foster RS, et al (Eds). St. Louis, CV Mosby Co, 1987, pp 3171-3211

31. Schraut WH, Lee KKW, Tsujinaka Y: Intestinal preservation of small bowel grafts by vascular washout and cold storage. *In*: Small Bowel Transplantation. Deltz E, Thiede A, Hamelmann H (Eds). New York, Springer Verlag, 1986, pp 65-73

32. Ricour C, Revillon Y, Pletynex M, et al: Conservation hypothermique et autotransplantation du grele chez le porcelet. *Gastroenterol Clin Biol* 1981; 5:977

33. Toledo-Pereyra LH, Simmons RL, Najarian JS: Comparative effects of chlorpromazine, methylprednisolone, and allopurinol during small bowel preservation. *Am J Surg* 1973; 126

34. Croitoru DP, Sybicki M, Grand RJ, et al: Lidoflazine protects against reperfusion injury during small bowel transplantation. Presented at the Pediatric Surgery Residents Conference. Toronto, Canada, 1987

35. Jamieson NV, Sundberg R, Lindell S, et al: Successful 24 hour liver preservation: A preliminary report. Proceedings of International Organ Transplant Forum, 1987. *Transplant Proc* (In Press)

36. Toledo-Pereyra LH, Najarian JS: Small bowel preservation: Comparison of perfusion and nonperfusion systems. *Arch Surg* 1973; 107:875

37. Schraut WH, Abraham VS, Lee KKW: Portal versus systemic venous drainage for small bowel allografts. *Surgery* 1985; 98:579

38. Koltun WA, Madara JL, Smith RJ, et al: Metabolic aspects of small bowel transplantation in inbred rats. *J Surg Res* 1987; 42:341

39. Kimura K, Money SR, Jaffe BM: The effects of size and site of origin of intestinal grafts on small bowel transplantation in the rat. *Surgery* 1987; 101:618

40. Levine GM, Deven JJ, Steiger E: Role of oral intake in maintenance of gut mass and disaccharide activity. *Gastroenterology* 1974; 67:975

41. Kirkman RL: Small bowel transplantation. *Transplantation* 1984; 37:429

42. Okumura M, Fujimara I, Ferrari AA, et al: Transplante del intestino delgrado: Aspresentacao de um caso. *Rev Hosp Clinc Fac Med Sao Paulo* 1969; 24:39

43. Olivier CL, Rettori R, Olivier CH, et al: Interruption of the lymphatic vessels and its consequences in total homotransplantation of the small intestine and right side of the colon in man. *Lymphology* 1972; 5:24

44. Alican F, Hardy JD, Cayirli M, et al: Intestinal transplantation: Laboratory experience and report of a clinical case. *Am J Surg* 1971; 121:150

45. Starzl TE, Iwatsuki S, Shaw Jr BW, et al: Pancreaticoduodenal transplantation in humans. *Surg Gyencol Obstet* 1984; 159:265

46. Goulet O, Revillon Y, Jan D, et al: Small intestinal transplantation in children using cyclosporine. Presented at the Second International Congress on Cyclosporine. Washington, DC, Nov 4-7, 1987

47. Starzl TE, Kaupp HA, Brock DR, et al: Homotransplantation of multiple visceral organs. *Am J Surg* 1961; 103:219

Chapter 9

Immune System Dysfunction in Multiple Organ Failure

Nicolas V. Christou, MD, PhD, FRCS(C), FACS

Outline

Educational Objectives

In this chapter the reader will learn:

1. about the immune system and how the specific and nonspecific host defense mechanisms help defend against invading pathogens.

2. about the humoral immune mediators interleukin-1, interleukin-2, and cachectin/tumor necrosis factor, and how they may be involved in multiple organ failure.

3. about the defects in humoral, cell-mediated, and nonspecific immune deficits in the surgical ICU patient and how these may contribute to the multiple organ failure seen in such patients.

Introduction

Multiple organ failure (MOF) is a state of profound organ collapse in surgical patients. Although failure of organs such as the lung and the liver have been recognized in the past, recent evidence also points to failure of the immune system in these patients. The patient with multiple organ failure (MOF) is commonly suffering from the systemic effects of postsurgical or post-traumatic sepsis. An understanding of the role of the systems that mediate infection and produce much of the clinical picture is an important base for management and for future research. The use of the term "immunity" in relation to this process refers to two general response systems which differ in some important aspects. The so-called *cellular immune system,* which embodies specific and pre-programmed responses, centers on the various populations of lymphocytes. Conversely, there is less known about the mediator systems, which seem to be more closely involved in the patient with MOF. The so-called *nonspecific immune system,* which includes the relatively nonspecific responses of the circulating fixed macrophages and of granulocytes and monocytes, together with complement and other opsonins, clearly needs considerable further investigation to define its critical role.

In this chapter we will discuss the immunologic processes and mediators responsible for immune system dysfunction in MOF. There are many such mediators including the interleukins, cachectin/tumor necrosis factor, platelet-derived growth factor, alpha and beta interferons, and the complement system. MOF is usually associated with inflammation and activation of macrophages. These changes are brought about by signals mediated by monokines — regulatory proteins secreted by macrophages and monocytes in response to phagocytic stimulation. Monokines function locally as paracrine mediators and/or systemically as endocrine-like mediators to provide nonspecific local and systemic host-defense mechanisms; they also initiate immunologic, metabolic, and endocrine changes in preparation for specific immune responses. Monokines result in the release of lymphokines — nonimmunoglobulin polypeptide factors secreted by activated lymphocytes that have a broad range of pathophysiological effects on immunologically mediated reactions. Monokines are also called cytokines because they can be produced by other cell lines such as epidermal fibroblasts, and mesangial and neural tissues. Cytokines can act in a genetically unrestricted manner and can often function across species barriers. Cytokines are extremely potent in stimulating target cells and are active at concentrations of 10^{-10} to 10^{-15} M.

Overview of the Immune System

The task confronting the natural defense system can be described by seven key words: encounter, recognition, activation, deployment, discrimination, eradication, and regulation. The final outcome, i.e., elimination of an invader (be it a virus, a microbe, or a foreign protein), occurs via the inflammatory response. Failure of the last component, regulation, may be responsible for immune system dysfunction in MOF. Indeed, the whole MOF process may be mediated and possibly propagated by altered regulation of the nonspecific immune system, especially the macrophage with excessive production of cachectin (1).

Specific Immunity

Specific immunity refers to that part of the immune defense system associated with responses that are antigen-specific, i.e., they are targeted to only one particular antigen. Thus, an antibody produced to an *E. coli* bacterial antigen will interact with that particular antigen and none other. Strictly speaking, the immune system is degenerate and redundant; thus, one antibody may cross-react with a similar antigen and one antigen may unite with many antibodies, but in general a very high degree of specificity is maintained. Before a specific

144

immune response can begin, the invading microbe and antigens derived from it must encounter cells capable of responding. There exist in the body accessory cells, such as monocytes, macrophages, fixed tissue histiocytes, dendritic cells, and Langerhans cells, all of which can capture and break down a microbe and expose its antigens (epitopes) on their surface in a form that can be recognized by memory T cells that migrate past. This is the *encounter* component of immune defense. Accessory cells are most concentrated in the spleen and lymph nodes, places where lymphocytes are abundant; thus, the chance for the next step, recognition, is amplified. Both B cell differentiation in the bone marrow and T cell differentiation in the thymus occur via gene translocations that result in surface receptors of a particular specificity. These germ-line repertoires are created through essentially antigen-independent differentiation or lymphoneogenesis. When antigen activates a particular lymphocyte, antigen-driven processes initiate a second cycle of multiplication and differentiation in which lymphocytes multiply and stimulate B cells with the same antigen code to produce antibodies to the specific antigen. The T cells which carry this out are the CD4 or T_4-positive helper/inducer T cells. Accessory cells secrete interleukin-1, which amplifies this response. The stimulated helper/inducer cell produces interleukin-2 and divides to form a clone. The B cell, thus activated by a combination of signals produced by binding of antigen and further signals from T cell products, enlarges, divides, and differentiates to antibody-secreting status.

Deployment of the immunologic message is mediated by lymphocytes and their lymphokines. In health, immune responses to autologous constituents are kept within very strict bounds. Only an event such as organ transplantation will lead to the cataclysmic immune responses which lead to rejection of the organ. Autoaggression-prevention mechanisms are covered under the term of immunologic tolerance. Immunologic tolerance is but one facet of the complex regulatory loops of the immune response. The dysfunction of these regulatory mechanisms in MOF leads to the observed alterations in host defense.

Nonspecific Immunity

In contrast to specific immunity discussed above, this component of the immune system does not discriminate on the basis of antigen-antibody specificity. It is directed against a wide variety of invaders. For example, a macrophage will phagocytose and kill an *E. coli* organism, just as easily as it will kill a Staphylococcus, or a virus or a fungus, without regard to surface antigen expression other then appropriate opsonization.

Phagocytic Cells

The phagocytic cells of the body can be found fixed in such areas as the spleen, bone marrow, lung, and liver parenchyma, grouped under the name of the reticuloendothelial system. They are also found in the circulation in the form of monocytes and polymorphonuclear neutrophils. This system guards against bacterial invasion of the body through the three most common portals of entry: the skin, the respiratory tract, and the peritoneal cavity. Once the environmental or mechanical barrier of the skin or the intact bowel mucosa is damaged, bacteria gain access to the subcutaneous space or the peritoneal cavity. The phagocytes in the skin and the peritoneal cavity, together with circulating humoral factors such as antibodies and the complement system, provide the first line of defense. If this defense barrier is unsuccessful in containing the infection, the infection becomes established and sets up processes that involve the specific immune system discussed above.

Complement

The prime function of the complement system is to mediate some aspects of inflammation and to facilitate ingestion of pathogens by phagocytes (opsonization) (2). This action is nonspecific only in the immunologic sense, i.e., antibodies to many types of antigens will trigger complement activation. The biochemical steps that comprise the sequence of complement interactions are highly specific. Most complement component proteins are present in serum in small amounts and are easily denatured (Table 1). There is also the alternate complement pathway which is phylogenetically older than the antibody recognition mechanism and appears to play an important role in host defense, particularly before antibody synthesis begins. The classical complement pathway is activated by antigen antibody complexes which lead to the generation of biologically important effector proteins.

Table 1. Molecular weights and serum concentrations of the various complement components

Classical Pathway	Molecular Weight	Concentration (μg/ml)
C1q	410,000	70
C1r	90,000	34
C1s	85,000	31
C2	117,000	25
C3	190,000	1,200
C4	206,000	600
C5	180,000	85
C6	128,000	60
C7	120,000	55
C8	150,000	55
C9	179,000	60
Alternate Pathway		
Properdin	190,000	25
Properdin factor B	100,000	225
Properdin factor D	25,000	1

The early components of the complement cascade circulate as inactive precursors until they are activated sequentially by highly specific, biochemical reactions. In many cases, this activation involves limited proteolytic cleavage with the formation of two fragments of unequal size. The smaller fragment often contributes to the development of the inflammatory process (e.g., C3a and C5a). The larger fragment continues the sequence of complement reactions. To produce their immunopathologic effects, complement proteins must react in precisely the right sequence. For example, the sequence of the classical pathway is C1, C4, C2, C3, and C5 through C9 in numerical order. Absence of any of the proteins in the sequence will interrupt the succession of reactions at that point.

Humoral Immune Mediators

Interleukins

Macrophages and some macrophage cell lines can be stimulated by a wide variety of agents to secrete a monokine that was initially called "lymphocyte activating factor," but was renamed interleukin-1 (IL-1) because of the multiplicity of its effects on lymphocytic cells. Resting macrophages produce little or no IL-1. Stimulation of macrophages, either directly or indirectly, leads to an increased production of IL-l. Interleukin-1 has a multiplicity of effects on the afferent limb of the immune response, such as enhancing the proliferation of T lymphocytes, promoting antibody production by B lymphocytes, augmenting lymphokine production, promoting thymocyte differentiation, and inducing receptor expression on T lymphocytes. IL-1 is closely related to endogenous pyrogen and it is also indistinguishable from the monocyte-derived factor that stimulates synovial cells of inflamed joints to produce considerable amounts of prostaglandin and collagenase. IL-1 stimulates prostaglandin-mediated bone resorption by osteoblasts, muscle cells to undergo proteolysis, and chondrocytes to degrade cartilage tissue in vitro. IL-1 also promotes the growth of dermal fibroblasts in culture. IL-1 is chemotactic for polymorphonuclear leukocytes and monocytes, and also stimulates the metabolic activities and lysosomal enzyme release by neutrophils. In vitro administration of IL-1, in addition to causing fever, also drastically affects the activities of hepatocytes which convert from producing albumin and pre-albumin to producing a battery of acute-phase proteins such as serum amyloid.

IL-1 produced by a human tumor cell line has been purified to homogeneity by a three-step chromatographic method. Purified IL-1 stimulates the proliferative response of the D10.G4.1 cell line, a mouse IL-1 indicator T cell, causes the release of prostaglandin E_2 and prostacyclin from cultured human foreskin fibroblasts and from primary human umbilical vein endothelial cells and elicits characteristic endogenous pyrogen fever in rabbits. Further work has shown that IL-1 exists in two forms: a neutral form with pl = 7 called IL-1 beta, and an acidic form with pl = 5 called IL-1 alpha. Both come from 30 to 35-kilodalton (kd) precursor molecules, which may exist as transmembrane proteins and require processing to form the mature 23-kd proteins with biologic activity. Fragments as small as 4 kd may be active. IL-1 beta is the major IL-1 produced by human cells, and in general has a higher specific activity then IL-1 alpha in bone resorption and other assays. There is about 26% homology of the two near the carboxy terminus.

The IL-1 receptor seems to be a protein 80 kd in weight in the murine LBRM cells, or a 41-kd protein with autophosphorilating properties in the human k562 cells. Recombinant human IL-1 is now available, and studies have shown that it mediates some of the changes in inflammation and shock. A universal component of inflammation is the increased synthesis of a series of plasma proteins by the liver, termed acute-phase proteins. The liver response to injury and sepsis is one of the many facets of the acute-phase reaction which includes a febrile response, leukocytosis, and altered cellular metabolism of numerous tissues.

The liver responds to trauma with increased uptake of amino acids, iron, and zinc. This is followed by intracellular increases in certain enzymes such as sialyltranferase and increased transcription of mRNA for various proteins such as alpha-1-acid glycoprotein. Subsequently there is a characteristic change in the plasma levels of a series of proteins synthesized by the liver, commonly known as acute-phase reactants. IL-1 is thought to play a major role in the mediation of these changes (3).

Interleukin-2 (IL-2) is a lymphokine released by lymphocytes following stimulation by IL-1. IL-2 plays an essential role in triggering proliferation of activated T cells, a response mediated by interactions of the factor with a high-affinity membrane receptor. IL-2 also influences a number of other cellular responses, including natural killer cell activity and antibody secretion. Thus, directly or indirectly, IL-2 has the properties of both a growth factor and a differentiation signal. Both IL-2 and its receptor have been purified to homogeneity and extensively characterized at the molecular level. IL-2, originally termed T-cell growth factor, represents one element in a cascade of lymphokines released during an immune response. IL-2 is released by T cells in response to two signals provided by antigen-pulsed accessory cells. The first signal is antigen, presented in the context of proteins of the major histocompatibility complex, and the second signal is IL-1.

Although all subclasses of T cells have been shown to release IL-2 under the appropriate conditions, helper T cells appear to be the major source. Once released, IL-2 promotes the proliferation of any IL-2 receptor-positive T cell, regardless of its subclass and antigenic specificity. The specificity of the immune system is instead maintained at the level of induction of IL-2 receptor expression. Receptor induction is also dependent on antigen-presentation by accessory cells and may, in addition, require one or more lymphokine signals. The concentration of IL-2, the number of IL-2 receptors per cell, and the continued expression of receptors together determine the level and duration of the response. IL-2 has a molecular weight of 15,400. Human IL-2 consists of a 133-amino-acid polypeptide containing a single intramolecular disulfide bridge. The gene for IL-2 was recently shown to be located on human chromosome 4q. IL-2 is immunogenic, and an antibody against human IL-2 has been obtained which inhibits its biological activity. Human IL-2 has been cloned using recombinant DNA techniques (4).

Cachectin/Tumor Necrosis Factor

In recent years, there has been a growing awareness that endogenous mediators are essential elements in the pathogenesis of shock and cachexia alike. The role of bacterial endotoxin in the pathogenesis of septic shock illustrates this principle. Endotoxin does not exert most of its effects on the host's metabolism directly, nor is it highly toxic to most mammalian tissues. On the contrary, endotoxin elicits the production of a host factor (or factors) that may in turn lead to shock and death. These factors appear to be produced by cells of hematopoietic origin. Transplantation studies in which marrow from endotoxin-sensitive (C3H/HeN) mice was infused into endotoxin-resistant (C3H/HeJ) recipients have shown that sensitivity is conferred by cells of the donor. The macrophage is suspected to be the cell responsible for endotoxin-induced injury and death, since various facultative intracellular bacteria, capable of eliciting reticuloendothelial hyperplasia, greatly enhance the endotoxin sensitivity of infected ani-

148

mals. Moreover, endotoxin-induced macrophages produce, in vitro, a mediator capable of killing endotoxin-resistant mice.

Identification of the mediators that confer endotoxin sensitivity would seem to be essential in the design of a specific strategy to arrest the development of shock in sepsis. Cachectin is the name applied to a macrophage hormone originally isolated in the course of studies aimed at delineating basic mechanisms of cachexia in chronic disease. Cachectin has been purified to homogeneity and is a polypeptide hormone with a subunit size of approximately 17 kd. Cachectin is produced in considerable abundance, accounting for 1% to 2% of the total secretory product of endotoxin-activated mouse peritoneal macrophages. Very small amounts of the hormone are made by circulating monocytes, unless the latter are primed with interferon-gamma, which greatly augments synthesis.

The hormone can bind by means of a high-affinity receptor to adipocytes and myoblasts, as well as to a wide variety of other tissues. After injection of endotoxin, cachectin appears in the circulation within minutes, reaches peak levels after 2 h, and then rapidly declines in concentration. The half-life of the hormone in the circulation is approximately 6 min.

The role of cachectin as a mediator of endotoxic shock was suggested by studies where this was infused into rats in quantities similar to those produced endogenously in response to lipopolysaccharide. Cachectin caused piloerection, diarrhea, and an ill, unkempt appearance. Hemoconcentration, shock, metabolic acidosis, and transient hyperglycemia followed by hypoglycemia and hyperkalemia were observed. Severe end-organ damage was apparent on both gross examination and light microscopy. The major arteries of the lungs became plugged with thrombi composed primarily of polymorphonuclear leukocytes, and a severe interstitial pneumonitis was present. Acute renal tubular necrosis, as well as ischemic and hemorrhagic lesions of the GI tract, followed the administration of relatively low doses of the hormone (100 to 200 mg/kg body weight in rats). In addition, adrenal and pancreatic hemorrhages were commonly noted. These events are not unlike those of MOF in man.

Early in 1985, it was noted that the amino terminal sequence of mouse cachectin was strongly homologous to that reported for human tumor necrosis factor (TNF). It was also observed that cachectin and TNF possessed an identical spectrum of bioactivities and were immunologically indistinguishable, suggesting that they were in fact the same molecule. This assumption was soon confirmed by genetic sequence analysis.

TNF was found to be a product of mononuclear phagocytes and was observed in several different species. Interestingly, the factor was found to be cytotoxic to selected tumor-cell lines in vitro. The L-929 cell cytotoxicity assay allowed purification of TNF/cachectin. Both tumor necrosis and endotoxic shock arise through the action of the same macrophage hormone, cachectin/TNF. Cachectin is produced as a prohormone, which appears to be biologically inactive in in vitro assays of lipoprotein lipase suppression and cytotoxicity. The propeptide, which like cachectin itself is extensively conserved, is cleaved at several sites to yield the mature polypeptide.

In addition to exerting this direct effect, cachectin is known to induce release of IL-1 by monocytes and endothelial cells. IL-1, in turn, may elicit some of the features that characterize endotoxin poisoning, contributing to the fever, hypotension, neutropenia and thrombocytopenia that prevail. Cachectin is an endogenous pyrogen, capable of inducing fever both through a direct effect on hypothalamic neurons and through the peripheral induction of IL-1, which in turn elicits fever. Hence, administration of lipopolysaccharide-free preparations of cachectin to rabbits evokes a biphasic febrile response. The initial rise in temperature is attributable to the direct effect of the hormone, whereas the second rise results from IL-1 release.

Cachectin activates polymorphonuclear leukocytes, stimulating their adhesion to endothelial-cell surfaces and enhancing their phagocytic activity. A separate effect of the hormone on the endothelial cells themselves also promotes neutrophil adhesion. The range of stimuli known to evoke cachectin production is incompletely known at present. Endotoxin remains the most potent stimulus known (5).

Immune System Function (Dysfunction) in Multiple Organ Failure

Humoral or B Cell Dysfunction

Most data concerning evaluation of antibody response to new (primary antibody response) or previously encountered (secondary or anamnestic response) antigens have been collected in burn patients. Alexander and Moncrief (6) were able to show that the primary response to a new antigen, alligator erythrocytes, was depressed following burns, whereas the secondary response to tetanus toxoid was enhanced. Using a rat burn model, they correlated the degree of burn to the depressed primary response. Support for an intact secondary response has been presented by Balch (7). Such findings become significant when one examines Pseudomonas infections in the ICU (8). Patients that survived had normal serum titers of antitoxin-A, the most lethal toxin of Pseudomonas, but those patients who died had very low levels of this antibody, implying an inability in severely ill patients to generate antibody to the de novo exposure of the antigen presented by the infection. Data by Volenec et al. (9) indicate that immediately following a burn injury there are immature mononuclear cells released in the circulation, and the numbers of B-lymphocytes are decreased in nonsurvivors. This would support the thesis of a depressed humoral response in the burned ICU patient. Miller and Trunkey (10) found decreased ability to generate de novo antibody-forming cells in vitro in mice receiving 10% scald burns, further supporting this thesis.

Anergy to recall skin test antigens (discussed later) identifies patients likely to become septic and die from sepsis. The B cell function or the ability of the anergic patient to synthesize antibodies to antigens presented by an invading organism is not known. The only statement which can be made is that immunoglobulin levels of all five classes are not different in preoperative anergic patients compared to reactive controls of equal disease or the laboratory personnel. Complement levels, either C_3 or total hemolytic complement, are similarly alike. Similar studies in the ICU patient are not valid due to the need for aggressive fluid replacement with crystalloids, plasma, and blood. This may change the in vivo native values of these substances. One study (11) showed that bluntly traumatized patients admitted to the ICU had no significant differences in plasma IGG, IGA, IGM, and C_3 levels. Nearly all patients had elevated acute-phase proteins as measured by C-reactive protein, irrespective of skin test response. Studies by Nohr et al. (12) of the secondary or anamnestic response of ICU patients indicates that there is a defect in antibody synthesis to tetanus toxoid. Sixty-six subjects, including laboratory controls (n = 21), hospitalized reactive patients (n = 15, responding to two or more of five skin test antigens), and hospitalized anergic patients (n = 30, not reacting to skin test antigens) were given a standard booster dose of adsorbed tetanus toxoid. Exclusion criteria were: trauma, burns, radiotherapy, steroid or antineoplastic therapy, administration of blood products, failure to survive 14 days, or a history of recent booster (<2 yr). Immunization history was similar in all groups. Plasma IgG antibody content was determined in IU/ml using a solid-phase radioimmunoassay. A positive response was defined as greater than a ten-fold increase in serum antibody content, which was maximal at 14 days. As can be seen from Table 2, the anamnestic humoral immune response to tetanus toxoid is reduced in surgical patients. This reduction is more severe and more frequent in anergic patients. Humoral immune dysfunction of this magnitude is likely to be important in the response to bacterial challenge in the ICU patient.

Table 2. Antibody synthesis response of control subjects, and reactive and anergic patients following tetanus toxoid administration

	n	Geometric Mean Antibody Response	Positive Response (%)	Negative Response (%)
Lab Controls	21	27.0	15 (71)	6 (29)
Hospital Reactive	15	12.7	8 (53)*	7 (47)
Hospital Anergic	30	2.0	5 (17)	25 (83)

* X^2 2df = 16.11; $p < .01$

Similar work has shown an abnormality in antibody production to tetanus toxoid from burn patients (13). Because most bacterial antigens are polysaccharides, not proteins, we studied in vivo and in vitro antibody responses to a relatively T cell independent polysaccharide antigen, 23 valent Pneumovax® (PPS). Subjects were classified by skin testing. There were five reactive patients, seven anergic patients, and eight laboratory control subjects. Blood lymphocytes taken before and after immunization with 0.5 ml PPS were cultured in vitro. Quantities of total and anti-PPS IgG, IgM, and IgA in culture supernatants and serum were measured by radioimmunoassay. There was no difference in in vivo anti-PPS production in the three groups. Positive response rates (>2-fold increase) for all classes of immunoglobulin were also similar in the three groups. In in vitro studies, peak quantities of IgA anti-PPS produced by anergic patients were significantly less than laboratory controls (0.64 x: 0.41 vs. 2.03 x: 0.6, $p < .04$, Wilcoxon rank sum test). Synthesis of all other classes of Ig anti-PPS and simultaneous measurement of total Ig (ng/culture) produced in vitro were not significantly different among all groups. Peak in vitro isotype specific anti-PPS production correlated with the magnitude of the in vivo serum response (Spearman rank correlation = 0.53, 0.60 and 0.59 for IgG, IgM and IgA, $p < .05$). Thus, we found a normal in vivo antibody response to a relatively T cell-independent bacterial polysaccharide antigen in surgical patients, and a good correlation of

151

in vivo to in vitro specific antibody responses. The data imply that a T cell defect is responsible for reduced humoral immunity to protein antigens. Because most bacterial antigens are polysaccharides, not proteins, active immunization of surgical patients with bacterial vaccines may produce effective immunity (14).

Cell-Mediated Immune Dysfunction

The Delayed Type Hypersensitivity Response as a Clinical Tool

Delayed type hypersensitivity (DTH) is a name applied by Hans Zinsser (15) to the erythematous indurated reactions elicited in specifically sensitized subjects by intracutaneous challenge with bacterial antigens. The basis of the DTH response is the ability of the host, in particular the T-lymphocyte, to recognize an antigen as foreign. A sensitized lymphocyte (long-lived T cell that has been modified by a macrophage to recognize the antigen because of previous exposure) encounters the antigen in the dermis. This cell releases lymphokines (mostly proteins) which attract nonsensitized lymphocytes (short-lived T-lymphocytes), macrophages, and PMNs to the skin test site. These cells release other proteins, resulting in fluid accumulation. The end result of the inflammatory reaction is the eradication of the antigen which could very well have been an invading pathogen. The above reaction produces the induration which one measures in assessing the DTH response.

Technique of Skin Testing to Assess the DTH Response of a Patient

The technique we presently use to evaluate the DTH response is as follows: An experienced nurse is best to administer the recall test antigens in the skin of the arm, forearm, or thigh. The sites are rotated for sequential testing, usually once a week. The antigens used are the ones most likely to have provided previous exposure for the endemic area of the country. We use Candida (Candidin 1:100 dilution), mumps skin test antigen (undiluted), purified protein derivative (PPD, 5 TU/0.1 ml), Trichophyton, and streptokinase-streptodornase (Varidase, 100 U/ml). They are injected intradermally so that a raised wheel is visible. The resulting area of induration at 24 and 48 h is then delineated by means of delicately approaching the lesion from the normal skin toward its center with a felt-tip pen. The pen stops at the edge of the induration with some practice. The two greatest diameters are then measured, summed, and divided by two; the resulting mean sum is recorded. The erythema is ignored. A positive response is defined as a mean diameter of induration equal to or greater than 5 mm. A reactive subject (R) is defined as one with two or more responses. A relatively anergic subject (RA) responds to only one antigen. An anergic subject (A) has no responses at any time. A commercially available device (MULTITEST CMI, Antigen Supply House, Northridge, CA) can also be used. We found that the antigen concentrations with this device are such that it leads to a higher proportion of anergic patients compared to the method described above (16).

Correlation Between Skin Test Results and Outcome in Patients Admitted to the Surgical ICU.

The data presented here involve the analysis of skin tests on 486 patients admitted to the surgical ICU (SICU) of the Royal Victoria Hospital, McGill University, Montreal, Quebec. Many of these patients went on to develop MOF. Patients were skin tested upon admission to the SICU and then once weekly until discharge, or more often under certain protocols.

In skin tests on over 200 laboratory healthy control subjects, we found >95% positive DTH reactions. Repeated weekly skin tests were not shown to augment the DTH response. The overall data relating SICU admission, DTH skin test response to clinical outcome of 486 patients is shown in Table 3. Clearly, there is a correlation between the DTH response and major sepsis and mortality in this group of patients. Development of major sepsis was at a rate of 50% in patients who were anergic upon admission to the SICU compared to reactive patients ($X^2 = 11.5, p = .003$). Mortality was 35% in anergic patients upon admission to the SICU compared to 15% in reactive patients ($X^2 = 20.8, p < .0001$).

Table 3. Skin test response upon admission to the SICU and clinical outcome in 486 surgical patients

	DTH Response	n	Sepsis	Mortality
	R	164	55 (34%)	24 (15%)
	RA	94	34 (36%)	23 (24%)
	A	228	113 (50%)	80 (35%)
Sepsis outcome	$X^2 = 11.5; p = .003$			
Death outcome	$X^2 = 20.8 \ p < .001$			

The septic "load" of these patients indicated a similar distribution of bacteremias, abscesses, or both abscess and bacteremias in the three groups. Similarly, the numbers of different bacteria per bacteremic episode were the same. Approximately 50% of bacteremias were due to a single organism, 35% due to two organisms, and 15% were due to three or more organisms. Sepsis is known to suppress systemic host defense, and this was further supported by this data. Thirty-three of 44 patients (75%) with admission diagnosis of sepsis (positive blood cultures, proven intra-abdominal abscess, or suppurative peritonitis) were anergic compared to eight of 24 (33%) of those with no sepsis. Trauma, which is also known to suppress host resistance, led to 16 of 23 (70%) of severely traumatized patients (mostly blunt trauma) to be anergic upon admission to the SICU.

A hypothesis proposed was that once major sepsis becomes established in an anergic patient, that patient does not handle the bacterial challenge as well as a reactive patient. Support for this hypothesis comes from patients who were admitted to the SICU because of established major sepsis, and who subsequently died. Table 4 lists the outcome data. These 115 patients were diagnosed to have either suppurative peritonitis or intra-abdominal abscess(es), bacteremia, or a combination of these. The distribution of these types of sepsis was equal among the three groups. The rates of subsequent additional septic episodes following admission were high in all three groups. There was no significant difference between septic challenge of reactive versus anergic patients (44% vs. 66%). The mortality of the anergic patients was four-fold greater compared to the reactive patients with an $X^2 = 8.8$ and $p = .0122$.

Table 4. Skin test response of patients admitted to the ICU with the diagnosis of major sepsis and their clinical outcome (n =115)

DTH Response	n	Further Sepsis	Mortality
R	27	12 (44%)	3 (11%)
RA	18	11 (61%)	7 (39%)
A	70	46 (66%)	30 (43%)

Summary of the Royal Victoria Hospital Experience

Research into antibacterial host defense mechanisms over the past 10 yr in our laboratory using preoperative, postoperative, post-trauma, and septic surgical patients has shown the following: Patients who are anergic, i.e., no (DTH) skin test response to five ubiquitous antigens upon admission to the hospital, have a 33% mortality rate, over 80% of which can be attributed to sepsis, compared to 4% in those patients who are reactive, i.e., respond to two or more antigens (17). These data have been confirmed in studies of over 3,000 patients in our institution. Many other laboratories throughout the world concur with these findings (18-28) with one exception (29). Even this group of researchers, who categorically state that DTH responses are not useful in the clinical setting, have shown mortality rates of 35% in anergic patients compared to 0% in the reactive patients. Since prevention of infection is the job of the immune system, the correlation between sepsis and failure of the DTH reaction suggested that a cause-and-effect relationship may exist between the two. Because the organisms identified in these septic patients were Gram-positive and Gram-negative extracellular bacteria normally handled by humoral and nonspecific local host defense, not DTH, it was reasoned that anomalies seen in DTH may in fact signal broader immune deficits.

For these reasons, various parameters of the immune response were studied, starting with the DTH reaction and its in vitro correlate, the proliferative reaction to alloantigens and to skin test antigens. In vitro lymphocyte studies from anergic patients showed normal mixed lymphocyte culture reactions, normal response to lymphokines, normal generation of cytotoxic T cells, and normal proliferative reactions to mitogens and antigens. The in vitro lymphocyte proliferative reaction to PPD is normal despite in vivo anergy to PPD skin tests. This indicates that lymphocyte and macrophage function, as reflected in in vitro tests, are normal in anergy, and these cells are unable to respond to antigen in vivo. The failure to obtain a DTH reaction might be due to an "anergic environment" in the host, preventing in vivo lymphocyte activation. In fact, when patients' lymphocytes were activated with a skin test antigen (PPD) in vitro, such cells returned to the patients' skin, set in motion an antigen-specific DTH reaction (30). Not only the activated cells, but culture supernatants (lymphokines) derived from them, duplicated these results. Except in the case of serum of anergic patients which may have been occasionally inhibitory to lymphocyte activation, we could not demonstrate this in vivo anergic environment effect in vitro. With this constraint, we directed our further studies in vivo, selecting as the vehicle the noninvasive tape strip skin window technique (31). Using normal subjects, we found that attraction of mononuclear cells to the skin window 24 and 48 h after injection of antigen yielded a faithful, quantitative, antigen-specific correlate of the DTH reaction. In anergic patients, a negligible cell delivery without additives to the window was seen to be corrected by injection of antigen and lymphokine, thus confirming our previous observations of the restoration of the DTH response. In addition, the evaluation of the DTH response in terms of the number of mononuclear cells attracted to the reaction site, and their paucity in windows placed on anergic patients alerted us to the possibility that the immune deficit in anergy might be due in part to abnormal cell chemotaxis.

At the level of nonspecific local antibacterial host defense, our studies showed that patients with anergy seen immediately following trauma, major surgery, or severe sepsis were different from those with anergy seen in elective surgical patients who walk into the hospital with no focus of infection, a condition we term walk-in anergy. The first group, in addition to anergy, have stickier PMNs determined from in vitro adherence measurements to nylon fiber. The in vitro chemotaxis of such PMNs is always reduced, measured both in filter-type assays or under agarose. The reduced PMN chemotaxis is inversely related to the adherence, i.e., the cells are stickier and they move slower than controls in in vitro studies (32). These in vitro abnormalities have in vivo significance in that the accumulation of PMNs to Rebuck-type window chambers over a skin abrasion (different from the tape stripping window) is much reduced in anergic patients with increased adherence and decreased chemotaxis compared to laboratory controls or reactive patients with normal PMN function (33). We were surprised, however, to find that in some patients there is divergence of anergy and local nonspecific host defense. By this we mean that some patients who remained reactive following trauma showed abnormalities in local nonspecific host defense, albeit of lesser magnitude compared to those with anergy (34). The reverse does not occur. Anergic patients after trauma always have abnormal local nonspecific host defense. Patients with walk-in anergy have normal adherence and chemotaxis and cannot be distinguished from laboratory controls on the basis of these measurements (35). Furthermore, delivery of PMNs to skin windows in these walk-in anergic patients is not reduced compared to reactive patients. In the postoperative period, the walk-in anergic patients (along with the reactive patients) develop increased adherence, decreased chemotaxis, and decreased delivery of PMNs to skin windows, i.e., they demonstrate decreased local nonspecific host defense in addition to decreased DTH. Like the T cell defects, these abnormalities in local nonspecific host defense are due to an in vivo "suppressive environment": there are factors in the plasma of patients with increased PMN adherence that increase the adherence of normal control PMNs following treatment in vitro; thus, in the case of PMN the decreased chemotaxis is mediated by factors in the serum (36). Cell transfer experiments with thermally injured rats have confirmed this suppressive environment effect on local nonspecific host defense, in particular PMN localization. Normal unburned PMNs injected into burned rats accumulate in inflammatory sites at the same rate as burn PMNs in burned rats. Burned rat PMNs injected into unburned rats accumulate in inflammatory sites at the same rate as unburned PMNs into normal rats.

The injection of culture supernatants from cells activated with the specific antigen PPD, or supernatants raised in mixed leukocyte cultures, i.e., with unrelated antigens, when injected along with PPD could restore an antigen-specific DTH response in anergic patients. Keyhole Limpet Hemocyanin (KLH), is an antigen to which prior sensitization has not occurred, and for immunization this was injected alone, or together with lymphokine. Injection of KLH with lymphokine, but not without it, induced a cell-mediated immunity in the majority of patients as assessed by DTH and by a lymphocyte proliferative assay 1 and 2 wk after immunization, testifying to a systemic immune response induced to a neoantigen during the anergic state. These measures, however, did not elicit an antibody response to KLH for reasons that are not yet clear.

The various components of the immune system are elegantly integrated in vivo and, along with local nonspecific host defense, provide for control of bacterial infections. We studied how some of these components interact in the host by multivariate logistic regression analysis. We chose septic-related mortality as the dependent variable. DTH expressed as a skin test score (the sum of the diameters of induration of each of the individual five antigens), PMN function, serum albumin, Hgb, sex, and age were used as independent variables. The analysis showed that DTH score, age, and serum albumin were the strongest predicting variables (37). The following equation can be used to calculate the probability of septic related mortality of any patient given his preoperative DTH score, age, and serum albumin:

$$P|\text{death}| = 1 - \{1 + \exp(1.343 - 1.372(\text{albumin}) - 0.173(\log[\text{DTH score}]) + 0.026(\text{age}))\}^{-1}$$

This equation can give an *objective measure* of preoperative patient risk for a postoperative adverse outcome. It has been tested in a prospective manner, and the predicted and expected mortalities are similar. The contribution of the serum albumin is an interesting observation. Although it is tempting to attribute this to malnutrition in the host, we do not believe this to be the case. A variable such as the Acute Physiology Score, which measures the degree of physiologic stress on the host, displaces the albumin from the predictive model. We interpret this to mean that the reduced albumin indicates a condition of physiologic stress that exists in the host. This stress results in a redirection of protein synthesis by the liver, with suppression of albumin synthesis in favor of acute-phase proteins which may be needed for survival. The mediator may be IL-1, which together with its breakdown product, Proteolysis Inducing Factor, is present in the host undergoing any form of stress such as trauma or sepsis (38). Cachectin or another as yet unidentified macrophage monokine may also be involved. In fact, this observation may indicate a possible modulating control of macrophages on the immune system, both at the specific and local nonspecific host-defense level. We found that rats who had their Kuppfer cells activated by an intraportal injection of bacteria exhibited suppressed DTH responses in the skin, whereas when Kuppfer cells were ablated with intraportal carrageenan, there was an enhancement of the DTH response. Keller et al. (39) have also found evidence that Kuppfer cells modulate hepatocyte function. This modulation of hepatocyte function by an endotoxin-stimulated Kuppfer cell preparation may, in part, represent the mechanism of hepatic insufficiency associated with the MOF syndrome.

In Vitro Assessment of Cell-Mediated Immunity

Wolfe et al. (40) reported on skin tests with four recall antigens performed serially in 21 patients after a major thermal burn. They looked for a correlation between the occurrence of anergy, the presence of immunosuppressive serum, and the impairment of the lymphocyte-proliferative response to phytohemagglutinin (PHA). When anergy developed, it became apparent early in the course of the illness. It did not correlate closely with the severity of the burn, but was associated with mortality. There was a good correlation between anergy and coexisting serum suppression of lymphocyte activation in vitro. This serum immunosuppressive activity was not related to serum cortisol, PGE_2, or plasma endotoxin levels. Anergy also correlated with coexistent impairment of patient peripheral blood lymphocyte activation by PHA. These results suggest that both immunosuppressive serum and an impaired lymphocyte response to mitogens are associated with anergy in burn patients, and confirm that the development of anergy is an index of poor prognosis.

Serial blast transformation in vitro was measured in peripheral lymphocytes from 38 patients with major thermal injury by Munster et al (41). Lymphocytes were tested with the antigens streptokinase-streptodornase (SKSD), mumps, PPD, the mitogens concanavalin A and PHA, and in the one-way mixed lymphocyte reaction. Statistically significant suppression by the burn injury was noticed in all measurements except response to PHA. One-time measurements were not significantly different between the patients who survived and the patients who did not survive their burn injuries. However, serial determinations of responsiveness to the three natural antigens SKSD, mumps, and PPD, as well as the mixed lymphocyte reaction, accurately reflected prognosis. Ninnemann (42) has also shown that a significant number of patients with severe thermal injuries are profoundly immunosuppressed. This immunosuppression is mediated by substances which circulate in the serum which could be easily detected using in vitro lymphocyte assays. The suppressive material is not present in normal serum, and exerts its effects through the activity of a specific (suppressor) subpopulation of lymphocytes. There is evidence linking suppressive activity in serum to the presence of endotoxin, prostaglandin E, interferon, and "cutaneous burn toxin." Patients with severe thermal injuries who often display an impaired cell-mediated immune response have an increased susceptibility to infection. Experimentally, patient serum suppressive to the PHA response of normal human lymphocytes does so through B cell participation in the generation of suppressor T cells. Bacterial endotoxin can also produce these effects, both in vivo and in vitro. It is felt by these authors that normal human lymphocytes isolated by cotton column adherence should be used to obtain a reliable assay of immunosuppression of PHA-induced blastogenesis by serum from patients with burn injuries.

Summary

There remains much work to be done in the area of MOF and immune system function. The data presented here have not been confined exclusively to those patients with MOF, since this syndrome is new and immune dysfunction in MOF has been realized only recently. It would appear that the central cell is the macrophage. This presents a paradox in that this cell plays a pivotal role in combating infection, yet if overstimulated, the monokines it produces (such as IL-1 and cachectin) can lead to septic shock and if prolonged, to MOF. A complete understanding of the regulatory mechanisms of macrophage function during sepsis should lead to ways and means of preventing MOF in surgical patients and improving their clinical outcome.

References

1. Keller GA, West MA, Cerra FB, et al: Macrophage-mediated modulation of hepatic function in multiple-system failure. *J Surg Res* 1985; 39:555

2. Frank MM: Complement in Current Concepts Monograph. Kalamazoo, MI, Upjohn Co, 1985

3. Dinarello CA: Interleukin-1 and the pathogenesis of the acute phase response. *N Engl J Med* 1984; 311:1413

4. Robb RJ: Interleukin 2: The molecule and its function. *Immunology Today* 1984; 5:203

5. Beutler B, Cerami A: Cachectin: More than a tumor necrosis factor. *N Engl J Med* 1987; 316:379

6. Alexander JW, Moncrief JA: Alterations of immune response following severe thermal injury. *Arch Surg* 1966; 93:75

7. Balch HH: The effect of severe battle injury and post-operative renal failure on resistance to infection. *Ann Surg* 1955; 142:145

8. Cross AS, Sadoff JC, Iglewski BH, et al: Evidence for the role of toxin-A in the pathogenesis of infection with *Pseudomonas aeruginosa* in humans. *J Infect Dis* 1980; 142:538

9. Volenec FJ, Wood GW, Mani MM, et al: Mononuclear cell analysis of peripheral blood from burn patients. *J Trauma* 1979; 19:86

10. Miller CL, Trunkey DD: Thermal injury: Defects in immune response induction. *J Surg Res* 1977; 22:621

11. Christou NV, McLean APH, Meakins JL: Host defense in blunt trauma: Interrelationships between kinetics of anergy and depressed neutrophil function, nutritional status and sepsis. *J Trauma* 1980; 20:833

12. Nohr CW, Christou NV, Broadhead M, et al: Failure of humoral immunity in surgical patients. *Surg Forum* 1983; 34:127

13. Wood JJ, O'Mahony ML, Rodrick R, et al: Abnormalities of antibody production following thermal injury. An association with reduced interleukin 2 production. *Arch Surg* 1986; 121:108

14. Nohr CW, Latter DA, Meakins JL, et al: In vivo and in vitro humoral immunity in surgical patients: Antibody response to pneumococcal polysaccharide. *Surgery* 1986; 100:229

15. Zinsser H: Delayed hypersensitivity. *J Exp Med* 1921; 34:495

16. Christou NV, Boisvert G, Broadhead N, et al: Two techniques of measurement of the delayed hypersensitivity skin test response for the assessment of bacterial host resistance. *World J Surg* 1985; 9:798

17. Christou NV: Host defense mechanisms in surgical patients: A correlative study of the delayed hypersensitivity skin test response, granulocyte function and sepsis in 2202 patients. *Can J Surg* 1985; 28:39

18. Adami GF, Terrizzi A, Vita M, et al: The assessment of skin tests in surgery. *Surgery in Italy* 1980; 10:297

19. Casey J, Flinn WR, Yao JS, et al: Correlation of immune and nutritional status with wound complications in patients undergoing vascular operations. *Surgery* 1983; 93:822

20. Gertner MH, Mullen JL, Buzby GP, et al: Implications of malnutrition in the surgical patient. *Arch Surg* 1979; 114:121

21. Griffith CDM, Ross AHM: Delayed hypersensitivity skin testing in elective colorectal surgery and relationship to postoperative sepsis. *JPEN* 1984; 8:279

22. Johnson WC, Ulrich R, Meguid MM, et al: Role of delayed hypersensitivity in predicting postoperative morbidity and mortality. *Am J Surg* 1979; 137:536

23. Harvey KB, Moldawer LL, Bistrian BR, et al: Biological measures for the formulation of a hospital prognostic index. *Am J Clin Nutr* 1981; 34:2013

24. Kienlen J, Chardon P, Nury G, et al: Study of delayed skin hypersensitivity using the multitest in an intensive care unit. *Annals Anesthesiologie France* 1981; 22:285

25. Tasseau F, Gaucher L, Nicolas F: Cell-mediated immunity studied by skin tests in patients receiving intensive care. Prognostic value of repeated tests. Study of some factors predisposing towards anergy. *Seminars Hospital Paris* 1982; 58:781

26. Morath MA, Miller SF, Finley RK: Nutritional indicators of postburn bacteremic sepsis. *JPEN* 1981; 5:488

27. Jensen TG, Long JM III, Dudrick SJ, et al: Nutritional assessment indications of postburn complications. *J Am Diet Assoc* 1985; 85:68

28. Fletcher JP, Little JM, Walker PJ: Anergy and the severely ill surgical patient. *Aust NZ J Surg* 1986; 56:117

29. Brown R, Bancewicz J, Hamid J, et al: Failure of delayed hypersensitivity skin testing to predict post-operative sepsis and mortality. *Br J Surg* 1982; 284:851

30. Rode HN, Christou NV, Bubenik O, et al: Lymphocyte function in anergic patients. *Clin Exp Immunol* 1981; 47:155

31. Mass MF, Dean PB, Weston WL: Leukocyte migration in vivo: A new method of study. *J Lab Clin Med* 1975; 86:1040

32. Christou NV: The delayed hypersensitivity response, granulocyte function and sepsis in surgical patients. *J Burn Care Res* 1985; 6:157

33. Morris JS, Meakins JL, Christou NV: In vivo neutrophil delivery to inflammatory sites in surgical patients: Correlation with in vitro neutrophil chemotaxis and adherence. *Arch Surg* 1985; 120:205

34. Christou NV, McLean APH, Meakins JL: Host defense in blunt trauma: Interrelationships of kinetics of anergy and depressed neutrophil function, nutritional status, and sepsis. *J Trauma* 1980; 20:833

35. Christou NV, Rode HN, Larson D, et al: The walk-in anergic patient: How best to assess the risk following elective surgery. *Ann Surg* 1984; 199:438

36. Christou NV, Meakins JL: Neutrophil function in surgical patients: Two inhibitors of granulocyte chemotaxis associated with sepsis. *J Surg Research* 1979; 26:355

37. Christou NV: Predicting septic related mortality of the individual surgical patient based on admission host defense measurements. *Can J Surg*, In Press

38. Clows GHA Jr, George BC, Villee CA, et al: Muscle proteolysis induced by a circulating peptide in patients with sepsis or trauma. *N Engl J Med* 1983; 308:545

39. Keller GA, West Ma, Cerra FB, et al: Multiple systems organ failure. Modulation of hepatocyte protein synthesis by endotoxin activated Kupffer cells. *Ann Surg* 1985; 201:87

40. Wolfe JH, Wu AV, O'Connor NE, et al: Anergy, immunosuppressive serum, and impaired lymphocyte blastogenesis in burn patients. *Arch Surg* 1982; 117:1266

41. Munster AM, Winchurch RA, Birmingham WJ, et al: Longitudinal assay of lymphocyte responsiveness in patients with major burns. *Ann Surg* 1980; 192:772

42. Ninnemann JL: Immunosuppression following thermal injury through B cell activation of suppressor T cells. *J Trauma* 1980; 20:206

SELF-ASSESSMENT QUESTIONS

1. Antigen presentation to lymphocytes on the surface of cells occurs during the recognition phase of the immune response. Which of the following cells can act as antigen-presenting cells?
   A. monocytes/macrophages
   B. dendritic cells
   C. fixed tissue histiocytes
   D. Langenhans' cells
   E. red blood cells

2. Interleukin-1 exerts multiple effects on the afferent limb of the immune response. From the list below, choose those specifically influencing T cells:
   A. production of interleukin-2
   B. augmentation of hemopoiesis
   C. prostaglandin production in joint fluid
   D. proliferation of dermal fibroblasts
   E. stimulation of metabolism of polymorphonuclear neutrophils

3. Cachectin administration into rats produces which of the following:
   A. piloerection, diarrhea, and an ill appearance
   B. hemoconcentration
   C. shock
   D. metabolic acidosis, hypoglycemia, hyperkalemia
   E. severe end-organ damage

4. Anergy to skin test antigens upon admission to the surgical ICU indicates an increased risk of mortality. Choose the item below which best estimates this risk:
   A. 15%
   B. 25%
   C. 35%
   D. 50%
   E. 85%

5. Logistic regression techniques utilizing several variables indicating various alterations in host defense allow for estimating the probability of mortality of a particular patient based on which of the following variables?
   A. age
   B. serum albumin
   C. circulating lymphocyte count
   D. delayed type hypersensitivity skin test score
   E. serum immunoglobulin levels

6. An anergic patient who subsequently develops major life-threatening sepsis in the surgical ICU, such as an intra-abdominal abscess, has a higher chance of dying from this infection compared to a reactive patient.
   A. true
   B. false

SELF-ASSESSMENT ANSWERS AND RATIONALE

1. A-D.   The red cell membrane lacks the Ia surface proteins and cannot serve as an antigen-presenting cell. All other cells contain this protein and, thus, can serve as antigen-presenting cells in the body.

2. A.   Stimulated macrophages produce IL-1, which in turn stimulates lymphocytes to produce interleukin-2 and lead to clonal expansion of lymphocytes. None of the other processes is mediated via lymphocytes or their products.

3. A-E.   Cachectin/tumor necrosis factor, when administered to rats, will produce all of the listed changes, which lead to multiple organ failure and death.

4. C.   Several studies quoted in this review have shown that a patient who is anergic upon admission to a surgical ICU runs a risk of 50% for subsequent major life-threatening sepsis and 35% for mortality.

5. A, B, D. An extensive logistic regression analysis carried out by the author examined age, serum albumin, DTH skin test score, circulating lymphocyte and polymorphonuclear (PMN) count, PMN adherence to nylon wool, PMN chemotaxis, and circulating Hgb count as independent variables with septic-related mortality as the dependent variable. Only age, serum albumin, and the DTH skin test score were significantly related to outcome and could be used in an equation which could be used to calculate the septic-related mortality of an individual patient.

6. A.   An anergic patient who develops life-threatening sepsis has a 71% chance of dying from this sepsis compared to a reactive patient in whom the chance of mortality is 45% (calculated from Table 3).

Chapter 10

Pharmacokinetics in Multiple Organ Failure

James R. Jacobs, PhD and W. David Watkins, MD, PhD

Outline

Educational Objectives

In this chapter the reader will learn:

1. that multiple organ failure may result in a complex array of pharmacokinetic aberrations that depend on the disease state, the drug, and concurrent therapies.

2. that modern analytical and computational techniques could and should be applied to further the study of pharmacokinetics in multiple organ failure.

Introduction

Although data quantifying drug disposition in multiple organ failure (MOF) are virtually nonexistent, it is generally assumed that the pharmacokinetics of a particular drug in the critically ill patient are likely to be significantly different than those in the "healthy young volunteer" from whom most published pharmacokinetic parameters, and many standard dosing schemes, are derived. Pharmacokinetics under the conditions of combined renal and hepatic failure have been determined for a few drugs, but for the most part qualitative and quantitative descriptions of the pharmacokinetics of MOF, defined here as the functional insufficiency of two or more pharmacokinetically important organ systems, do not exist. Recently, Mann et al. (1) presented an excellent review of pharmacokinetics and pharmacodynamics in critically ill patients, but they had to consider the consequences of failure of each of the individual organ systems — cardiac, renal, hepatic — separately because pharmacokinetic data from the

patient suffering MOF are so rare. We will, in this summary, attempt to complement rather than duplicate Mann and colleagues' introduction to this important
subject. Basic pharmacokinetic principles will be emphasized. Note that this
chapter deals with the consequences of diminished function of pharmacokinetically significant organs and not with the multiple organ system
failure (MOSF) syndrome per se.

Route of Administration

The pharmacokinetic characterization of a particular drug encompasses the
processes of absorption, distribution, biotransformation, and elimination. Since
drugs must be physically absorbed from their site of application before the other
pharmacokinetic processes and pharmacological effects (pharmacodynamics)
can occur, alterations in drug absorption precipitated by MOF should influence
decisions regarding the route of drug administration.

Renal failure (2) can impair GI absorption because of higher gastric pH due to
ammonia buffering, solute (e.g., antacids) binding, impaired transport secondary to 1,25 vitamin D deficiency, or bowel edema; absorption of drugs administered at peripheral sites (e.g., subcutaneously) may be delayed if chronic renal
failure has resulted in edema formation at the site. If the efficiency with which
hepatic enzymes irreversibly remove drug (first-pass metabolism) from the
blood is decreased, as it may be in liver failure, systemic availability of orally
(peroral) administered drugs may be increased (3). The effect of liver disease on
the bioavailability of a drug is dependent on the class to which the drug belongs.
The systemic availability of flow-limited (i.e., high hepatic extraction ratio)
drugs may be increased considerably in liver disease. Another factor leading to
the increase in bioavailability of flow-limited drugs is the shunting of portal vein
blood past functioning hepatocytes in response to the portal hypertension that
may result from liver disease (3). The bioavailability of enzyme-limited (low
hepatic extraction ratio) drugs is high in normal subjects and remains relatively
unaffected in liver disease. In cardiac failure, hypoperfusion of peripheral
tissues due to decreased cardiac output and regional vasoconstriction may result
in slowed or erratic absorption (4, 5) from intramuscular, subcutaneous, rectal,
transdermal, and sublingual sites of administration. Cardiac failure may also
impede the rate and extent of intestinal drug absorption by decreasing GI
motility due to sympathetic stimulation, causing edematous changes in the
intestinal wall, and by reducing intestinal blood flow (6). Although pulmonary
disease does not in itself dramatically influence drug absorption kinetics (other
than those of the inhalational route), the tissue hypoxia and acid-base derangements that may result from pulmonary failure can alter blood flow distribution
and thereby affect drug absorption as in cardiac failure (7). Finally, conditions
that produce nausea and vomiting are likely to delay gastric emptying and
thereby delay the absorption of orally administered drugs (8).

Thus, when multiple organs are in various stages of failure, drug absorption
from all routes other than intravenous injection is likely to be abnormal, or at
best, unpredictable. That most drugs given to critically ill patients are administered by the intravenous route is a pharmacokinetically sound practice in that
the alterations in drug absorption caused by organ failure are completely
avoided. Intravenous administration ensures not only complete and rapid bioavailability (amount of, and rate at which, drug enters the systemic circulation

164

from an administered dosage form), but also a degree of predictability and relia-bility not possible through any other route; in the pharmacological management of critically ill patients, such control may be vital. It is also recognized, however, that altered blood flow distribution patterns in the presence of cardiac failure may cause intravenously administered drugs to reach critical organs, such as the heart and brain, in unexpectedly high concentrations (5). This may lead to acute toxicity. Nevertheless, the remainder of this chapter will be based on the assumption of intravenous administration.

Mann et al. (1) suggest that exceptions to the caveat of intravenous admin-istration are drugs that have a local effect on the GI tract and agents with a wide therapeutic index. They also exclude agents with a pharmacodynamic response that is easy to monitor. We do not necessarily agree with this final assertion, as a measurable response does not necessarily permit safe and efficient administra-tion if the delivery of drug cannot be carefully regulated.

Basic Pharmacokinetic Principles

The classic reference on pharmacokinetic principles is the text by Gibaldi and Perrier (9); a more clinically oriented treatment is given by Wartak (10). The pharmacokinetics of intravenous infusion have been reviewed by Hug (11). Of particular relevance to critical care medicine is the chapter by Thompson (12), which provides an excellent review of clinical pharmacokinetics and dosage optimization, and includes many enlightening graphic simulations of phar-macokinetic concepts.

The three-compartment model shown in Figure 1 is often used to schematize the pharmacokinetic processes that occur following intravenous administration. This model consists of a central compartment and two peripheral compartments where $C_i(t)$ in ng·ml^{-1} represents the drug concentration in each of the respec-tive compartments as a function of time. The disposition of some drugs can be adequately described by a one or two-compartment structure, and for some drugs it is necessary to use complex nonlinear, nonparametric models; however, the diagram in Figure 1 is sufficiently general for our purposes here.

Based on similarities in blood flow and affinity for a given drug, various tissues and organs may be grouped and assigned to either the central or peripheral compartments. The central compartment represents a distribution volume of V_1 l·kg^{-1} and is usually assumed to include the blood, extracellular space, and well perfused organs. Most significantly, it is assumed that the phar-macodynamic effect of the drug is related in some way to the concentration of free drug in the central compartment, the blood or plasma being the only reasonable window into this compartment. $K_o(t)$ in µg·kg^{-1}·min^{-1} represents the rate of administration (intravenous) of drug into the central compartment and may, over the course of time, represent any combination of bolus injections and con-tinuous infusions.

The peripheral compartments can be thought of as those tissues and organs showing a time course and extent of drug accumulation (or dissipation) different than that of the central compartment. In the three-compartment model, for example, the two peripheral compartments may correspond roughly to fat stores and muscle tissue, respectively; however, it is important to realize that the model is merely a mathematical abstraction of the time course of drug

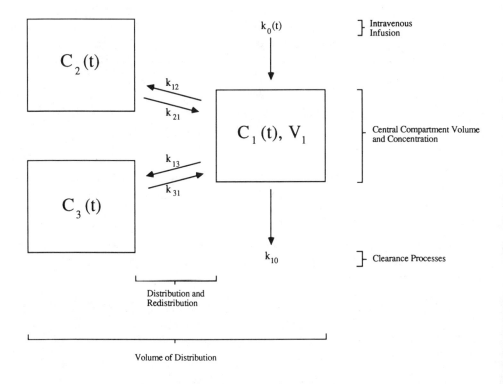

$k_0(t)$

Intravenous Infusion

$C_2(t)$

k_{12}
k_{21}

$C_1(t), V_1$

Central Compartment Volume and Concentration

k_{13}
k_{31}

$C_3(t)$

k_{10}

Clearance Processes

Distribution and Redistribution

Volume of Distribution

Fig. 1. Three-compartment model schematizing the basic pharmacokinetic processes that occur following intravenous drug administration. Explanation of symbols: V_1 ($l \cdot kg^{-1}$) is the central compartment volume; $C_i(t)$ ($ng \cdot ml^{-1}$) is the drug concentration in compartment i at time t; $k_0(t)$ ($\mu g \cdot kg^{-1} \cdot min^{-1}$) is the rate of intravenous drug administration; and k_{ij} (min^{-1}) are intercompartmental rate constants.

concentration in blood or plasma as a function of infusion rate, and that no physiological reality is implied. The sum of the calculated (but not necessarily real) compartment volumes is known as the apparent volume of distribution and represents the proportionality constant relating drug concentration in blood or plasma to the total amount of drug in the body.

The k_{ij}, in units of reciprocal minutes, are the rate constants describing the flow of drug from compartment i into compartment j. The value k_{10} reflects all of those processes acting through biotransformation or elimination to irreversibly remove drug from the central compartment; these processes are collectively known as drug clearance. The rate constants and central compartment volume are generally determined by nonlinear least-squares analysis of the drug blood or plasma concentration resulting from a known bolus or infusion. The more familiar distribution (alpha) and elimination (beta) half-lives are hybrid functions of the k_{ij} constants.

Of the total amount of drug in the body at any point in time, some will exist as free (not protein-bound) drug in the central compartment, some will be bound to plasma proteins, and some will have distributed into those tissues comprising the peripheral compartments. The rate and extent of drug distribution, and the subsequent redistribution back into the central compartment, depend on the extent of binding to plasma and tissue proteins, the rate and distribution of tissue blood flow, lipid solubility, extent of ionization, molecular size, and possibly active transport processes. It is only the free drug which equilibrates between plasma and tissues that is pharmacologically active and which is subject to elimination from the body. For most drugs, reversible binding to serum albumin is quantitatively the most important drug-protein interaction (13, 14). For drugs that are extensively bound to plasma proteins, a small change in the conditions affecting binding can dramatically alter the fraction of free drug. Additionally, the albumin-drug complex serves as a circulatory drug reservoir that releases drug while free drug is being metabolized or excreted. The greater the lipid solubility, the more rapidly the drug penetrates all types of membranes. For drugs which penetrate membranes rapidly, tissue perfusion can be the rate-limiting factor in the exchange of drug between plasma and tissues (11). Thus, there is an intimate, but not necessarily rigid, relationship between rate of distribution and extent or volume of distribution.

The clearance processes acting to rid the plasma of unbound drug are predominantly renal excretion and hepatic metabolism. There is a complex interaction between volume of distribution and clearance in that a drug molecule that has distributed into a peripheral tissue or which is bound to a plasma protein cannot, in general, be eliminated or biotransformed. If an alteration in the drug's total volume of distribution changes the concentration of free drug in the central compartment, a corresponding change in the clearance of that drug will result. If both distribution volume and clearance are decreased proportionally, no change in elimination half-life will be observed, but loading and maintenance dosages will certainly require adjustment (15).

The motivation for this chapter is the supposition that the distribution volumes and rate constants for a particular drug in the patient with MOF are likely to be much different than they are in the relatively healthy population in whom they are usually calculated. The central compartment concentration resulting from a drug dosage based on "normal" kinetics may consequently be lower or higher than expected.

Pharmacokinetic Implications of Organ Failure

Recent reviews on an organ-by-organ basis of pharmacokinetics in single organ failure have been presented by Mann et al. (1), Paxton (15), and Kato (16). The rationale for studying pharmacokinetics in disease states is to avoid, if possible, overly conservative dosing schemes that result in inadequate serum drug concentrations and overly ambitious dosing schemes that may result in drug accumulation and an increased incidence of toxicity.

Protein Binding

Changes in drug distribution seen with various disease states are frequently the result of a decreased binding of the drug to plasma protein. This effect is most prominent for drugs that exist as anions (17).

Renal failure can alter protein binding through a number of mechanisms. Among these are reduced plasma albumin or total protein levels, changes in the molecular structure of the binding protein, or competition with the endogenous binding substances accumulated in uremia. Plasma protein binding of acidic drugs tends to decrease in uremia, with much variability seen in the effects on the binding of basic drugs (18, 19). Uremia also decreases binding to intracellular proteins (2).

In chronic liver failure there can be a decreased production of plasma proteins (albumin in particular) and increased production of defective plasma proteins. Both occurrences will decrease drug protein binding. For drugs characterized by a high hepatic extraction ratio, decreased plasma protein binding can cause a decreased hepatic drug clearance. Conversely, the hepatic clearance of drugs with a low hepatic extraction ratio may increase when protein binding decreases (10). Both renal and hepatic failure can lead to the accumulation of exogenous (e.g., drug metabolites) and endogenous substances that may compete for protein binding sites. As an example, some forms of liver failure can lead to elevated bilirubin levels; the increased bilirubin concentration, along with the strong affinity of bilirubin for protein binding sites on albumin, will displace acidic drugs from this protein (3).

There is little information on the influence of cardiac failure on drug protein binding, except that the concentration of alpha-1 acid glycoprotein, which plays an important role in the binding of several basic drugs, has been shown to be elevated during acute myocardial infarction, thereby decreasing the free drug fraction (4, 15). Competition for binding sites between the many drugs typically given to cardiac patients probably has a greater influence on protein binding of a particular drug than the direct effects of cardiac disease.

There is some evidence that the free fraction of basic drugs is decreased in pulmonary failure (20). Pulmonary disease has little direct effect upon volume of distribution (7).

Other Factors Influencing Rate and Volume of Distribution

The primary determinants of the rate and volume of distribution of a particular drug are plasma protein binding and the physiochemical properties of the drug. There are, however, several additional pathophysiological factors that have been demonstrated to be relevant in organ failure.

Uremia may increase capillary permeability, which would increase the distribution rate of drugs that disperse by diffusion. Extracellular fluid and total body water ordinarily constitute a higher fraction of body mass in uremia patients, another factor acting to increase potential distribution volume (18). Cirrhotic patients may sometimes have a decreased effective plasma volume due to sequestration of blood in the splanchnic circulation, resulting in retention of drug in the tissues and a larger apparent volume of distribution (17). In states of circulatory insufficiency, the rate of presentation of drug to tissues and therefore, the rate of overall tissue uptake, may be slowed (5); serum concentrations of drugs that normally distribute rapidly after a dose may be transiently much higher than expected. With chronic circulatory failure and third spacing of fluids, the volume of distribution of water-soluble drugs increases (1). Ambient (blood) pH, relative to the drug's pK_a, can markedly influence lipid solubility; if

168

the blood pH becomes more acidic, which may be common in renal, circulatory, or respiratory failure, the nonionized form of weak acids is favored, and lipid permeability increases (21).

Clearance

The liver and kidneys are the major organs responsible for removing drug from the blood. When these organs are diseased, there will be direct and obvious alterations in drug clearance. In the patient with MOF there is also a variety of other direct and indirect factors that may concomitantly alter clearance, in addition to the dependence of clearance on free drug fraction and volume of distribution.

For drugs eliminated by the kidney, the decreased elimination caused by renal failure overrides any fractional increase in availability for elimination that may occur due to decreased protein binding (18). Acidosis secondary to renal disease can decrease renal tubular reabsorption and slow the degradation of some drugs (1, 22). The accumulation of active or toxic metabolites produced through other functional routes of biotransformation can be as troublesome as the primary inability of the kidneys to eliminate parent drug compounds.

Drugs with a high extraction ratio are usually not affected by hepatic impairment because the metabolic capacity is much greater than the rate at which the drug is presented to the liver, making their clearance dependent on hepatic blood flow. The clearance of low extraction ratio drugs is dependent on protein binding (1, 23). Reduction in the intrinsic drug metabolizing ability of the liver would be expected to reduce the systemic clearance of a poorly extracted drug. However, this might be offset by an increase in the free fraction in plasma secondary to decreased protein binding (15).

In cardiac failure, drugs with a high hepatic extraction ratio will experience a decrease in clearance, as will drugs primarily eliminated by the kidneys. Cardiac failure might decrease the metabolic capacity of the liver either through hepatocellular damage resulting from hepatic congestion or hypoperfusion, or through hypoxemia with impaired microsomal drug oxidation (5). Decreased hepatic blood flow and increased hepatic venous pressure are the major causes of hepatic dysfunction in cardiac failure, while arterial hypoxemia is a minor cause. The most likely final common pathway through which these factors cause hepatic damage is cellular hypoxia (24). Cardiac failure may affect renal clearance by decreasing glomerular filtration rate secondary to hypoperfusion, and increasing tubular reabsorption owing to redistribution of intrarenal blood flow and reduced urine flow (5).

Although the lung has remarkable properties affecting the accumulation and metabolism of drugs, and despite substantial evidence that some of these functions are impaired in disease, the lung should not be regarded as a significant modulating factor in drug disposition (25). There has been one report (26) directly linking pulmonary failure with changes in drug clearance, but it was not clear that lung clearance itself was involved. The clearance of flow-dependent drugs can be decreased in pulmonary failure due to decreased perfusion of the kidney and liver (15), possibly as a result of blood gas disturbances and increased pulmonary vascular resistance.

169

Exceptions

To this point, no specific drug names have been mentioned. We conclude this section by recognizing esmolol and atracurium as two new drugs for which very little of the preceding applies — their metabolism is relatively independent of organ function, and they are fast-acting and short-lived enough to be rapidly titratable, making them pharmacokinetically ideal for patients with MOF. The introduction of additional drugs designed with the critically ill patient in mind can be expected.

Pharmacokinetic Implications of Critical Illness and Intensive Care

Almost by definition, patients with MOF are critically ill and will be receiving intensive medical care. These circumstances may require use of one or more therapeutic modalities which may in themselves have significant pharmacokinetic implications independent of, and in addition to, diminished organ function.

The effects of hemodialysis on drug pharmacokinetics have been reviewed recently (27). Hemodialysis may alter protein binding in a multifactorial manner, the net effect of which is not easily predicted. Hemodialysis does not seem to appreciably alter distribution volume, but obviously there is the potential for a substantial transient increase in the clearance of water-soluble drugs. No pharmacokinetic alteration could be more literal than the direct removal of free drug from the plasma by the artificial kidney; this must be considered when a patient receiving dialyzable drugs undergoes dialysis.

Cardiopulmonary bypass is another short-lived perturbation that can result in a complex progression of acute, and occasionally prolonged, pharmacokinetic changes (28). Although pharmacokinetics in this setting have been determined for only a few drugs, one relatively consistent trend is reduced drug clearance during the early postbypass period.

Mechanical ventilation may decrease regional blood flow, hepatic blood flow in particular. Hepatic elimination of flow-limited drugs might thus be reduced during mechanical ventilation (29).

It is well documented that malnutrition and starvation can alter the disposition of certain drugs (16, 30). In fact, nutritional/pharmacologic interactions are very complex and have the potential to disrupt virtually all pharmacokinetic processes, including GI absorption, hepatic microsomal enzyme activity and protein synthesis, renal concentrating ability, and cardiac function (31). Of particular interest may be a decline in serum albumin concentration. A recent review (32) discusses the biochemical basis for many of the interactions seen between nutritional status and drug metabolism.

Other pharmacokinetically relevant interventions to consider are blood and fluid replacement, parenteral alimentation, organ transplantation, and sepsis, but possibly the most pharmacokinetically important aspect of intensive care medicine is the polypharmacy approach to treatment of the critically ill patient, which may lead to the well known plethora of drug-drug interactions. MOF is likely to exacerbate the potential for, and consequences of, these drug-drug interactions, and further complicates the pharmacokinetic and pharmacodynamic approach to caring for these very sick patients. Additionally, the pharmacodynamic results of pharmacological treatment may themselves alter kinetics. For instance, vasopressors will cause blood flow redistribution and hypoperfusion of some tissues, and drugs given to increase cardiac output might improve renal elimination.

Clinical Implications, Therapeutic Drug Monitoring, and Population Kinetics

Listed in the preceding sections are many of the pharmacokinetic aberrations that might occur in various stages and combinations of organ failure. The degree to which any of these will alter the disposition of a particular drug in an individual patient will depend on the extent of organ failure, the clinical condition of the patient, and the clinical circumstances under which the drug is being administered. The fate of the drug under "normal" physiological conditions offers the greatest insight into the possible significance of specific pharmacokinetic insults, but even, for example, if a drug is normally cleared exclusively by renal elimination, concomitant hepatic and cardiac failure threaten to markedly alter its clearance even when renal function is normal.

With the possible exception of rapid-acting, short-lived drugs that can be quickly titrated to achieve the desired effect, virtually all dosing regimens are based directly or indirectly (empirically) on the pharmacokinetic characteristics of the agent being administered. This may often be transparent to the prescribing physician, but in the patient with organ failure pharmacokinetics become a very real consideration. In MOF, the pharmacokinetic consequences of single organ failure are likely to be additive and probably supra-additive, and pharmacokinetic parameters may change from day to day and even hour to hour.

The scenario is further complicated by the many pharmacodynamic changes that are also known to accompany organ failure (for example, see reference 33). Due to altered pharmacokinetics, a dose of drug given to produce a serum concentration of X may result in a concentration of 2X. After gaining an appreciation for the patient's pharmacokinetic state, the dose is adjusted and a concentration of X is achieved. However, due to pharmacodynamic sensitization, X is associated with toxicity and X/2 is the level actually required to achieve the desired effect.

Given the myriad of potential pharmacokinetic actions and interactions in MOF, one is tempted, in exasperation, to conclude that pharmacokinetic analysis in critically ill patients is too complex and intractable to be of any practical relevance. We disagree, for two reasons. First, pharmacodynamics can only occur as a consequence of pharmacokinetics. If for no other reason than to guide the initial dosing (therapeutic drug level monitoring would be expected to guide subsequent dosing; see below) of a particular drug, it is vital that the physician has some feel for the disposition of that drug in the patient population, if not the individual patient, being cared for. Second, although it is disease that is causing these pharmacokinetic aberrations, it is possible that quantitative analysis of pharmacokinetic changes would provide novel insight into the underlying pathologies. Thus, systematic serial appraisal of pharmacokinetic parameters may have diagnostic and prognostic value that has yet to be exploited.

Therapeutic drug level monitoring of total serum drug concentrations is now commonplace in many institutions (34). Most recent reviews of the pharmacologic management of the critically ill patient suggest that therapeutic drug level monitoring is a necessity to effect the optimal care of this population. Even when a satisfactory pharmacodynamic response is apparent, measurement of serum drug levels helps to ensure that pharmacodynamics are not occurring at the price of toxic concentrations; likewise, when a response is not apparent, such measurements ensure that theoretically therapeutic levels have indeed been achieved. However, plasma protein concentrations and binding characteristics are likely to be altered in MOF. This dictates that for drugs that are normally extensively protein-bound, it is free drug levels that should be monitored (35, 36); therapeutic ranges should be defined in terms of free rather than total serum concentration, since it is usually the free fraction that interacts with the effector substrate to produce the pharmacological effect. Inexpensive techniques for measuring the unbound concentration of a variety of drugs are slowly becoming widely available.

We submit that therapeutic drug level monitoring provides not only the data necessary to guide safe and effective drug dosing, but also offers the means to answer many scientific questions about the pharmacokinetics of MOF and critical illness. Starting with average pharmacokinetic parameters for a given drug, the data from several serial plasma concentration measurements can be used to characterize the pharmacokinetics (e.g., V_1 and k_{10}) of that drug in the individual patient through the mathematical technique of Bayesian estimation (37, 38). With each additional plasma level measurement, this process can be repeated throughout the course of the patient's treatment. In so doing, not only does the clinician know the current concentration of drug in the patient's blood, but if a change in plasma level is required, knowing the patient's actual kinetics allows the concentration to be adjusted most efficiently (39) (recalling, for example, that approximately three elimination half-lives are required for a constant infusion to achieve relatively steady levels). This approach has been realized by several groups (40-44). Moreover, the potential exists to construct a comprehensive picture of pharmacokinetics and pharmacodynamics in various disease states by creating a computerized database into which detailed data quantifying a patient's medical condition, drug therapy, therapeutic drug level measurements, and medical interventions are entered. Through the use of appropriate statistical techniques, including Bayesian estimation of pharmacokinetic parameters, innumerable questions could be addressed regarding dynamic changes in individual patients across time and as a function of various therapeutic modalities, population kinetics (45, 46) within well defined classes of patients, and the possible relationship between pharmacokinetics and outcome measures. Certainly, one explanation for the sparsity of pharmacokinetic data in MOF is a reluctance to perform research on critically ill patients; one of the attractions of the scheme that we propose is that no unusual or hazardous interventions are required to collect the desired data, as it is all gathered in the routine care of the patient. This would be a monumental undertaking, but one which offers great promise to yield exciting and useful results.

Despite the complexity, known and unknown, of pharmacokinetics in MOF, dosing practices based on clinical experience, generalized guidelines, an occasional plasma level measurement, and actual patient response are generally effective. Dosing recommendations for numerous drugs when given to patients with single organ failure have been established and published. Recent and comprehensive reviews of the pathophysiology and pharmacokinetics of renal failure, and dosing guidelines for patients with renal failure, are given by Anderson et al. (47) and Maher (18), and for hepatic failure by Wedlund and Branch (3). Dosing recommendations for patients with cardiac failure are given by Benowitz and Meister (5), and likewise by Watson (7) for patients in pulmonary failure.

Conclusion

Stanski and Watkins (48) have (under)stated that, "It is not possible to make generalizations about the effect of liver disease on drug pharmacokinetics." It is even more difficult to make generalizations about the pharmacokinetic implications of MOF. These patients are at great risk for a dangerous pharmacokinetic event and can seldom tolerate suboptimal pharmacologic management, yet the pharmacokinetics of MOF have been poorly studied! For many of the drugs utilized in the treatment of critically ill patients, the analytical, mathematical, and computational tools are presently available to facilitate rapid progress in this field. This research would result not only in better patient care, but probably also would yield new insight into the complex disease processes encompassing MOF.

References

1. Mann HJ, Fuhs DW, Cerra FB: Pharmacokinetics and pharmacodynamics in critically ill patients. *World J Surg* 1987; 11:210

2. Maher JF: Pharmacokinetics in patients with renal failure. *Clin Nephrol* 1984; 21:39

3. Wedlund PJ, Branch RA: Adjustment of medications in liver failure. *In:* The Pharmacologic Approach to the Critically Ill Patient. Chernow B, Lake CR (Eds). Baltimore, Williams & Wilkins Co, 1983, pp 84-114

4. Williams RL, Benet LZ: Drug pharmacokinetics in cardiac and hepatic disease. *Annu Rev Pharmacol Toxicol* 1980; 20:389

5. Benowitz NL, Meister W: Pharmacokinetics in patients with cardiac failure. *Clin Pharmacokinet* 1976; 1:389

6. Benet LZ, Greither A, Meister W: Gastrointestinal absorption of drugs in patients with cardiac failure. *In:* The Effect of Disease States on Pharmacokinetics. Washington, DC, American Pharmaceutical Association, 1976, pp 33-50

7. Watson CB: Adjustment of medications in pulmonary failure. *In:* The Pharmacologic Approach to the Critically Ill Patient. Chernow B, Lake CR (Eds). Baltimore, Williams & Wilkins Co, 1983, pp 115-132

8. Nimmo WS: Drugs, disease, and altered gastric emptying. *Clin Pharmacokinet* 1976; 1:189

9. Gibaldi M, Perrier D: Pharmacokinetics. Second Edition. New York, Marcel Dekker, 1982

10. Wartak J: Clinical Pharmacokinetics: A Modern Approach to Individualized Drug Therapy. New York, Praeger Publishers, 1983

11. Hug CC: Pharmacokinetics of drugs administered intravenously. *Anesth Analg* 1978; 57:704

12. Thompson WL: Pharmacodynamic and pharmacokinetic relationships for dosage optimization. *In:* Textbook of Critical Care. Shoemaker WC, Thompson WL, Holbrook PR (Eds). Philadelphia, WB Saunders Co, 1984, pp 833-866

13. Koch-Weser J, Sellers EM: Binding of drugs to serum albumin: Part 1. *N Engl J Med* 1976; 294:311

14. Koch-Weser J, Sellers EM: Binding of drugs to serum albumin: Part 2. *N Engl J Med* 1976; 294:526

15. Paxton JW: Elementary pharmacokinetics in clinical practice. 5: The effect of pathological condition on pharmacokinetics. *NZ Med J* 1982; 95:116

16. Kato R: Drug metabolism under pathological and abnormal physiological states in animals and man. *Xenobiotica* 1977; 7:25

17. Gonzalez G, Arancibia A, Rivas MI, et al: Pharmacokinetics of furosemide in patients with hepatic cirrhosis. *Eur J Clin Pharmacol* 1982; 22:315

18. Maher JF: Adjustment of medications in renal failure. *In:* The Pharmacologic Approach to the Critically Ill Patient. Chernow B, Lake CR (Eds). Baltimore, Williams & Wilkins Co, 1983, pp 65-83

19. Reidenberg MM, Drayer DE: Alteration of drug-protein binding in renal disease. *Clin Pharmacokinet* 1984; 9(Suppl 1):18

20. deSouich P, McLean AJ, Lalka D, et al: Pulmonary disease and drug kinetics. *Clin Pharmacokinet* 1978; 3:257

21. Brater DC: Pharmacokinetics. *In:* The Pharmacologic Approach to the Critically Ill Patient. Chernow B, Lake CR (Eds). Baltimore, Williams & Wilkins Co, 1983, pp 1-21

22. Gibaldi M, Levy G, Hayton WL: Tubocurarine and renal failure. *Br J Anaesth* 1972; 44:163

23. Rowland M: Protein binding and drug clearance. *Clin Pharmacokinet* 1984; 9(Suppl 1):10

24. Dunn GD, Hayes P, Breen KJ, et al: The liver in congestive heart failure: A review. *Am J Med Sci* 1973; 265:174

25. Camus P, Jeannin L: The diseased lung and drugs. *Arch Toxicol* 1984; 7:66

26. Vozeh S, Powell R, Riegelman S, et al: Changes in theophylline clearance during acute illness. *JAMA* 1978; 240:1882

27. Lee CC, Marbury TC: Drug therapy in patients undergoing hemodialysis: Clinical pharmacokinetic considerations. *Clin Pharmacokinet* 1984; 9:42

28. Holley FO, Ponganis KV, Stanski DR: Effect of cardiopulmonary bypass on the pharmacokinetics of drugs. *Clin Pharmacokinet* 1982; 7:234

29. Richard C, Berdeaux A, Delion F, et al: Effect of mechanical ventilation on hepatic drug pharmacokinetics. *Chest* 1986; 90:837

30. Krishnaswamy K: Drug metabolism and pharmacokinetics in malnutrition. *Clin Pharmacokinet* 1978; 3:216

31. Ross LH, Grant JP: Parenteral nutrition. *In:* The Pharmacologic Approach to the Critically Ill Patient. Chernow B, Lake CR (Eds). Baltimore, Williams & Wilkins Co, 1983, pp 728-756

32. Bidlack WR, Brown RC, Mohan C: Nutritional parameters that alter hepatic drug metabolism, conjugation, and toxicity. *Fed Proc* 1986; 45:142

33. Fabre J, Balant L: Renal failure, drug pharmacokinetics and drug action. *Clin Pharmacokinet* 1976; 1:99

34. Taylor WJ, Diers Caviness MH (Eds): A Textbook for the Clinical Application of Therapeutic Drug Monitoring. Irving, TX, Abbott Laboratories, 1986

35. Levy RH, Moreland TA: Rationale for monitoring free drug levels. *Clin Pharmacokinet* 1984; 9(Suppl 1):1

36. MacKichan JJ: Pharmacokinetic consequences of drug displacement from blood and tissue proteins. *Clin Pharmacokinet* 1984; 9(Suppl 1):32

37. Kelman AW, Whiting B, Bryson SM: OPT: A package of computer programs for parameter optimization in clinical pharmacokinetics. *Br J Clin Pharmacol* 1982; 14:247

38. Sheiner LB, Beal SL: Bayesian individualization: Simple implementation and comparison with non-Bayesian methods. *J Pharm Sci* 1982; 71:1344

39. Wagner JG: A safe method for rapidly achieving plasma concentration plateaus. *Clin Pharmacol Ther* 1974; 16:691

40. Jelliffe RW: Clinical application of pharmocokinetics and adaptive control. *IEEE Trans Biomed Eng* 1987; BME-34:624

41. Whiting B, Kelman AW, Bryson SM, et al: Clinical pharmacokinetics: A comprehensive system for therapeutic drug monitoring and prescribing. *Br Med J* 1984; 288:541

42. Gilman TM, Muir KT, Jung RC, et al: Estimation of theophylline clearance during intravenous aminophylline infusions. *J Pharm Sci* 1985; 74:508

43. Vozeh S, Muir KT, Sheiner LB, et al: Predicting individual phenytoin dosage. *J Pharmacokin Biopharm* 1981; 9:131

44. Vozeh S, Hillman R, Wandell M, et al: Computer-assisted drug assay interpretation based on Bayesian estimation of individual pharmacokinetics: Application to lidocaine. *Ther Drug Monit* 1985; 7:66

45. Whiting B, Kelman AW, Grevel J: Population pharmacokinetics: Theory and clinical application. *Clin Pharmacokinet* 1986; 11:387

46. Maitre PO, Vozeh S, Heykants J, et al: Population pharmacokinctics of alfentanil: The average dose-response plasma concentration relationship and interindividual variability in patients. *Anesthesiology* 1987; 66:3

47. Andersen RJ, Bennett WM, Gambertoglio JG, et al: Fate of drugs in renal failure. *In:* The Kidney. Second Edition. Brenner BM, Rector FC (Eds). Philadelphia, WB Saunders Co, 1981, pp 2659-2708

48. Stanski DR, Watkins WD: Drug Disposition in Anesthesia. New York, Grune and Stratton, 1982

Chapter 11

Acute Renal Failure

Alan S. Tonnesen, MD

Outline

Educational Objectives

In this chapter the reader will learn:

1. to understand current theories of the pathogenesis of ARF and their clinical implications.

2. to recognize groups of patients at high risk of developing ARF.

3. to be familiar with investigational means of preventing ARF.

4. to be familiar with indications for and complications of various management methods for patients with ARF.

Introduction

Acute renal failure (ARF) is a dreaded complication in critically ill patients, carrying high rates of morbidity and mortality. Management of the patient becomes significantly more complicated and expensive. In the setting of critical illness, acute tubular necrosis (ATN) is the most common cause of ARF. Hence, this review will concentrate most heavily on ATN and largely ignore other categories of ARF such as glomerulonephritis and papillary necrosis.

Little space will be devoted to pre-renal failure because this state represents the renal response to hemodynamic and fluid abnormalities and critical care physicians are intimately familiar with management of the latter. Second, conditions which lead to the pre-renal state will lead to parenchymal renal failure if allowed to persist. Third, identification of a condition as pre-renal may lead to a relaxation of pursuit of the underlying abnormality. Fourth, it is not possible to distinguish patients with irreversible renal failure from the pre-renal state with certainty until hours or days after dysfunction is identified. Fifth, if parenchymal damage has occurred, it is probably even more important that every effort should be made to limit further damage by continuous efforts to eliminate any pre-renal factors.

Most of our current concepts of the pathogenesis of ARF have been derived from animal models which are poor analogues of ARF as seen in the ICU population. The most popular model of ARF is clamping of the renal artery for 40 to 180 min with various interacting, prophylactic, or therapeutic modalities applied. Although no one doubts that total cessation of renal circulation will cause renal damage, the relevance of conclusions from this model to explaining how the non-hypotensive patient with an intact renal circulation develops ARF over a period of a few hours to a few days is open to question. Until more realistic models are developed, it is unlikely that we will make significant progress in reducing the incidence of ARF or shortening its course.

Finally, numerous reviews of ARF are available; thus, I have devoted disproportionately more space to newer concepts and raised questions for further research than to old and more established practices, without ignoring the latter.

Diagnosis

Definition

ARF is defined as a loss of renal function, occurring over a period of hours to days, in the presence of previously stable function. A common clinical categorization consists of pre-renal, intrinsic, or parenchymal, renal, and postrenal causes. Detection of postrenal causes is critical because therapy is radically different than for intrinsic disease. Discrimination of pre-renal from intrinsic renal causes is more difficult and, as discussed above, less useful. ARF should be considered in the framework of normal renal physiology. Although renal function is classically discussed in terms of filtration, reabsorption, and secretion, all three components are critically dependent on adequate renal blood flow. Of these, filtration is the sine qua non of renal function, and is the most important functional loss in ARF. Tubular dysfunction is an important component of ARF, and tubular damage is probably intimately related to maintenance of filtration failure after ARF is established.

Filtration Failure

Creatinine is considered to be the best available physiologic substrate for estimating the glomerular filtration rate (GFR). Most clinical studies of acute renal failure have utilized serum creatinine as a marker of GFR (1). This is true primarily because most studies of human ARF have been retrospective and more complete data are simply unavailable to the investigators. Use of creatinine concentration as an estimate of GFR is associated with several major problems: a) Creatinine is secreted as well as reabsorbed and the degree of secretion increases as the plasma level rises. Thus, the measurement of serum creatinine or creatinine clearance (Ccr) will overestimate GFR. b) The rate of creatinine production is roughly proportional to muscle mass (15 $mg \cdot kg^{-1} \cdot day^{-1}$ for women and 20 $mg \cdot kg^{-1} \cdot day^{-1}$ for men), with a gradual fall with age. Not only does muscle mass vary with age, sex (2), and physical conditioning, it falls rapidly in critically ill patients. Thus, the normal range of production is wide, and it changes rapidly in the ICU patient. c) Because the plasma level varies inversely with GFR and volume of distribution, and directly with muscle mass, rapid changes in GFR will not be reflected rapidly in the plasma creatinine level. Thus, if the plasma level is used to monitor GFR, the recognition of declining or improving renal function will be delayed (2, 3). d) Creatinine concentration is falsely elevated by the presence of noncreatinine chromogens such as ketones, flucytosine, and some cephalosporins (e.g., cephalothin, cefoxitin, ceforanide) when measured using spectrophotometric methods. e) Creatinine secretion is impaired by some drugs (e.g., cimetidine and trimethoprim-sulfamethoxazole) (4), leading to changes in creatinine when the GFR is unchanged.

Choice of a degree of loss of GFR for definition of significant renal dysfunction is somewhat arbitrary. A reduction in function which requires modification of diet or drug dosage would qualify for renal dysfunction, while a loss sufficient to result in acidosis, hyperkalemia, or fluid overload, despite a normal intake, would qualify for renal failure. Several drugs require dosage adjustment when the creatinine clearance falls below 40 ml/min (approximately 25 $ml \cdot m^{-2} \cdot min^{-1}$). This level of dysfunction also would narrow the range of potential compensation for variations in catabolism and intake of protein and electrolytes. When GFR falls to less than 15 ml/min (approximately 10 $ml \cdot m^{-2} \cdot min^{-1}$), ability to compensate is exhausted and any changes in intake or production result in abnormalities of extracellular fluid volume or composition and would qualify as a definition of renal failure. These GFR levels correspond to loss of 60% and 85% of a normal filtration rate, respectively. Table 1 shows the resulting equilibrium levels of creatinine for these levels of renal dysfunction given different normal creatinine levels. Of course, after the onset of renal dysfunction, but prior to establishment of equilibrium, lower creatinine values would be present. This broad range of normal and abnormal values seriously limits the diagnostic utility of the plasma creatinine level and argues strongly for monitoring of creatinine clearances as an estimate of GFR. Transient reductions in GFR may reverse with establishment of normal fluid volume status and hemodynamic parameters. In order to avoid classifying such fluctuations as cases of ARF, a duration parameter is usually included in the definition. A reasonable definition of filtration failure after adequate fluid and hemodynamic resuscitation might be: Ccr <10 ml$\cdot$m$^{-2}\cdot$min^{-1} for 2 days or more.

Table 1. Creatinine levels (mg/dl) following 60% or 85% loss of GFR

Normal Value	60% Loss	85% Loss
0.6	1.5	4.0
0.8	2.0	5.3
1.0	2.5	6.7
1.2	3.0	8.0

Tubular Abnormalities

Tubular Dysfunction

Filtration failure is virtually always accompanied by tubular dysfunction and damage. The latter is required to make a diagnosis of ATN, the most common form of ARF in critically ill patients. Tubular dysfunction is manifest by abnormalities in reabsorption and secretion, although the former have been better characterized (5). A number of tests based on abnormalities of tubular function aid in differentiating between oliguria due to pre-renal factors and that due to intrinsic renal damage. Reabsorption of Na and H_2O causes the concentration of creatinine in the tubular fluid to rise because it is not reabsorbed. When tubular functions are depressed, urinary creatinine concentration fails to increase normally and the ratio of urine to plasma concentration falls. The ability of the tubules to produce a concentrated medullary interstitium is impaired and results in an inability to concentrate or dilute the final urine. Impairment of Na reabsorption causes the proportion of filtered Na which is excreted to increase, i.e., the fractional excretion of Na (F_{ENa}) rises. Reabsorption of glucose, bicarbonate, and amino acids are impaired when proximal tubules are damaged, resulting in an increased excretion of these substances.

Tubular dysfunction can be defined as an inability to appropriately concentrate or dilute the urine, concentrate creatinine, or urea, and to reabsorb sodium. It is difficult to state specific values because they are clearly related to the balancing functions of the kidney. For example, if the plasma osmolality, plasma volume, and hemodynamic parameters are in the normal range, urine osmolality will be nearly isotonic and water clearance close to zero. If the plasma osmolality is high or low, the urine should be concentrated or dilute, respectively. If the reduction in GFR or urine flow rate is due to pre-renal factors, the sympathetic nervous system, the reninangiotensin-aldosterone systems, and antidiuretic hormone system will be activated and should lead to near-maximal sodium and water reabsorption. Typical values for urinary findings in ATN are shown in Table 2 (6).

Table 2. Urinary indices in oliguria

	Pre-Renal	Parenchymal Renal (Tubular dysfunction)
UNa (mEq/L)	<20	>40
FENa (%)	<1	>2
RFI	<1	>2
U/P creatinine ratio	>40	<20
U/P urea ratio	>8	<3
P urea/Pcr	>20	10
Uosm (% of plasma)	>120	80 to 120
CH_2O (ml/h)	<−15 >+15	−15 to +15
UChloride	<20	>20

U = urinary concentration, P = plasma concentration, FENa(%) = 100 × (UNa/PNa)/(Ucr/Pcr), RFI = renal failure index UNa/(Ucr/Pcr), CH_2O = clearance of water.

The FENa test and the related renal failure index are based on the presence of tubular dysfunction, and aid in classifying patients into pre-renal and intrinsic renal dysfunction (7, 8). With time it has been realized that the FENa test falls far short of its initial promise and that prognostication is not possible for an individual patient (9). FENa remains elevated during the first 1 to 2 wk of the diuretic phase, indicating persistent tubular dysfunction (10).

Tubular Damage

Evidence of tubular damage may be detected by examination of the urinary sediment and by the finding of abnormal cellular enzymes or basement membrane antigens in the urine.

When tubular damage is present, enzymes leak from the tubular epithelial cells into the tubular fluid and are excreted in increased amounts in the urine (11). Increased excretion of lactic dehydrogenase, 1-alanine-aminopeptidase, and ligandin have been observed (12). Beta-glucuronidase and N-acetyl-beta-D-glucosaminidase are lysozymal enzymes. Gamma-glutamyl-transpeptidase, leucine-amino-peptidase (LAP), and alkaline phosphatase (AP) are derived from the proximal tubular brush border. Healthy patients excrete very small quantities of these enzymes; increases in their absolute excretion rates, or excretion rate normalized for creatinine excretion, indicate tubular damage.

Beta-2 microglobulin (β_2MG) is a small protein which is normally removed from the filtrate by the proximal tubules and metabolized; thus, excretion is normally quite low (<500 ng/mg creatinine). Patients with ATN excrete increased amounts (13).

Adenosine deaminase binding protein (ABP) is an antigen derived from the basement membrane. Urinary ABP levels are elevated in acute pyelonephritis, during renal allograft rejection and pre-renal oliguria, and to very high levels in ATN (Table 3) (14). Currently, urinary enzyme, β_2MG, and ABP excretions are mostly of research interest.

Table 3. Frequency distribution of urinary ABP levels

Clinical Condition	Urinary ABP level (assay units)				
	<0.2	0.2-0.4	0.4-0.6	0.6-1.0	>1.0
Normal	100				
Glomerular	72.5	22.5	5		
Pre-renal		80.0	20		
ATN			6.3	29.1	64.6

Urinalysis

Examination of the urinary sediment gives useful information (Table 4). Tubular damage is accompanied by sloughing of tubular epithelial cells and formation of epithelial cellular and granular casts. White cells and white cell casts may be present. Tubular damage seen in cases of ATN is not associated with hematuria, red cell casts, or heavy proteinuria, all of which are associated with acute glomerular injury.

Scanning electron micrographs of the centrifuged urinary sediment from patients with ATN revealed ischemic changes in renal tubular epithelial cells. Patients without ATN displayed predominantly transitional epithelial cells or cells of extraurinary origin. The authors divided the sediments into three histologic grades: type I patients had a homogeneous population of severely damaged cells; type II patients had a homogeneous population of mildly damaged cells, and type III patients had a heterogeneous population of variably damaged cells. The outcome correlated with the histologic grading, with type I patients doing very poorly, type II doing well, and type III with an intermediate prognosis (Table 5) (15).

182

Table 4. Abnormalities observed in urinary sediment in acute kidney disease

Finding	ATN	Glomerulo-nephritis	Interstitial nephritis	Pyelo-nephritis
Red blood cells	0	+ + +	0	
Red cell casts	0	+ + +	0	0
White cells	0	0	+	+ + + +
White cell casts	0	+	+	+ + + +
Eosinophiluria	0	0	+	0
Epithelial cells	+		+	
Cellular casts	+ +	0	+ +	
Pigmented	+ +	+	0	0
Granular casts	+ + +	0	0	+
Protein	+	+ + +	+	+ +
Lipid	0	+ +	+	0
Crystals	0	0	0	0

0 indicates that the finding is generally absent. The plus signs indicate a semiquantitative estimate of the degree of abnormality likely to be seen. Blanks indicate an absence of good information.

Table 5. Correlation between scanning electron microscopic findings in urinary sediment and outcome

Clinical Finding	Sediment Type		
	I	II	III
Oliguria	100	12	50
Dialysis	88	13	50
Renal recovery	0	100	67
Survival	18	88	58

The figures represent the percent of patients with the given sediment type who manifest the clinical finding.

Thus, confirmation of ATN should be supported by a low urine/plasma creatinine ratio, a high F_{ENa}, a free water clearance near zero to document tubular dysfunction, and excretion of epithelial cells and cellular casts to indicate structural tubular injury. For research studies, excretion of tubular cellular enzymes or β_2MG add supportive evidence.

Urine Flow Rate

Cases of ARF are subclassified according to the amount of urine produced. This is partially a historical accident related to the fact that ARF was originally recognized by the presence of oliguria. It is now clear that many, if not most, cases of ARF are not oliguric. The classification retains its utility because non-oliguric patients have sustained a lesser insult and the prognosis is correspondingly better (16, 17).

It can be shown that the minimal urine output is related to maintenance of osmolar balance. Urinary osmoles consist mostly of electrolytes and urea. A healthy person consuming a normal diet is said to produce 12 $mOsm \cdot kg^{-1} \cdot day^{-1}$, or 0.5 $mOsm \cdot kg^{-1} \cdot h^{-1}$. Concentrated urine can excrete approximately 1 mOsm/ml, which is equivalent to a urine osmolality of 1,000 mOsm/kg H_2O. Thus, if urine is maximally concentrated, a urine output of 0.5 $ml \cdot kg^{-1}$ body weight $\cdot h^{-1}$ is necessary to maintain osmolar balance. If the urine osmolality is less than maximal, a higher urine output will be needed. In critically ill patients in one survey, the average excretion was 17 $mOsm \cdot kg^{-1} \cdot day^{-1}$, with a range from 10 to 40 $mOsm \cdot kg^{-1} \cdot day^{-1}$. Use of these figures would lead one to define oliguria as 840 to 1,176 ml/day, or less than 0.7 $ml \cdot kg^{-1} \cdot h^{-1}$, for a 70-kg person, but would have a very wide range of acceptable values. Most patients with a urine flow rate less than 0.5 to 0.7 $ml \cdot kg^{-1} \cdot h^{-1}$ will have a depressed GFR and should be considered at risk of developing ARF. Most clinical studies have defined oliguria as 400 ml/day or less (16), which would be equivalent to 0.24 $ml \cdot kg^{-1}$ body weight $\cdot h^{-1}$. Of all the definitions found in the renal failure literature, the use of 400 ml/day as the definition of oliguria is the most consistent. The physiologic or empiric rationale for this figure is weak. When this definition is used, however, the mortality rate for ARF with oliguria is nearly twice that for patients not having oliguria. Anuria is classically defined as a flow of less than 100 ml/day.

Classification

Thus, ARF secondary to ATN can be classified along three axes: filtration failure, tubular dysfunction, and urine output. This results in four subclasses of ARF as shown in Table 6. The utility of this classification remains to be demonstrated. The first two categories correspond to oliguric and nonoliguric ATN, respectively. The other categories are consistent with pre-renal dysfunction or glomerular injury. Rigorous application of this or similar classification to cases of ARF in critically ill patients should lead to a better understanding of the risk factors, pathogenesis, and prognosis than when all cases are lumped together. To facilitate such classification, monitoring of filtration by frequent, repetitive Ccr should be routine. When GFR appears to be falling, evidence of tubular and glomerular injury should be sought by measuring FeNa and water clearance, and by examining the urinary sediment.

Diagnostic Procedures

Application of more specific diagnostic tests follows initial evaluation and is designed to elucidate specific etiologies which have therapeutic implications unique to the etiology.

Renal uptake of technetium 99m dimercaptosuccinic acid, intravenous urography (18), CT scans, and retrograde pyelography have limited value in

184

Table 6. Filtration failure

Tubular injury present		Tubular injury absent	
Oliguric	Nonoliguric	Oliguric	Nonoliguric

evaluating ARF patients. Radionuclide flow scans are useful in documenting vascular patency in cases of suspected occlusion. Angiography is utilized when arterial or venous occlusion is suspected, and vascular repair is contemplated.

In ATN, dynamic CT scanning following injection of iothalamate produces a series of curves from selected areas of the kidney and the aorta. The density of cortical and medullary regions of the kidney are compared with each other and to the density of the aorta. In severe ATN, the cortical and medullary curves are indistinguishable. The reappearance of a differential density of the cortex and medulla predicted the onset of diuresis (19).

Ultrasonography is highly useful for eliminating urinary tract obstruction and assessing kidney size, which is reduced in chronic renal disease and may be increased with ATN (20).

Biopsy is reserved for cases with evidence of glomerular injury or interstitial nephritis and is rarely performed in critically ill patients who are far more likely to suffer from ATN.

Pathogenesis

The pathogenesis of ARF must be related to disruptions in normal physiology for maximal understanding of the disease. Filtration is the first and absolutely necessary process in excretion, and is the most important loss in ARF. Thus, a first approach to understanding ARF will be to review potential mechanisms whereby filtration may be reduced. The amount filtered is best described by the modified Starling equation:

$$GFR = Kf\,(Pgc - Pt) - R(COPgc - COPt)$$

where Kf is the ultrafiltration coefficient, Pgc is the glomerular capillary pressure, Pt is the proximal tubular pressure, and COPgc and COPt are the colloid osmotic pressure in the glomerular capillary and the proximal tubule, respectively.

A critical point in understanding the pathophysiology of ARF is that the events initiating the disease are not necessarily the same as those which maintain it.

Pathophysiology

A variety of physiologic disturbances could result in failure of filtration as shown in Table 7.

185

Table 7. Potential pathophysiologic mechanisms for reduced filtration

Reduced Kf
  Reduced permeability
    Endothelial damage
    Basement membrane
    Epithelial cell damage
  Reduced surface area
    Lost nephrons
    Occluded capillary bed
    Shunt channels

Reduced ultrafiltration pressure gradient
  Reduced glomerular capillary pressure
    Reduced MAP
    Increased afferent tone
    Decreased efferent tone
  Increased tubular pressure
    Tubular obstruction
    Intraluminal material
        Casts
        Cellular debris
    Luminal narrowing
        Tubular cell swelling
        Tubular compression
            Interstitial edema
            Extra-renal compression
            (tubular contraction)
      Extra-renal obstruction
      (increased tubular fluid viscosity)
  Increased glomerular plasma COP
    Increased arterial COP
    Reduced renal plasma flow
    Reduced MAP
    Increased renal venous pressure
    Increased RVR
        Contraction
  Interlobar, arcuate arteries
            Efferent arteriolar resistance
            Afferent arteriolar resistance
        Compression of lumen
            Endothelial edema
            Interstitial edema
            Extra-renal compression
        Intraluminal material
  Fibrin, WBC, platelet plugs
        Increased blood viscosity

Table 7. (Continued)

Increased reabsorption
    Tubular backleak
    Tubular transport
    Extra-renal backleak

MAP = mean arterial pressure.

Reduced Glomerular Ultrafiltration Coefficient

Glomeruli are usually reported to be normal or to have minimal abnormalities in animal models and human ARF (21), although this has been challenged (22). Solez (23) has reported that during the initiation phase of ARF the epithelial cell bodies and podocytes flatten and increase the degree of coverage of the glomerular capillary bed. This rapidly reverses with reperfusion and is not apparently important during the maintenance phase of ARF. Angiotensin-II (A-II) may induce similar changes in glomerular ultrastructure. Mannitol and clonidine blunt these changes in some animal models of ARF and provide some GFR protection (23). The Kf is generally found to be low, but this may be due to a reduction in the surface area available for filtration rather than a change in permeability. This could result either from preferential shunting of blood through short capillary loops or by contraction of the mesangium of the glomerulus, a phenomenon known to be caused by A-II and arginine vasopressin (AVP).

Reduced Glomerular Ultrafiltration Pressure Gradient

The net ultrafiltration pressure gradient is determined by the difference between the hydrostatic pressure gradient and the oncotic pressure gradient between the glomerular capillary and proximal tubule.

Reduced Glomerular Capillary Hydrostatic Pressure

A reduction in mean arterial pressure (MAP), renal blood flow (RBF) or an increase in the ratio of afferent/efferent arteriolar resistance will decrease hydrostatic pressure in the glomerular capillary bed.

Blood Flow

A reduction in RBF has been described in ARF even after full hemodynamic resuscitation. However, by use of volume loading and vasodilators, total RBF can be restored to normal without restoration of filtration. Thus, although a reduction in RBF may be crucial for induction of ARF, the maintenance phase is not critically dependent on global renal ischemia. Injection of radioactive xenon into the renal artery and analysis of the washout curve allows an estimate of RBF. The technique revealed a reduction in RBF to about one-third of normal, with absence of the early rapid washout component, indicating a reduction in cortical blood flow. These changes were independent of the etiology of ARF. Flow was only 10% of normal in patients with cortical necrosis. Patients with hepatorenal syndrome show severe reductions in mean blood flow, absence of a cortical component, and marked irregularity and instability of the washout curve, consistent with active, phasic vasoconstriction (24). RBF was reduced to about 60% of control in patients in shock, most due to sepsis. The low RBF was due almost entirely to hypotension, as renal vascular resistance (RVR) was not elevated. Infusion of low-molecular-weight dextran resulted in increases in MAP, CVP, RBF, cardiac output, and reductions in RVR and systemic vascular resistance (25). The deficit in RBF, as compared to normal, after volume expansion was due to the much lower MAP in the shock patients, not elevated RVR.

Vascular Occlusion

The site of ischemia during induction of ARF has recently been re-interpreted by Mason (26). During ischemia, superficial nephron cells swell, but rapidly return to normal after restoration of perfusion. Despite this, total renal function remains depressed. Therefore, the deeper nephrons must be nonfunctioning. This is consistent with the pathology observed in ischemic animal models of ARF. The outer medullary vasculature is congested with erythrocytes (27). By increasing renal perfusion pressure, medullary congestion is improved and renal function improves concomitantly. Mason believes that cell swelling during ischemia is responsible for extracting fluid from the extracellular and vascular space, thus obstructing blood flow with subsequent loss of plasma fluid, leaving behind the erythrocyte-rich blood congesting the vasculature. This hypothesis would explain the greater damage to the pars recta of the proximal tubule, not by any greater susceptibility to anoxia but to its position in an area in which blood flow is more markedly impaired for a longer period of time. Solez (23) also believes that vasa recta blood flow is impaired. He has noted accumulation of white blood cells in the vasa recta and believed that this was accompanied by endothelial damage to the vasa recta early in the initiation phase. The loss of deeper nephrons might also explain the early and nearly universal loss of concentrating ability in ischemic ARF. The therapeutic implications of this hypothesis do not suggest major changes from current practices. The more rapidly substrate delivery to the cells is restored, the more rapidly cell swelling will be reversed, the less necrosis will occur, and the more rapidly vascular congestion will be cleared. The congested vessels can be flushed out by raising perfusion pressure. Hyperosmotic solutions may aid in reducing cell swelling and cause hemodilution by volume expansion, which should reduce the tendency to sludging.

The impairment of perfusion of the deeper cortex and outer medulla also may result in damage to the thick ascending limb. The medullary thick ascending limb of Henle's loop has a high metabolic rate due to its high rate of Na reabsorption. During the initiation phase of ARF, proximal tubular dysfunction results in delivery of increased amounts of solute to Henle's loop. This increases pumping activity by the thick ascending limb, increasing its susceptibility to anoxia. Ischemic damage to the thick ascending limb is worse when renal perfusion is only impaired, as compared to totally occluded. This may occur because the thick ascending limb of the nonfiltering kidney is not reabsorbing Na, and thus has a lower metabolic rate and is less susceptible to anoxia. Inhibition of electrolyte transport by ouabain or furosemide can protect against ischemic injury to the thick ascending limb, providing support for this hypothesis. Similarly, amphotericin B increases membrane permeability to Na. The rise in intracellular Na stimulates the sodium pump and metabolic rate, and thus mimics an ischemic injury. Selective damage of the thick ascending limb produces a concentrating defect prior to the onset of ARF. Defective reabsorption at this site and in the proximal tubule will release renin, activate the tubulo-glomerular feedback loop, and result in a reduced glomerular plasma flow and GFR (28).

Mediators of Vasoconstriction

Vasoconstriction may play a role in reducing RBF, especially during the initiation phase of ARF. Maintenance, or rapid restoration, of RBF is probably important in preventing or minimizing renal damage and reduction in GFR. Vasoconstrictor candidates include catecholamines, AVP, A-II, TBX, a deficiency of the renal vasodilator prostaglandins, or atrial natriuretic factor (atriopeptin or ANF).

Angiotensin-II

Many clinical situations associated with ARF (e.g., shock, hypovolemia) would be expected to cause renin release. It also has been postulated that dysfunction of the proximal tubules allows delivery of an excessive amount of solute to the juxtaglomerular apparatus, stimulating renin release and subsequent generation of A-II (28, 29). A great deal of research into the role of A-II as a mediator of the constriction has failed to reveal a consistent role. In addition, vasoconstriction in ARF, demonstrated by angiography, primarily affects the arcuate and segmental arteries, but A-II fails to constrict these vessels (23), which are more likely to be constricted by catecholamines or vasopressin. Interpretation of these findings is confused by the fact that the major damage in both human and animal models occurs in the inner cortex and outer medulla, not in the superficial cortex. A-II preferentially increases efferent arteriolar resistance. This leads to a fall in RBF, but a rise in filtration fraction. Thus, the blood leaving glomeruli would have higher concentrations of protein and cells, increasing viscosity.

Prostaglandins

Prostaglandins in the kidney are predominantly vasodilators and play little role in regulation of the vasculature under normal circumstances. When vasoconstrictor agents are activated, prostaglandins are released and blunt the resulting rise in resistance. Inhibition of prostaglandin synthesis potentiates a variety of renal insults. Infusion of PGE_2, a vasodilating prostaglandin, following 180 min of renal artery clamping (RAC) quickly restored RBF to near-normal levels and the decrement in GFR was halved (30). Conversely, thromboxane, a vasoconstrictor, is produced by the kidney and stimulates platelet aggregation. After RAC or glycerol injection, thromboxane rises rapidly. Inhibition of thromboxane synthesis protected against RAC-induced and glycerol-induced ARF, but prostaglandin synthesis inhibition combined with inhibition of thromboxane synthesis was not protective. These findings led to the conclusion that maintenance of a high ratio of vasodilator prostaglandins to thromboxane was important in maintaining RBF after ischemic insults (31). A protective effect of thromboxane synthesis inhibition is not always seen (32-34).

Alpha-Adrenergic Stimulation

Alpha-adrenergic stimulation causes vasoconstriction and reduced RBF. Blockade of these receptors results in improved renal perfusion and can be protective against renal failure in models utilizing norepinephrine infusion to induce renal ischemia. In theory, blockade of these receptors coupled with maintenance of MAP could result in better maintenance of RBF. During the maintenance phase, alpha-receptor stimulation appears to play little role.

Vasopressin

Vasopressin is a potent vasoconstrictor, but its role in inducing ARF has not been well studied. Animals deficient in AVP are susceptible to ARF in a variety of ischemic models.

Dopamine, Bradykinin, Acetylcholine, Atrial Natriuretic Factor

These agents all have the potential for causing renal vasodilation. The possibility that deficiencies of these agents could result in enhanced ischemia during the initiation phase has not been well studied to date. Their use after establishment of ARF appears to have little effect.

Tubular Backleak

The pathologic picture, especially in animal models, reveals extensive tubular necrosis with denudation of the basement membrane. This, coupled with the apparently normal glomeruli, suggests that filtrate may be formed and then leak back through the damaged tubules to be reabsorbed into the circulation. This mechanism would be applicable only during maintenance of ARF, not initiation. Studies in most animal models have not revealed a quantitatively important amount of backleak (35). In human, nonoliguric renal failure, the clearance of dextran molecules, which are not secreted, exceeds unity. This could be explained by backleak of inulin molecules, which are smaller than the dextrans, through damaged tubules. Calculations revealed that 44% of the filtrate was reabsorbed (36). While this may be true, the GFR in these patients was depressed to an average of 5.0 ml·min^{-1}·1.73 m^{-2}. Even if no backleak had occurred, GFR still would have been depressed by 90%. Thus, the quantitative contribution of backleak to the reduction of GFR was minimal.

Tubular Obstruction

The sequence of events in ARF of a variety of causes may be explained on the basis of obstruction of tubules. Cellular anoxia or toxins may cause dysfunction of membrane Na pumps. Swelling and death of the tubular cells, usually proximal tubular in origin, results. The susceptibility of the proximal tubular cells is related to their high metabolic rate and the exposure of these cells to any filtered toxin. The cellular swelling and subsequent sloughing of necrotic debris causes obstruction, resulting in elevation of the proximal tubular pressure which causes slowing and finally cessation of filtration. In addition, interstitial edema or extrinsic compression could lead to obstruction.

In opposition to this view, most authors have stated that there is a lack of correlation between the histologic damage and the degree of dysfunction. Solez (23) has critically reviewed the literature dealing with the pathology of AFR in humans and animal models, and concluded that there is a strong correlation between the degree of tubular necrosis and the degree of functional impairment. He also mustered evidence correlating the degree of tubular obstruction, initially by cellular debris and later by casts, and the severity of failure. The hallmarks of ATN include injured and necrotic proximal tubular cells, casts, interstitial edema, and accumulation of WBCs in the vasa recta. He believed that this was accompanied by endothelial damage to the vasa recta early in the initiation phase. Sluggish blood flow in this area would impair oxygenation of the pars recta of many proximal tubules as well as the thick ascending limbs. Tubular dilation due to obstruction may impinge on the peritubular capillaries leading to vascular congestion. He postulated that the initial phase of ischemia leads to sloughing of the brush border of the proximal tubular cells, followed by impaction of the sloughed vesicles in Henle's loop. This blocks flow to the thick ascending limb where casts are formed. The vesicles formed by sloughed brush border membranes lyse within several hours, but the casts, which have formed in the interim, maintain the obstruction. This secondary obstruction will persist until urinary proteolytic enzymes digest the casts or the intratubular pressure rises to a level sufficient to dislodge the casts. Micropuncture studies revealed that injection of fluid into the proximal tubules caused very high pressures. Continued injection resulted in a reduction of high pressures and a flushing of debris from the tubule with restoration of filtration in that nephron. When the proximal tubule of a nonfiltering nephron was punctured and tubular fluid vented, filtration resumed, lending further support to the role of tubular obstruction in maintaining ARF.

After renal ischemia in animal models, the surface nephrons vary greatly in their measured filtration rate. Some nephrons, with high tubular pressures, manifest dysfunction due to obstruction, while others, with low tubular pressures, malfunction due to glomerular dysfunction (35).

Mechanisms of Ischemic Damage

Loss of ATP

Renal O_2 consumption ($\dot{V}O_2$) is directly related to sodium reabsorption and, thus, to GFR which determines the filtered load of sodium. When blood flow to the proximal tubule or thick ascending limb is impaired significantly, ATP levels fall, followed by impaired pumping by the Na-K-ATPase membrane pump. Procedures which replace ATP (37) or improve RBF support cellular energy stores and protect against functional and histologic changes of ARF (37-41).

Calcium

The role of Ca in cell dysfunction and death has received considerable attention. This was prompted by recognition of the deposition of intracellular Ca in necrotic tissue. Ca is distributed in a pool bound to plasma membranes (10% to 20%), a pool within intracellular organelles, and a cytosolic pool. Sixty percent to 70% of the organelle pool is within the mitochondria, and 10% to 20% in the endoplasmic reticulum. Free cytosolic Ca ranges between 0.05 and 0.50 mM. The total Ga concentration is over 100 times higher due to binding to soluble proteins, phosphate, and citrate. The mitochondria serve to protect against rising free cytosolic intracellular Ca. Ca activates membrane phospholipases and directly changes membrane permeability. The increase in tissue Ca during cell injury is predominantly due to increases in mitochondrial Ca accumulation. Most of this increase occurs after reperfusion. Verapamil is not protective against RAC, but does protect against norepinephrine-induced ARF, probably by blunting vasoconstriction. Lack of protection is probably related to the presence of abundant intracellular Ca stores. In toxic models of ARF, Ca accumulation occurs late in the course of ARF. In fact, CA loading protects against aminoglycoside toxicity. Humes (42) believes that Ca overload is not an early mediator of ARF and that its role in ischemic ARF is unclear.

Risk Factors of ARF

The incidence of ARF is estimated to be between 0.1% and 4.9% (43) of hospitalized patients (44). Identification of factors which are associated with an increased risk of ARF would serve several purposes. Risk factors may be related to the pathogenesis of ARF and may thus give clues for new avenues of investigation into both etiology and protection. ARF is a relatively uncommon event, even in critically ill patients, and would necessitate enrollment of numerous patients in any prospective clinical trial. Such prospective studies of ARF could include fewer patients if the high-risk group alone could be studied. Risk factors have utility only if they clearly precede the onset of a reduction in GFR. Surprisingly, few data are available to define these risk factors. A list of potential and reported risk factors for ARF is presented in Table 8.

Table 8. Potential risk factors for ARF

Chronic disease states
    Advanced age
    Hypertension
    Diabetes mellitus
    Renal disease
    Hyperuricemia
    Generalized vascular disease

Acute disease states
    Sepsis syndrome
    Jaundice
    Liver dysfunction
    Muscle injury
    Hemolytic transfusion reaction
    Disseminated intravascular coagulation
    Increased abdominal pressure
    Renal trauma
    Soft tissue injury
    Soft tissue ischemia
    Thermal burn
    Electric burn

Physiologic or metabolic abnormalities
    Advanced age
    Tachycardia
    Hypotension
    Elevated CVP
    Reduced RPP
    Hemodynamic profile abnormalities
        Low or high CI
        High or low O_2 extraction
        High or low $\dot{V}o_2$
        High or low systemic vascular resistance index

Table 8. (Continued)

Oliguria or polyuria
Free water clearance
Uosm, U/P osm ratio
Osmolar excretion
Fractional excretion of potassium
F_{ENa}
Positive fluid balance
Edema
Protein intake
Hyperuricemia

Chronic drug therapy

Nonsteroidal anti-inflammatory drugs
Diuretics

Acute drug therapy

ATN
Aminoglycosides
Amphotericin
Cephalosporins
Diuretics
Radiocontrast agent
Rifampin
Lithium
Cisplatin
Mithramycin
Acute interstitial nephritis
Penicillin
Sulfonamides
Rifampin
Cephalosporins
Furosemide
Thiazides
Nonsteroidal anti-inflammatory drugs
Triamterene
Cimetidine

Procedures

Aortic/renal artery clamp, renal vascular interruption
Transfusion
Intracranial
Intrathoracic
Intra-abdominal
Major orthopedic (pelvis, femur, lumbar or thoracic spine, tibia)
Somatic soft tissue
Peripheral

In war casualties, risk factors were considered to be massive muscle injury, visceral trauma, shock, severe sepsis, and hypoxia (Table 9). Sixty of 1147 (5.2%) severely injured patients developed ARF. Injuries of more than one site were associated with a significantly increased risk of ARF: 3.2% with a single major injury, compared with 18% of those with more than one major injury. Oliguria occurred in 25.9% of multiply injured and 13.8% of single-injury ARF patients. Isolated injuries to the face, scalp, noncervical spine, shoulder, axilla, hand, foot, pelvis, abdominal wall, back, or perineum were considered noncritical. Injuries to the abdomen, thigh or leg, head, or cervical spine were considered critical injuries. The incidence of ARF was related to the presence of these critical injuries, especially intra-abdominal injury. Sixty percent of the abdominal injury patients suffering ARF were septic, and 30% were in shock (45).

Table 9. War injuries

Site of Injury	Incidence of ARF (%)
Single noncritical injury	0.8
Single critical injury	6.7
Head or cervical spine	4.5
Thigh or leg injury	4.6
Major abdominal injury	35.6
Multiple noncritical injuries	14.3
Single critical plus noncritical injury	16.9
Two critical injuries	39.1
Head or cervical spine plus another	26.5
Thigh or leg plus another	21.7
Abdominal plus another	29.3

Obstructive jaundice is associated with a significant risk of postoperative ARF (16% to 18%) (46, 47). Cardiac and vascular surgery are generally considered to represent high-risk situations (48, 49). Plasma fibronectin deficiency was more common in patients who developed multiple organ failure after operation for intra-abdominal infection (50).

Physiologic Abnormalities

Certain physiologic abnormalities may be related to ARF. Ischemic ARF should be related to a reduction in delivery of critical metabolic substrates such as O_2 to the kidney in relation to their consumption by the kidney. Renal O_2 delivery is dependent on RBF and arterial O_2 content. The latter is primarily determined by Hgb concentration and P_{O_2}. The primary determinant of renal $\dot{V}_{O_2}$ is sodium reabsorption. Thus, the higher the GFR and the lower the FE_{Na}, the higher $\dot{V}O_2$ will be. RBF is determined by renal perfusion pressure (RPP) divided by RVR. RPP is determined by MAP and renal venous pressure. Although clinical measurement of renal venous pressure is not often performed, it must be higher than CVP. Thus, RPP may be estimated as being less than MAP minus CVP. Thus, hypotension (44), elevated CVP, and reduced RPP may be risk factors. RVR is known to be influenced by sympathetic nervous system (SNS) activation, A-II, prostaglandins, ANF, and vasopressin. Activation of the SNS produces some readily observable physical signs: sweating, tachycardia, and peripheral vasoconstriction manifest by cool skin. A-II produces vaso-constriction, release of aldosterone which results in hypokalemia, decreased urinary sodium loss, and thirst. Renal prostaglandins are predominantly vasodilators and protect against excessive vasoconstriction. They do not produce any readily observable signs, but inhibition of production by nonsteroidal anti-inflammatory drugs potentiates many forms of ARF. ANF causes relaxation of preconstricted arteries, especially if produced by A-II, and natriuresis and diuresis. Suppression of ANF by hypovolemia (44) would be associated with a fall in urine and sodium output. In addition to causing vasoconstriction, vas-opressin causes urine flow rate to fall, urinary concentration to increase, and a negative free water clearance.

The SNS, renin-angiotensin and vasopressin systems are activated by numerous hemodynamic aberrations including hypovolemia, hypotension, car-diac failure, low cardiac index (CI), hypercarbia, and evidence of low perfusion such as an increased O_2 extraction ratio (O_2 Extr) and low $\dot{V}O_2$ and high sys-temic vascular resistance index (SVRI). Sepsis is also associated with develop-ment of ARF and multiple organ failure. Sepsis causes a marked fall in SVRI and O_2 Extr with an increase in CI and either low or high $\dot{V}O_2$.

Hypokalemia, high protein intake (51, 52), and hypophosphatemia have been associated with impaired resistance to various models of ARF. High protein intake is associated with an increase in thromboxane production and arteriolar resistance following release of ureteral obstruction (51).

Chronic Disease States

Hypertension (44) is associated with chronic vascular disease and causes a shift of the autoregulatory range to higher values. Diabetes mellitus (53) causes chronic renal insufficiency and generalized vascular disease. While smoking has not been associated with ARF, it has been associated with cardiac and vascular disease and may be a potential risk factor.

Chronic Drug Therapy

Chronic use of diuretics is associated with a variety of abnormalities which may predispose to ARF including hypovolemia, activation of the renin-angioten-sin axis, hypokalemia, and reduced RBF, as well as hypertension. Nonsteroidal anti-inflammatory drugs were discussed above.

Acute Drug Therapy

Certain drugs may cause tubular necrosis in uniquely susceptible patients or in toxic doses. They may be considered risk factors because of the variable expression of their toxicity or because they may potentiate the effects of other injurious factors such as sepsis (1, 54) or ischemia. For example, aminoglycoside toxicity (55, 56) is enhanced by concurrent administration of other nephrotoxins, diuretics, cephalosporins, volume depletion, and potassium depletion (4, 44, 57).

One might predict that the incidence of ARF would be higher in patients housed in ICUs, but this has received little attention. In one study of all patients with ARF, 63% were in ICUs, but it is not entirely clear that ARF began in critically ill patients in ICUs or whether these patients were placed in an ICU because of renal failure (58).

Etiologies of ARF

Ideally, the risk factors for, and etiology of, ARF should be related to the theories regarding pathogenesis which in turn should be soundly based in renal physiology. In ARF, this chain of understanding has been only partially constructed. Parenchymal, or intrinsic, ARF may be caused by anoxia, toxic chemicas, metabolic abnormalities, immunologic disorders, infiltration of parenchyma, and acute infection (Tables 10-16). In many cases, the etiology is multifactorial and one abnormality potentiates the effects of another. Among patients cared for by the critical care physician, however, the majority of cases will be related to renal anoxia, toxic chemicals, and metabolic factors. Postrenal causes must always be considered (59).

Parenchymal Renal Failure

Anoxia

Hypotension per se can reduce RBF sufficiently to halt filtration, but rarely results in ARF unless accompanied by significant soft tissue damage or infection. Hypotension also stimulates the SNS, renin release, and vasopressin release, which further reduce blood flow. Hypotension is a potent contributor to the production of ARF in conjunction with a variety of other renal insults.

Acute renal arterial occlusion may result from thrombosis, arterial trauma, as a manifestation of a generalized arteritis, or an embolism of atheromatous material, especially during aortic surgery.

Sepsis is believed to be associated with multiple organ failure and ARF. This correlation with ARF has not been explored fully in clinical or experimental studies. RBF has been reported to fall in septic patients (25), to fall after endotoxin administration (60), to fall with a lethal dose of endotoxin (61-64), not change (65, 66), or to rise (61, 67). RVR may fall (25, 64, 67), not change (65), or rise (60, 62). GFR has generally been reported to fall (63, 65, 68), or rise transiently followed by a fall (68). Urine flow rate may increase (54) or decrease (68), but urine concentration has been reported to fall (54). The explanation of these differences remains to be elucidated. One factor which requires better control in such studies is RPP. There is a suggestion in current data that RVR falls during endotoxin challenge and in septic patients, and that RBF then is dependent on MAP. There seem to be differences in renal response depending on the dosage (lethal vs. sublethal) of endotoxin and the method of administration (bolus vs. infusion) in addition to well recognized species differences in general response to endotoxin. Furthermore, the renal response may be biphasic. The results then depend on the stage at which studies are performed.

196

Table 10. Etiologic classification of ARF

Parenchymal Renal Failure

Anoxic

Toxic

Metabolic

Immune

Infiltrative

Infectious

Postrenal Failure

Obstruction

Disruption

Table 11. Anoxic causes of ARF

Hypotension

Renal arterial occlusion

Renal vasospasm

Shock

Hepatorenal failure

Endotoxin

Malignant hypertension

Renal venous occlusion

Thrombosis

Elevated intra-abdominal pressure

Intravascular coagulation

Hemolytic-uremic syndrome

Disseminated intravascular coagulation

Table 12. Toxic causes of ARF

Therapeutic
- Acetaminophen
- Allopurinol
- Aminoglycosides
- Amphotericin
- Cancer chemotherapeutic agents
- Cephalosporins
- EDTA
- Hydralazine
- Lithium
- Mannitol
- Methoxyflurane
- Penicillamine
- Probenecid
- Procainamide
- Propylthiouracil
- Radiocontrast
- Rifampin
- Sulfonamides
- Thiazides
- Vitamin D intoxication

Nonmedicinal
- CCl_4
- Ethylene glycol
- Heroin
- $HgCl_2$
- Metals
- Methanol
- Organophosphates
- Toluene
- Uranyl nitrate

Table 13. Metabolic causes of ARF

Hypercalcemia

Hypokalemia

Hyperuricemia

Pigmenturia

   Bilirubin

   Myoglobin

   Hemoglobin

Hyperphosphatemia

Elevated COP

Table 14. Immune causes of ARF

Acute allergic interstitial nephritis

   Acetaminophen

   Aspirin

   Methicillin

   Penicillin G

   Phenacetin

   Rifampin

   Cimetidine

   Furosemide

   Captopril

Glomerulonephritis

Systemic disease with renal involvement

Table 15. Other causes of ARF

Infiltrative Causes of ARF

   Amyloidosis

   Malignancy

Infectious Causes of ARF

   Pyelonephritis

   Endotoxemia

Table 16. Postrenal causes of ARF

    Obstruction

        Urethral obstruction

        Bladder neck obstruction

        Bilateral ureteral obstruction

        Stones, clots, tumor, papillary necrosis, retroperitoneal fibrosis, surgical ligation

    Disruption

        Bladder rupture

        Ureteral or renal pelvic trauma

Additional renal actions have be attributed to endotoxin. Endotoxin may cause sequestration of leukocytes in peritubular capillaries with stasis of erythrocytes (62, 69). In addition, endothelial lesions appear, resulting in peritubular capillary disruption (69). Endotoxin markedly potentiated the effect of 25 min of RAC in rats without affecting BP or RBF (66). The latter conforms to the suspicions of many clinicians that even brief hypotensive episodes in toxic patients may result in rapid loss of renal function, while prolonged hypotension is often well tolerated by the kidney of nonseptic patients. Bacteremia may potentiate the nephrotoxicity of aminoglycoside antibiotics (70).

The mechanism of the changes induced by endotoxin are equally unclear. The effects may be the result of direct actions of endotoxin, or endotoxin may stimulate other physiologic systems directly (e.g., sympathetic, prostaglandins, renin-angiotensin systems) or indirectly as a result of other vascular actions (e.g., hypotension). Many of the effects of endotoxin can be reproduced by infusion of cachectin, an endogenous mediator of inflammation. Cachectin has major vascular actions promoting vasoconstriction of many vascular beds and damaging the endothelium (71). Its role in ARF will undoubtedly receive attention in the future.

Hepatorenal syndrome (HRS) is generally defined as oliguria, rising serum creatinine, low urine Na and F_{ENa}, and a bland urinalysis in a patient with established liver disease, most commonly cirrhosis. The prognosis is uniformly bad and depends primarily upon the reversibility of the hepatic lesion. The evidence of intact tubular function, without evidence of casts, suggests a functional lesion. Pathological examination often fails to reveal anatomic lesions in the glomeruli, vessels, or tubules. Others have reported that classical ATN changes are found in cases of HRS. In addition to the usual finding of tubular cellular necrosis, large leucine crystals and bile-stained casts surrounded by polymorphonuclear leukocytes have been observed. The JG apparatus was hypertrophied, and proximal convoluted tubule cells contained coarse vacuoles of bile in the cytoplasm. There was marked heterogeneity of cellular morphology even within a single nephron (23). Further evidence for the presence of tubular damage is provided by the finding of enzymuria in cirrhotic patients with HRS (Table 17). Cirrhosis with ATN (C + ATN) was differentiated from HRS alone by the presence of elevated β_2MG excretion in the former group. There were no differences in enzyme excretion between the patients with cirrhosis and ATN and those with ATN alone. For each of the enzymes, excretion was higher in the patients with cirrhosis and ATN or ATN alone than among the HRS patients (13). Unfortunately, data were not analyzed in relation to the degree of depression of GFR or urinary output, nor to the outcome of the renal failure.

Table 17. Significance of elevations in enzyme excretion as compared to control patients

Group	GGT	F_{EGGT}	LAP	F_{ELAP}	AP	F_{EAP}	β-Glu	F_{EGlu}
HRS		*	*	*	*	*		*
C + ATN	*	*	*	*	*	*	*	*
ATN	*	*	*	*	*	*	*	*

*Represents a statistically significant elevation of the enzyme excretion as compared to the normal patients.
C + ATN = cirrhosis coincident with ATN, GGT = gamma-glutamyl-transpeptidase, F_{EGGT} = fractional excretion of gamma-glutamyl-transpeptidase, F_{ELAP} = fractional excretion of leucine-amino-peptidase, F_{EAP} = fractional excretion of aminopeptidase, β-Glu = Beta-glucuronidase, and F_{EGlu} = fractional excretion of β-Glu.

Evidence for renal vasospasm is present on analysis of washout curves of radioactive xenon injected into the renal artery and on renal arteriograms (24). The most dramatic demonstration of the reversibility of the lesion was the successful function of kidneys transplanted from patients with HRS into anephric patients (72).

Despite the apparent functional nature of the lesion, efforts to unravel the pathophysiology (73) of the dysfunction and to design effective management strategies have met with limited success. The potential contributing factors include functional hypovolemia, maldistribution of RBF, relative hypotension, inability of the diseased liver to either produce or remove a critical substance (e.g., aldosterone, false neurotransmitters), elevated intra-abdominal pressure, or chronic endotoxemia. The relative hypovolemia may result from hypoalbuminemia and vasodilation with splanchnic and peripheral venous pooling. The endotoxemia may result from collaterals which drain the GI tract without passing through the reticuloendothelial system of the liver, and to the absence of bile salts (74). The aldosterone levels do not correlate with the degree of Na retention (75-79). Patients with HRS have reduced blood volumes, increased intra-abdominal pressure, and decreased plasma renin substrate concentration. Correction of these resulted in improved renal function. Infusion of stored and fresh frozen plasma (FFP) each led to improvements of renal plasma flow and GFR, although the latter improved more after FFP. Filtration fraction fell after stored plasma, rose after FFP, and rose markedly after A-II infusion. A reduction in intraperitoneal pressure by a 2-L paracentesis resulted in improved para-aminohippurate clearance, and Ccr. Placement of a peritoneo-venous shunt resulted in sustained improvement in para-aminohippurate clearance and Ccr (80). It appears that hypovolemia and increased intra-abdominal pressure contribute to HRS in at least some patients.

Increased intra-abdominal pressure has been associated with impending ARF (81). Although the mechanism has not been completely clarified, elevation of renal venous pressure or direct renal compression seem the most likely. Elevated pressures may be seen with tense ascites or postoperatively, and renal function responds to measures which reduce the tension (80-83).

Toxic

The list of drugs and nontherapeutic chemicals associated with ARF is impressive, but for many the association is not proven or the mechanism is poorly understood. A few examples with relevance to critical care physicians are discussed, and readers are referred to more extensive reviews (84).

Aminoglycosides accumulate in the proximal tubules, causing necrosis (56, 85). The accumulation is probably an active process which occurs predominantly from the luminal border. The drug accumulates progressively because the tissue half-life is very long (100 h) in relation to the plasma half-life (2 to 4 h) and dosing interval (6 to 12 h). There is controversy regarding the role of ultrastructural changes in the glomerular endothelial cells. A reduction in the size and number of endothelial fenestrae (86, 87) may result from prolonged fixation times and thus, not by aminoglycosides themselves (21, 23). The toxicity may be potentiated by hypokalemia (55, 57), Gram-negative bacteremia (70), volume depletion, magnesium depletion, increased frequency of dosage, and in males (55). Protection is afforded by saline-loading, blockade of the renin-angiotensin system, castration of males, and hypercalciuria produced by dietary calcium loading (55). Gentamicin toxicity in females may often result from interstitial nephritis rather than tubular necrosis (23).

Nonsteroidal anti-inflammatory drugs inhibit the production of prostaglandins that in the kidney are predominantly vasodilators which are released in states characterized by renal vasoconstriction (88-91). Thus, nonsteroidal anti-inflammatory drugs lead to unimpeded vasoconstriction and have been associated with the production of ARF or potentiation of ARF caused by other factors (92).

Captopril, an angiotensin-converting enzyme inhibitor, has been associated with ARF. Most of these cases have occurred in patients with renal arterial stenosis, and reversed when captopril was withdrawn. In patients with arterial stenosis, GFR is dependent on an increase filtration fraction caused by an increase in efferent tone secondary to A-II stimulation. It is believed that a reduction in efferent arteriolar tone due to a lack of A-II leads to a reduction in glomerular ultrafiltration pressure (93).

ARF may follow oral, intravenous, intra-arterial, or transhepatic injection of a variety of contrast agents (94, 95). Risk factors include pre-existing renal disease, diabetes mellitus, type of study (53), volume of contrast injected, heart disease, and perhaps dehydration (96). When creatinine clearance is measured, a significant reduction in clearance is more likely to be found than when serum creatinine is used to identify cases (97). Mannitol infusion may be protective (98), but intentional hydration does not have a major protective effect (96, 99).

Injection of radiocontrast media causes osmotic nephrosis, transient albuminuria, and increased excretion of β_2MG, lactate dehydrogenase, N-acetyp-beta-D-glucosaminidase, alanine-aminopeptidase, LAP, AP, alpha-glucosidase, and gamma-GT (98), indicating tubular injury. Early albuminuria may correlate with later evidence of renal dysfunction. Oliguria occurs in only about 10% of these cases. The hyperosmolality of these agents leads to an osmotic diuresis which may cause hypovolemic hypotension (100). This is important because contrast agents appear to potentiate renal damage caused by renal ischemia (101).

Metabolic

Myoglobinuria due to rhabdomyolysis has been associated with alcohol intoxication, heroin and phencyclidine abuse (102), and viral pneumonia (103), as well as muscle ischemia and severe exertion, especially with hyperthermia (heat stroke), seizures, carbon monoxide poisoning, hypokalemia, hypophosphatemia, head injury (104), methanol poisoning (105), improper intraoperative positioning (106), succinylcholine administration, meningitis, and electrical burns. Rhabdomyolysis has been suggested as a cause of ARF in sickle cell disease (107).

Myoglobinuria results from rhabdomyolysis and is associated with a rise in creatine phosphokinase and lactate dehydrogenase, in a ratio of about 10:1 (108). Patients with myoglobinuria are at risk for ARF, although the exact mechanism is unclear as myoglobin itself is not a potent nephrotoxin. It seems likely that the combination of hypovolemia and tissue destruction with activation of inflammatory mediators leads to reductions of RBF and GFR. The filtered myoglobin may then precipitate in the tubules, sustaining the reduction in GFR. The best animal model of the disease would appear to be the glycerol injection model which produces hypovolemia, myoglobinuria, and hemoglobinuria. Significant protection is afforded by saline loading or mannitol infusion, and enhancement of injury is caused by dehydration. Solubility of myoglobin falls in acidic solutions, leading to use of $NaHCO_3$. Because most precipitation is observed in proximal tubules, plasma pH should be kept normal or alkaline to ensure a nonacid proximal tubular fluid. A brisk solute diuresis with a diuretic with proximal tubular action, such as mannitol, is rational. Although rational, clinical studies supporting an improved outcome following these interventions are not available.

Hyperuricemia, hyperkalemia, hyperphosphatemia, hypocalcemia, and disproportionately elevated plasma creatinine levels are common with rhabdomyolysis-induced ARF. Patients with rhabdomyolysis have hypocalcemia which is transient in the absence of ARF, but persists during the oliguric phase of ARF. Rhabdomyolysis is associated with positive pyrophosphate scans, indicating tissue Ca deposition (103). Hypercalcemia commonly develops during the diuretic phase of ARF induced by rhabdomyolysis. Serum parathyroid hormone levels are usually elevated in ARF, but were undetectable during hypercalcemia occurring during the diuretic phase. The 25-hydroxyvitamin D (25-OH-D) levels were low with rhabdomyolysis but rose during the diuretic phase of ARF. 1,25-dihydroxy-vitamin D (1,25-[OH]2-D) levels were initially normal, but rose during the diuretic phase of rhabdomyolysis-induced ARF and rose higher in those who developed hypercalcemia. Thus, the hypercalcemia during the diuretic phase of rhabdomyolysis-induced ARF is related to the elevation of 1,25-(OH)2-D.

Hemoglobinuria results when hemolysis outstrips the body's ability to bind and degrade Hgb. The most common setting in the ICU is ABO or Rh transfusion incompatibility due to clerical error. As with myoglobin, Hgb per se is not a significant nephrotoxin, but when combined with dehydration and hemo-dynamic instability, is associated with ARF. Comments relative to the patho-genesis and management of myoglobinuric ARF are applicable in hemoglobinuria.

Obstructive Jaundice. The risk of ARF following biliary surgery for obstructive jaundice is related to the level of bilirubin. It has been suggested that renal dysfunction is related to absorption of excessive amounts of endotoxin due to a deficiency of bile acids in the GI tract. Establishment of diuresis prior to surgery by administration of mannitol appears to protect against the reduction in GFR (46, 109-114).

Immune. Allergic interstitial nephritis has been associated with a variety of drugs (Table 14). About half the patients will have a rash, 75% fever, 80% eosinophilia, and many will have eosinophiluria. The latter finding is highly suggestive, but not pathognomonic, of acute interstitial nephritis (115, 116).

Management

Prevention

A number of agents have been used in animal models in attempts to amelio-rate the degree of dysfunction, including vasodilators, renin-angiotensin system blockade, and adrenergic blocking drugs. None of these has been consistently better than simple volume loading, although individual reports show some pro-tection for each. Nonsteroidal anti-inflammatory drugs generally worsen the course of the disease, while some positive responses have been reported for spe-cific blockade of thromboxane synthesis. More recently, quite different avenues have been explored including thyroid hormone manipulations, adenosine-blocking experiments, calcium channel blockers, and ATP infusion.

Volume Loading

Volume loading with saline before a renal insult has been one of the most consistently protective maneuvers in a variety of animal models and in per-ioperative fluid management in man (117, 118). The mechanism of its protective value has not been fully elucidated. In early studies, it was believed that sup-pression of the renin-angiotensin axis was responsible, but this probably plays little, if any, role. Protection seems to correlate best with solute excretion rate.

Diuretics

While mannitol is protective in a variety of animal models (119), the exact mode of protection is not yet clear and negative results are sometimes reported (120). Several lines of evidence suggest that mannitol might protect against ARF. Mannitol is a renal vasodilator (121), a scavenger of O_2 free radicals as well as a diuretic. The latter is important because most studies demonstrating pro-tection have correlated the protection with an increase in solute excretion rate prior to the renal insult. Its protective effect appears to correlate with an increase in solute excretion. Most of the pathology occurs in the proximal tubules and mannitol has most of its effect in this segment of the nephron. Hypertonic mannitol will aid in volume expansion, another protective pro-cedure. Cell swelling has been postulated to be important in the pathogenesis, and hypertonic agents may reduce cell swelling. If sludging of RBC and WBC in peritubular capillaries is important in pathogenesis, hemodilution provided by mannitol may be protective. Mannitol elevates proximal tubular pressure and should facilitate flushing of partially obstructing debris from the nephron. Despite these rationalizations and the fact that mannitol has performed better than furosemide in most animal models, there are very few well controlled clinical studies of its use in preventing or treating ARF. Mannitol may be protective in jaundiced patients perioperatively and during therapy with amphotericin B, radiocontrast agents, and cisplatin (4).

Furosemide is a weak renal vasodilator which increases solute excretion through the distal nephron because its major site of action is in the thick ascending limb of Henle's loop. Furosemide may be somewhat protective in ischemic models, but is not useful or even detrimental in nephrotoxic models. Its protective effects seem to correlate with an increase in solute excretion. Controlled clinical trials documenting improvement in renal function have been few and have failed to demonstrate any benefit.

Thyroid Hormones

Thyroidectomy significantly protected rats from ARF after 60 min of RAC. It was postulated that protection was related to a higher glutathione content of the cortex (121). In contrast, T4 stimulated Na-K-ATPase activity and protected against uranyl nitrate-induced ARF (122). T4 also increased renal solute excretion, urinary calcium excretion, and reduced the severity of gentamicin-induced ARF.

Reduced Protein Intake

The degree of rise in creatinine and mortality rate were directly proportional to the pre-ischemic protein content of the diet in rats subjected to 45 min of RAC. The postischemic diet did not appear to influence the outcome (52,123).

Calcium Channel Blockade

Ca channel blockers have been proposed as protective agents based on the observation of Ca accumulation in necrotic tissue and their ability to prevent Ca uptake by cells. In dogs subjected to RAC, pretreatment with verapamil failed to protect against ARF. When verapamil was infused for an hour after reperfusion of the kidney, urine output and GFR were better maintained (124). Verapamil infusion started before and continued during and after RAC was associated with better GFR and lower F_{ENa}. Infusion begun after reperfusion had no beneficial effect (125). Most studies to date suggest that any benefit is related to vasodilation and not to the blockade of Ca uptake by damaged cells.

Vasopressin Blockade

Agents such as clonidine, demeclocycline, and lithium, which block actions of vasopressin, reduce the severity of ARF in the RAC model in the rabbit (23). Specific AVP receptor blockers have not received much attention.

ATP Administration

Ischemia leads to rapid depletion of ATP stores. When ATP is given exogenously, it is capable of entering cells and substituting for endogenously produced energy. Pretreatment by flushing the rat kidneys with ATP-MgCl2 before 1 h of renal artery clamping completely prevented the functional and histologic changes seen in control subjects (119). ATP-MgCl2 after ischemia may hasten recovery, presumably by increasing energy availability to tubular cells (126).

Adenosine Blockade

Adenosine is released by the anoxic kidney; when administered exogenously, it causes a reduction in GFR and filtration fraction. Low cellular ATP levels activate 5-nucleotidase, which converts AMP to adenosine. Theophylline is an adenosine receptor antagonist with phosphodiesterase-inhibiting properties. The potent adenosine antagonist, 8-phenyl-theophylline, is without phosphodiesterase-inhibiting properties. Aminophylline protected against amphotericin B nephrotoxicity (127). In myohemoglobinuric ARF induced in the rat by intramuscular injection of glycerol, administration of aminophylline at the time of glycerol injection and for 3 days after the insult markedly improved renal function and survival. Single injections of aminophylline were also effective in ameliorating the degree of renal dysfunction, the efficacy declining rapidly with delay after glycerol injection (128). When 8-phenyl-theophylline was given after injection of glycerol, the degree of histologic damage, elevation of plasma creatinine, and kidney swelling were improved (129). It appears that the adenosine-blocking properties of these drugs rather than phosphodiesterase activity was the protective factor.

Antithrombin III

It is possible that intravascular coagulation could impede blood flow at either the glomerular or peritubular capillary level. Scald burns in rabbits caused renal dysfunction. Heparin plus antithrombin III replacement provided significant protection. The majority of this effect was produced by antithrombin-III alone (130).

Complications

After the development of ARF, the clinician must attempt to substitute for the functions normally performed by the kidney. Whereas in health the kidney compensates for wide variations in the intake water and electrolytes, in ARF this compensation must be accomplished by the physician. Thus, fluid and electrolyte administration must be matched to output, with steps taken to remove any excess.

Metabolic

Water balance is monitored by careful recording of intake and output and measurement of body weight, osmolality, and electrolyte concentrations. Estimation of water requirements in critically ill patients in ARF is nearly impossible without these measurements. Water requirements are directly proportional to the metabolic rate, which varies significantly in critically ill patients. These patients also have varying degrees of losses of other body fluids which may be difficult to measure, such as diarrhea, and insensible losses from wound surfaces and perspiration. Respiratory losses may be markedly increased in the dyspneic, febrile patient with an elevated respiratory dead space. Conversely, the ventilated patient may have no respiratory losses or may even gain water through the respiratory tract.

In addition, the clinician is frequently faced with obligatory administration of fluids to achieve other ends in the critically ill patient. Administration of multiple drugs, intravenous nutritional fluids, and maintenance of adequate intra-vascular volume all obligate a volume of fluid which is greater than the renal and extrarenal losses in many patients.

Water

The ideal plan is to limit administration of water to balance the amounts lost via urine and other routes. In the critically ill patient, this goal is rarely met because of other more pressing needs. Nutrition should be administered via the gut or parenterally in the most concentrated solutions. Drugs should be administered in small volumes. This usually results in the need for dialysis in oliguric ARF.

Sodium

Hyponatremia is common and usually results from water overload, not Na depletion. Careful attention to water balance should prevent or treat the problem. Sodium replacement is guided by serial measurements of plasma sodium concentration. When other losses, e.g., gastric or fistula drainage, are significant, it is best to measure the sodium content directly and plan replacement accordingly.

Potassium

Hyperkalemia can be combated by removing K from intravenous fluids, by administration of K-binding resins via the GI tract, and dialysis. Hyperkalemia is a greater problem in very catabolic patients, those with retained necrotic tissue, and anuric patients. A few medications contain significant amounts of K, e.g., aqueous penicillin. The electrophysiologic effects on the heart of severe hyperkalemia can be temporarily antagonized by the administration of calcium. Production of respiratory or metabolic alkalosis and insulin administration can cause a transient redistribution of potassium to the intracellular space. Once dialysis has begun, hypokalemia can also occur and can be dealt with by raising the K concentration in the dialysate or by K administration.

Acid-Base

The body normally produces about 1 mEq/kg body weight of nonvolatile acid per day. These acids are normally excreted by the kidney and accumulate in ARF, causing a metabolic acidosis. Adverse effects of acidosis include blunting of the actions of catecholamines, nausea, vomiting, CNS dysfunction, and glucose intolerance. Management includes prescription of a diet low in sulfur and phosphorous when possible, infusion of bicarbonate, and removal of acids by dialysis.

Calcium

Hypocalcemia is common and is multifactorial in origin. Hyperphosphatemia, hypoalbuminemia, and abnormalities in parathyroid hormone and vitamin D all may be important in individual cases. Correction of phosphate and protein levels is the mainstay of therapy. Measurement of ionized Ca levels is necessary to regulate Ca administration because the relation between total and ionized Ca is severely disturbed in critically ill patients. Hypercalcemia may be seen in the diuretic phase, especially when rhabdomyolysis occurred as a part of the initiating event. This appears to be related to tissue Ca deposition during the acute phase. It also occurs during the maintenance phase of ARF in some patients, and may require therapy with calcitonin.

Phosphorus

Hyperphosphatemia is common, and is associated with the same clinical states as hyperkalemia because both are major intracellular ions. Management consists of limitation of intake and enhanced removal via phosphate-binding agents in the GI tract and dialysis. Hypophosphatemia is sometimes seen after the patient stabilizes and adequate nutrition begins to establish positive nitrogen balance, at which time phosphate administration may be required.

Protein Catabolic Products

Lipids and carbohydrates are catabolized to CO_2 and water, which are excreted via the lungs. Proteins are degraded to urea, which is dependent on renal excretion. Nutritional considerations make administration of amino acids or protein mandatory, but as discussed with nutrition, some modification in the usual dietary prescription may limit the rate of accumulation of urea. Ultimately, removal depends on provision of dialysis.

Uric acid is the end product of nucleotide metabolism in man and is dependent on the kidneys for excretion. When excessive production of uric acid is anticipated, e.g., during lytic tumor therapy, allopurinol can be useful. Until dialysis is instituted, uric acid levels rise progressively.

Enzymes

Amylase is excreted in the urine and levels may increase during renal insufficiency. Amylase and lipase levels were elevated in 48% and 65% of patients, respectively, with ARF. Three patients with pancreatitis and ARF had elevations of 11 to 39 times the upper limit of normal (131).

Hormone Levels

The rates of production of several hormones, e.g., parathyroid hormone and growth hormone, are increased. Many polypeptide hormones are degraded to a significant degree by the kidney. Consequently, levels rise during ARF (132). The physiologic consequences of these elevations are less certain, making interpretation of the levels difficult.

Cardiovascular

Hypertension is relatively unusual during ARF unless a systemic disease has caused both hypertension and ARF, or the hypertension itself is the cause of ARF.

Hypervolemia is common during ARF in the critically ill patient as a result of attempts to reverse any hemodynamic contribution to the onset of ARF. This may result in pulmonary and systemic edema, high cardiac output with systolic flow murmurs and, rarely, hypertension.

Pericarditis and tamponade are related to the development of uremia and are rarely clinically significant in adequately dialyzed patients. The occurrence of pericarditis early in the course of ARF suggests a systemic disease as the cause of both, e.g., autoimmune disease or vasculitis.

Arrhythmias may result from K, Ca, Mg, acid-base abnormalities, pericarditis, drug toxicity, or underlying heart disease. Management consists of correction of the underlying disturbance whenever possible, coupled with antiarrhythmic agents.

Hematologic

Anemia results from a combination of a lack of production, iatrogenic losses from laboratory testing, losses to dialysis circuits, and hemorrhagic complications such as GI blood loss. In some cases, hemolysis may be a part of the underlying disease process. Provision of adequate nutrition, prophylaxis against GI hemorrhage, and transfusion as indicated by clinical indicators of O_2 delivery are the mainstays of therapy.

Infections

Wound infections, pneumonia, and other infections are commonly observed in these patients. Infection is probably the most common direct cause of death during ARF (133). Unique infections included infection of arteriovenous fistulas placed for dialysis and peritonitis in patients dialyzed via that route. The mechanisms leading to the increased susceptibility are currently speculative. Thus, management is based on general principles of infection control, monitoring for infection, and therapy based on culture results.

Pharmacologic

In general, drug dose is determined by the volume of distribution and the desired drug concentration in a particular body compartment. Interval is determined primarily by the rate at which the drug is eliminated either by excretion or metabolism to inactive metabolites. The excretion of many drugs or their metabolites is depressed when GFR is reduced. This will prolong the elimination half-life, the duration of action, and require a prolongation of dosage interval. The volume of distribution of hydrophilic drugs may be increased if ARF results in an increase in extracellular fluid volume, resulting in a need for a larger dose than normal. The interplay between dose and interval is complex, and depends on the therapeutic index (ratio of toxic to therapeutic drug level or dose) of the drug, volume of distribution, and contribution of nonrenal routes of elimination (134). Doses of drugs with a narrow therapeutic range, such as aminoglycosides, should be adjusted by individualized pharmacokinetic analysis. Nomograms relating dose schedules to creatinine or creatinine clearance are not useful after the first few doses.

Gastrointestinal

GI hemorrhage has been a frequent (up to 27%) and often fatal complication in the past (135), but its incidence has probably decreased in recent years. With azotemia there is anorexia, nausea, and vomiting, which are best controlled by adequate dialysis.

Mortality Rate

The prognosis for patients with ARF varies widely. Although a few generalities apply, the variability in outcome is so great that studies of interventions which use historical controls or nonrandomized designs are unlikely to give useful information. In general, the sicker the patient, the more likely is death (136-139). This is consistent with the findings that outcome in patients with multiple organ failure correlates with the number of organs failing. Death is rarely due to the immediate complications of ARF per se. For example, the occurrence of ARF does not influence outcome following renal transplantation (140). ARF may be seen, then, as a disease which complicates other frequently lethal diseases rather than as a major, direct cause of death.

A distressing finding is that mortality has not changed significantly since the introduction of hemodialysis. The reasons given for our lack of improvement include a more elderly patient population in more recent series, a sicker population, and elimination of ARF in many clinical situations associated with a better prognosis such as obstetrics due to better resuscitation skills. These explanations have not been critically tested and it has been suggested that mortality in truly comparable patients has not changed (141).

Cardiovascular disease is a very common accompaniment, if not a cause of, ARF. Hypovolemia (58, 141), cardiogenic shock (141), cardiovascular complications (141-143), cardiovascular surgery (138), hypotension (58, 137, 139), heart failure (137, 138), use of inotropic drugs (137), prior heart disease (142), tachycardia (58), hypervolemia (58), preoperative hypotension (138), and abdominal aortic surgery (138) have been related to an increased death rate in patients with ARF. In contrast, prior cardiovascular disease (137), chronic hypertension, cardiovascular surgery, abdominal aortic surgery, and duration of hypotension, dehydration, and bleeding have been reported to not influence prognosis (142).

Patients with respiratory disease and ARF may be at increased risk of death. Respiratory failure (58, 141-143) or prolonged ventilation (58, 137) seem to increase this risk. Chronic obstructive lung disease (137, 142) and acute respiratory illness (142) have been reported to not indicate a poorer prognosis.

Oliguric patients do worse than nonoliguric patients (16, 58, 141-144). Other factors related to the degree of ARF are less consistently related to outcome. A requirement for hemodialysis (141) and delayed onset of dialysis may be related to a higher mortality rate (138). The latter has been disputed (41). In general, the duration or number of times dialyzed, nor the intensity of dialysis do not relate to mortality rates (137, 138, 144). Prior renal disease may (137, 138) or may not (139, 142) worsen outcome. The influence of the delay between the onset of ARF and after the acute illness is unclear (138, 139).

The role of sepsis is of interest because infection appears to be the most common cause of death in ARF (133). Despite this, sepsis or bacteremia have not correlated with the death rate in some studies (137, 138, 142, 143), but have in others (58, 139).

CNS depression is consistently associated with poor outcome (137, 139, 141, 142). Underlying malignancy worsens prognosis (141, 142) and burned patients do very poorly with ARF (145). Jaundice has been associated with increased mortality (137, 141, 143) but pancreatitis has a variable influence (137, 142). The presence of malnutrition and use of parenteral nutrition are unfavorable signs (137), as is hypercatabolism (143), while enteral nutrition is unrelated to mortality (137). DIC correlates with mortality (143).

Male sex (138) and advanced age (137-139, 141, 143) may or may not (142) correlate with mortality rate. Some find no sex difference (142).

Certain administrative factors correlate with increased mortality in ARF. Surgical (58, 136, 141), cardiovascular surgery, trauma, general surgery, and aortic surgery have been associated with poorer outcome. Conversely, some find that medical patients do as poorly as surgical ones (137, 146). ICU patients may have a worse outcome (58, 141).

Dialysis

Hemodialysis

The application of hemodialysis (133, 147) has undoubtedly reduced mortality from ARF by reducing or nearly eliminating death due to acidosis, fluid overload, and electrolyte abnormalities. Unfortunately, since its clinical introduction there has been little further improvement in outcome. The role of intensity of dialysis has been debated with relatively few controlled data. Dialysis is indicated for hyperkalemia, acidosis, removal of drugs and toxins, fluid overload with pulmonary edema, and to maintain the BUN at a specified level, usually less than 100 mg/dl.

Hemodialysis in critically ill patients is often complicated by significant hypotension due to a reduction in cardiac output. The latter is caused by a reduction in stroke volume incompletely compensated by an increase in heart rate. Substitution of bicarbonate for acetate as the buffer may be associated with better preservation of cardiac output (147, 148). Dialysis is also accompanied by the sequestration of WBCs in the lungs and by hypoxia. The latter is also due to CO_2 removal by the dialysis membrane. Heparinization, even regionally, frequently results in anticoagulation of the patient after hemodialysis is completed. Measurement of partial thromboplastin time is necessary to regulate protamine administration.

Gillum et al. (144) prospectively matched 17 pairs of patients who had ARF; one group was dialyzed to maintain the BUN <100 mg/dl, and the BUN of the other group was <60 mg/dl (Table 18). The overall complications were similar between the groups and the mortality rate was not improved (Table 19). Thus, it appears that little benefit will be gained by more intense regimens of dialysis.

Table 18. Predialysis characteristics

	Intensive	Nonintensive
Number	17	17
Age (yr)	56.5	56.5
Nonoliguric	6	4
Delay until HD	5 days	7 days

HD = hemodialysis

Continuous Arteriovenous Hemofiltration (CAVH)

CAVH (133, 149-152) is an attractive alternative to intermittent hemodialysis because the equipment is simpler, and the rapid changes in volume status and substrate concentrations are avoided (153). Its ultimate role in ARF will depend on the results of appropriately controlled clinical trials. CAVH has generally been associated with greater hemodynamic stability and ability to freely administer fluid for nutrition (154). A more negative view has been reported (149). Both

Table 19. Outcome and complications

	BUN <60	BUN <100
Number	17	17
Number of HD	16	8
Duration of HD	23 days	22 days
Mortality	58.8%	47.1%
Sepsis	8	11
Hemorrhage	4	10
Cardiovascular	6	6
ARDS	3	2
Bowel infarct	1	1
Hepatic failure	2	1
Seizures	0	1

HD = hemodialysis; ARDS = adult respiratory distress syndrome.
Reprinted with permission from (144).
Within the total population, 71% of the oliguric and 20% of the nonoliguric patients died; these were not reported for the treatment groups separately.

hemodialysis and CAVH achieved fluid and electrolyte balance goals. When the two methods were compared on the basis of hours of therapy, acute hypotension was three times more likely with hemodialysis, but the incidence of arrhythmias was equal and bleeding was more common with CAVH. When compared on the basis of equivalent BUN removal, the incidences of hypotension and arrhythmias were higher with CAVH. Clotting of the filter, access problems, and low filtration rates are the major problems reported for CAVH (155). The role of CAVH in managing ARF remains to be clarified by appropriately designed comparative clinical studies.

By passing a dialysate fluid through the ultrafiltration cartridge, solute removal can be enhanced significantly, thus overcoming one of the limitations of CAVH (156).

Peritoneal Dialysis

Peritoneal dialysis (157) can be instituted rapidly to control acute hyperkalemia or acidosis, although it is not as efficient as hemodialysis. The equipment and access techniques are simple and most of the principles are straightforward. It can be used when anticoagulation is contraindicated (157). There is controversy regarding its use after abdominal surgery. If the peritoneum has not healed sufficiently, leakage of dialysate out of the abdomen into the abdominal wall or through the skin commonly occurs. When healing has progressed, adhesions may make distribution of the dialysate inadequate and, of course, increase the risk of bowel injury during catheter insertion. Its use in the presence of intra-abdominal infection is permissible and antibiotics may be delivered via the dialysate. The presence of an intra-abdominal vascular prosthesis is regarded by many as an absolute contraindication to use of peritoneal dialysis. The rate of fluid removal is related to maintenance of an osmotic gradient between the dialysate and the extra cellular fluid. The higher the dialysate osmolality and the more frequent the changes, the greater the rate of fluid removal. Control of electrolyte abnormalities is achieved by altering the electrolyte concentrations in the dialysate. Complications include bowel perforation or bleeding as a result of catheter insertion, peritonitis, and hyperglycemia, especially when concentrated dialysate solutions are used. Solutions with a dextrose concentration higher than 4.5% should rarely be used. The absorption of dextrose and other substances from the peritoneum is proportional to their concentration in the dialysate and can be used as a partial route of administration for nutritional purposes (158).

Nutrition

The role and particulars of nutrition management in the management of ARF remain controversial (159-162). Many believe that the provision of adequate nutrition is critical to survival (163), but animal studies suggest that intravenous amino acids may potentiate aminoglycoside nephrotoxicity and the effects of renal ischemia (52). At least 10 g/day of essential amino acids are required to maintain protein synthesis, and 30 to 40 g/day of amino acids are generally recommended. Dialysis clears a significant amount of amino acids, 10 to 20 g/day (164, 165), and patients aggressively dialyzed will need increased amounts of amino acids during dialysis. Fluid restriction is often a difficult problem in the critically ill ARF patient. Intravenous nutritional fluid can be based on a 70% dextrose solution which will allow administration of 40% more calories per ml of fluid, when compared to the traditional 50% dextrose base. Many clinicians prescribe standard nutritional fluids once dialysis has been established, reserving essential amino acid formulations for retarding the rate of the BUN rise prior to dialysis.

Translation of these findings to better survival has generally not been realized (166). Use of a parenteral or enteral diet rich in essential and branched-chain amino acids in conjunction with hemodialysis appeared to improve the negative nitrogen balance in a group of patients with post-traumatic ARF. Overall outcome was not affected, however (167).

Diuretics

Diuretics, predominantly furosemide and mannitol, have been used: a) to aid in differentiating parenchymal from pre-renal failure, b) to halt the progression to parenchymal renal failure, c) to convert oliguric to nonoliguric ARF, and d) to shorten the course of established ARF. Demonstration of any clinical value to the suggested uses is generally lacking, with uncontrolled trials tending to show some benefit and the few controlled trials showing no effect other than establishing a higher urine flow rate in some patients (168). A response in urine flow rate is seen in patients with well established ARF, and will not occur in the presence of pre-renal oliguria if the filtration rate is low. Thus, no diagnostic information is obtained. The only clinical situation which appears to benefit from prophylactic administration of mannitol is peri-operative administration in patients with obstructive jaundice. Diuretics have been suggested as a prophylactic measure during vascular surgery, but adequate volume resuscitation appears to be equally effective.

Diuretics have a limited role in established ARF and have not been demonstrated to modify the outcome in any significant way (168,169). Some patients will respond to diuretics, making administration of drugs and nutritional fluids easier.

References

1. Fry DE, Pearlstein L, Fulton RL, et al: Multiple system organ failure. The role of uncontrolled infection. *Arch Surg* 1980; 115:136

2. Bjornsson TD: Use of serum creatinine concentrations to determine renal function. *Clin Pharmacokinet* 1979; 4:200

3. Moran SM, Myers BD: Course of acute renal failure studied by a model of creatinine kinetics. *Kidney Int* 1985; 27:928

4. Hyneck ML: Current concepts in clinical therapeutics: Drug therapy in acute renal failure. *Clin Pharm* 1986; 5:892

5. Hori R, Takano M, Okano T, et al: Transport of p-aminohippurate, tetraethylammonium and D-glucose in renal brush border membranes from rats with acute renal failure. *J Pharmacol Exp Ther* 1985; 233:776

6. Corwin HL: Acute renal failure. *Med Clin North Am* 1986; 70:1037

7. Espinel CH: FENa test: Use in the differential diagnosis of acute renal failure. *JAMA* 1976; 236:579

8. Espinel CH, Gregory AW: Differential diagnosis of acute renal failure. *Clin Nephrol* 1980; 13:73

9. Zarich S, Fang LST, Diamond JR: Fractional excretion of sodium. Exceptions to its diagnostic value. *Arch Intern Med* 1985; 145:108

10. Lam M, Kaufman CE: Fractional excretion of sodium as a guide to volume depletion during recovery from acute renal failure. *Am J Kidney Dis* 1985; 6:18

11. Wanner C, Schollmeyer P, Horl WH: Urinary proteinase activity in patients with multiple traumatic injures, sepsis, or acute renal failure. *J Lab Clin Med* 1986; 108:224

12. Sherman RA, Feinfeld DA, Ohmi N, et al: A prospective study of urinary ligandin in patients at risk of renal tubular injury. *Uremia Invest* 1984; 8:111

13. Solis-Herruzo JA, Garcia-Cabezudo J, Diaz-Rubio C, et al: Urinary excretion of enzymes in cirrhotics with renal failure. *J Hepatol* 1986; 3:123

14. Tolkoff-Rubin NE: Monoclonal antibodies in the diagnosis of renal disease: A preliminary report. *Kidney Int* 1986; 29:142

15. Mandal AK: Transmission electron microscopy of urinary sediment in human acute renal failure. *Kidney Int* 1985; 28:58

16. Dixon BS, Anderson RJ: Nonoliguric acute renal failure. *Am J Kidney Dis* 1985; 6:71

17. Anderson RJ, Linas SL, Berns AS, et al: Nonoliguric acute renal failure. *N Engl J Med* 1977; 296:1134

18. Keeton GR, Pillay GP: Diagnostic role of intravenous urography in acute and chronic renal failure. *Urol Radiol* 1986; 8:72

19. Ishikawa I: Dynamic computed tomography in acute renal failure: Analysis of time-density curve. *J Comput Assist Tomogr* 1985; 9:1097

20. Chang VH, Cunningham JJ: Efficacy of sonography as a screening method in renal insufficiency. *JCU* 1985; 13:415

21. Bulger RE, Eknoyan G, Purcell DJ II, et al: Endothelial characteristics of glomerular capillaries in normal, mercuric chloride-induced, and gentamicin-induced acute renal failure in the rat. *J Clin Invest* 1983; 72:128

22. Williams RH, Thomas CE, Navar LG, et al: Hemodynamic and single nephron function during the maintenance phase of ischemic acute renal failure in the dog. *Kidney Int* 1981; 19:503

23. Solez K: Pathogenesis of acute renal failure. *Int Rev Exp Pathol* 1983; 24:277

24. Hollenberg NK, Mangel R, Fung HYM: Assessment of intrarenal perfusion with radioxenon: A critical review of analytical factors and their implications in man. *Semin Nucl Med* 1976; 6:193

25. Tristani FE, Cohn JN: Studies in clinical shock and hypotension. VII. Renal hemodynamics before and during treatment. *Circulation* 1970; 42:839

26. Mason J: The pathophysiology of ischaemic acute renal failure. *Renal Physiol* 1986; 9:129

27. Mason J, Torhorst J, Welsch J: Role of the medullary perfusion defect in the pathogenesis of ischemic renal failure. *Kidney Int* 1984; 26:283

28. Brezis M, Rosen S, Silva P, et al: Renal ischemia: A new perspective. *Kidney Int* 1984; 26:375

29. Hollenberg NK, Epstein M, Rosen SM, et al: Acute oliguric renal failure in man: Evidence for preferential renal cortical ischemia. *Medicine* 1968; 47:455

30. Neumayer H-H, Wagner K, Groll J, et al: Beneficial effects of long-term prostaglandin E_2 infusion on the course of postischemic acute renal failure. Long-term studies in chronically instrumented conscious dogs. *Renal Physiol* 1985; 8:159

31. Lelcuk S, Alexander F, Kobzik L, et al: Prostacyclin and thromboxane A_2 moderate postischemic renal failure. *Surgery* 1985; 98:207

32. Hatziantoniou C, Papanikolaou N: Renal effects of the inhibitor of thromboxane A_2-synthetase OKY-046. *Experientia* 1986; 42:613

33. Henrich WL, Brater DC, Campbell WB: Renal hemodynamic effects of therapeutic plasma levels of sulindac sulfide during hemorrhage. *Kidney Int* 1986; 29:484

34. Watson AJ, Stout RL, Adkinson NF Jr, et al: Selective inhibition of thromboxane synthesis in glycerol-induced acute renal failure. *Am J Kidney Dis* 1986; 8:26

35. Conger JD, Robinette JB, Kelleher SP: Nephron heterogeneity in ischemic acute renal failure. *Kidney Int* 1984; 26:422

36. Moran SM, Myers BD: Pathophysiology of protracted acute renal failure in man. *J Clin Invest* 1985; 76:1440

37. Stromski ME, Cooper K, Thulin G, et al: Postischemic ATP-MgCl2 provides precursors for resynthesis of cellular ATP in rats. *Am J Physiol* 1986; 250:F834

38. Ratcliffe PJ, Moonen CTW, Holloway PAH, et al: Acute renal failure in hemorrhagic hypotension: Cellular energetics and renal function. *Kidney Int* 1986; 30:355

39. Zager RA: Alterations of intravascular volume: Influence on renal susceptibility to ischemic injury. *J Lab Clin Med* 1986; 108:60

40. Sinsteden TD, O'Neil TJ, Hill S, et al: The role of high-energy phosphate in norepinephrine-induced acute renal failure in the dog. *Circ Res* 1986; 59:93

41. Lumlertgul D, Harris DCH, Burke TJ, et al: Detrimental effect of hypophosphatemia on the severity and progression of ischemic acute renal failure. *Miner Electrolyte Metab* 1986; 12:204

42. Humes HD: Role of calcium in pathogenesis of acute renal failure. *Am J Physiol* 1986; 250:F579

43. Hou SH, Bushinsky DA, Wish JB, et al: Hospital-acquired renal insufficiency: A prospective study. *Am J Med* 1983; 74:243

44. Rasmussen HH, Ibels LS: Acute renal failure. Multivariate analysis of causes and risk factors. *Am J Med* 1982; 73:211

45. Barsoum RS, Rihan ZEB, Baligh OK, et al: Acute renal failure in the 1973 Middle East war. Experience of a specialized base hospital: Effect of the site of injury. *J Trauma* 1980; 20:303

46. Dawson JL: The incidence of postoperative renal failure in obstructive jaundice. *Br J Surg* 1965; 52:663

47. Cahill CJ: Prevention of postoperative renal failure in patients with obstructive jaundice — The role of bile salts. *Br J Surg* 1983; 70:590

48. Porter GA, Kloster FE, Herr RJ, et al: Renal complications associated with valve replacement surgery. *J Thorac Cardiovasc Surg* 1966; 53:145

49. Kwaan JHM, Connolly JE: Renal failure complicating aortoiliofemoral reconstructive procedure. *Am Surg* 1980; 295:295

50. Richards WO, Scovill WA, Shin B: Opsonic fibronectin deficiency in patients with intra-abdominal infection. *Surgery* 1983; 94:210

51. Ichikawa I, Purkerson ML, Yates J, et al: Dietary protein intake conditions the degree of renal vasoconstriction in acute renal failure caused by ureteral obstruction. *Am J Physiol* 1985; 249:F54

52. Andrews PM: Dietary protein prior to renal ischemia dramatically affects postischemic recovery. *Kidney Int* 1986; 30:299

53. Grenfell A: Acute renal failure in diabetics. *Intensive Care Med* 1986; 12:6

54. Hermreck AS, Berg RA, Ruhlen JR, et al: Renal response to sepsis. *Arch Surg* 1973; 107:169

55. Bennett WM: Aminoglycoside nephrotoxicity. *Nephron* 1983; 35:73

56. Bennett WM: Aminoglycoside nephrotoxicity. Experimental and clinical considerations. *Miner Electrolyte Metab* 1981; 6:277

57. Brinker KR, Bulger RE, Dobyan DC, et al: Effect of potassium depletion on gentamicin nephrotoxicity. *J Lab Clin Med* 1981; 98:292

58. Frankel MC, Weinstein AM, Stenzel KH: Prognostic patterns in acute renal failure. *Clin Exper Dialysis Apheresis* 1983; 7:145

59. Mitchell JP: Trauma to the urinary tract. *N Engl J Med* 1973; 288:90

60. Rao PS, Cavanagh D, Marsden KA, et al: Prostaglandin D_2 in canine endotoxic shock. Hemodynamic, hematologic, biochemical, and blood gas analyses. *Am J Obstet Gynecol* 1984; 148:964

61. Hinshaw LB, Spink WW, Vick JA, et al: Effect of endotoxin on kidney function and renal hemodynamics in the dog. *Am J Physiol* 1961; 201:144

62. Kikeri D, Pennell JP, Hwang KH, et al: Endotoxemic acute renal failure in awake rats. *Am J Physiol* 1986; 250:F1098

63. Badr KF, Kelley VE, Rennke HG, et al: Roles for thromboxane A_2 and leukotrienes in endotoxin-induced acute renal failure. *Kidney Int* 1986; 30:474

64. Hinshaw LB, Bradley GM, Carlson CH: Effect of endotoxin on renal function in the dog. *Am J Physiol* 1959; 196:1127

65. Henrich WL, Hamasaki Y, Said SI, et al: Dissociation of systemic and renal effects in endotoxemia. Prostaglandin inhibition uncovers an important role of renal nerves. *J Clin Invest* 1982; 69:691

66. Zager RA: *Escherichia coli* endotoxin injections potentiate experimental ischemic renal injury. *Am J Physiol* 1986; 251:F988

67. Selmyer JP, Reynolds DG, Swan KG: Renal blood flow during endotoxin shock in the subhuman primate. *Surg Gynecol Obstet* 1973; 137:3

68. Sato T, Kono Y, Shimahara Y: The pathophysiology of septic shock: Acute renal failure in rats following live *E. coli* injection. A histochemical study of the proximal tubules. *Advances in Shock Research* 1982; 7:61

69. Richman AV, Okulski EG, Balis JU: New concepts in the pathogenesis of acute tubular necrosis associated with sepsis. *Ann Clin Lab Sci* 1981; 11:211

70. Zager RA, Prior RB: Gentamicin and Gram-negative bacteremia. *J Clin Invest* 1986; 78:196

71. Beutler B, Cerami A: Cachectin: More than a tumor necrosis factor. *N Engl J Med* 1987; 316:379

72. Koppel MH, Coburn JW, Mims MM, et al: Transplantation of cadaveric kidneys from patients with hepatorenal syndrome. Evidence for the functional nature of renal failure in advanced liver disease. *N Engl J Med* 1969; 280:1367

73. Wilkinson SP, Williams R: Renal failure in cirrhosis: Current views and speculations. *Adv Nephrol* 1977; 7:15

74. Richman AV, Gerber LI, Balis JU: Peritubular capillaries. A major site of endotoxin-induced vascular injury in the primate kidney. *Lab Invest* 1980; 43:327

75. Rosoff L Jr, Williams J, Molt P, et al: Renal hemodynamics and the renin-angiotensin system in cirrhosis. Relationship to sodium retention. *Dig Dis Sci* 1979; 24:25

76. Better OS, Schrier RW: Disturbed volume homeostasis in patients with cirrhosis of the liver. *Kidney Int* 1983; 23:303

77. Epstein M: Deranged sodium homeostasis in cirrhosis. *Gastroenterology* 1979; 76:622

78. Epstein M: Determinants of abnormal renal sodium handling in cirrhosis: A reappraisal. *Scand J Clin Lab Invest* 1980; 40:689

79. Skorecki KL, Brenner BM: Body fluid homeostasis in congestive heart failure and cirrhosis with ascites. *Am J Med* 1982; 72:323

80. Cade R, Wagemaker H, Vogel S, et al: Hepatorenal syndrome. Studies of the effect of vascular volume and intraperitoneal pressure on renal and hepatic function. *Am J Med* 1987; 82:427

81. Smith JH, Merrell RC, Raffin TA: Reversal of postoperative anuria by decompressive celiotomy. *Arch Intern Med* 1985; 145:553

82. Celoria G: Oliguria from high intra-abdominal pressure secondary to ovarian mass. *Crit Care Med* 1987; 15:78

83. Richards WO, Scovill W, Shin B, et al: Acute renal failure associated with increased intra-abdominal pressure. *Ann Surg* 1983; 197:183

84. Coggins CH, Fang LS-T: Acute renal failure associated with antibiotics, anesthetic agents, and radiographic contrast agents. *In:* Acute Renal Failure. Brenner BM, Lazarus JM (Eds). Philadelphia, WB Saunders Co, 1983, p 283

85. Kaloyanides GJ, Pastoriza-Munoz E: Aminoglycoside nephrotoxicity. *Kidney Int* 1980; 18:571

86. Luft FC, Aronoff GR, Evan AP, et al: The effect of aminoglycosides on glomerular endothelium: A comparative study. *Res Commun Chem Pathol Pharmacol* 1981; 34:89

87. Luft FC, Evan AP: Glomerular filtration barrier in aminoglycoside-induced nephrotoxic acute renal failure. *Renal Physiol* 1980; 3:265

88. Lifschitz MD: Renal effects of nonsteroidal anti-inflammatory agents. *J Lab Clin Med* 1983; 102:313

89. Carmichael J, Shankel SW: Effects of nonsteroidal anti-inflammatory drugs on prostaglandins and renal function. *Am J Med* 1985; 78:992

90. Dunn MJ: Nonsteroidal anti-inflammatory drugs and renal function. *Annu Rev Med* 1984; 35:411

91. Makhoul RG, Gewertz BL: Renal prostaglandins. *J Surg Res* 1986; 40:181

92. Reeves WB, Foley RJ, Weinman EJ: Nephrotoxicity from nonsteroidal anti-inflammatory drugs. *South Med J* 1985; 78:318

93. Coulie P, DePlaen JF, van Ypersele de Strihou C: Captopril-induced acute reversible renal failure. *Nephron* 1983; 35:108

94. Cramer BC, Parfrey PS, Hutchinson TA, et al: Renal function following infusion of radiologic contrast material. A prospective controlled study. *Arch Intern Med* 1985; 145:87

95. Kone BC, Watson AJ, Gimenez LF, et al: Acute renal failure following percutaneous transhepatic cholangiography. A retrospective study. *Arch Intern Med* 1986; 146:1405

96. Gomes AS, Baker JD, Martin-Paredero V, et al: Acute renal dysfunction after major arteriography. *AJR* 1985; 145:1249

97. Mason RA, Arbeit LA, Giron F: Renal dysfunction after arteriography. *JAMA* 1985; 253:1001

98. Golman K, Almen T: Contrast media-induced nephrotoxicity. Survey and present state. *Invest Radiol* 1985; 20(Suppl 1):S92

99. Mission RT, Cutler RE: Radiocontrast-induced renal failure. *West J Med* 1985; 142:657

100. Bettmann MA: Angiographic contrast agents: Conventional and new media compared. *AJR* 1982; 139:787

101. Cederholm C, Almen T, Bergqvist D, et al: Acute renal failure in rats. Interaction between a contrast medium and renal arterial occlusion. *Acta Radiol [Diagn]* 1986; 27:241

102. Akmal M, Bishop JE, Telfer N, et al: Hypocalcemia and hypercalcemia in patients with rhabdomyolysis with and without acute renal failure. *J Clin Endocrinol Metab* 1986; 63:137

103. Patel R: Technetium-99m pyrophosphate imaging in acute renal failure associated with nontraumatic rhabdomyolysis. *AJR* 1986; 147:815

104. Vertel RM, Knochel JP: Acute renal failure due to heat injury. An analysis of ten cases associated with a high incidence of myoglobinuria. *Am J Med* 1967; 43:435

105. Grufferman S, Morris D, Alvarez J: Methanol poisoning complicated by myoglobinuric renal failure. *Am J Emerg Med* 1985; 3:24

106. Leventhal I, Schiff H, Wulfsohn M: Rhabdomyolysis and acute renal failure as a complication of urethral surgery. *Urology* 1985; 26:59

107. Kelly CJ, Singer I: Acute renal failure in sickle-cell disease. *Am J Kidney Dis* 1986; 8:146

108. Fredericks MR, Dworkin R, Ward DM, et al: Antibiotic-induced acute renal failure associated with an elevated serum lactic dehydrogenase level of renal origin. *West J Med* 1986; 144:743

109. Wilkinson SP: Endotoxaemia and renal failure in cirrhosis and obstructive jaundice. *Br Med J* 1976; 2:1415

110. Wardle EN: Endotoxin and acute renal failure associated with obstructive jaundice. *Br Med J* 1970; 4:472

111. Pitt HA: Factors affecting mortality in biliary tract surgery. *Am J Surg* 1981; 141:66

112. Ozawa K: The mechanism of suppression of renal function in patients and rabbits with jaundice. *Surg Gynecol Obstet* 1979; 149:54

113. Allison MEM: Renal function and other factors in obstructive jaundice. *Br J Surg* 1979; 66:392

114. Bailey ME: Endotoxin, bile salts and renal function in obstructive jaundice. *Br J Surg* 1976; 63:774

115. Linton AK, Lindsay RM: Drug-induced acute interstitial nephritis. *Kidney* 1982; 15:1

116. Linton AL, Clark WF, Driedger AA, et al: Acute interstitial nephritis due to drugs: Review of literature with report of nine cases. *Ann Intern Med* 1980; 93:735

117. Bush HL Jr, Huse JB, Johnson WC, et al: Prevention of renal insufficiency after abdominal aortic aneurysm resection by optimal volume loading. *Arch Surg* 1981; 116:1517

118. Tiggeler RGWL, Berden JHM, Hoitsma AJ, et al: Prevention of acute tubular necrosis in cadaveric kidney transplantation by the combined use of mannitol and moderate hydration. *Ann Surg* 1985; 201:246

119. Andrews PM, Coffey AK: Protection of kidneys from acute renal failure resulting from normothermic ischemia. *Lab Invest* 1983; 49:87

120. Klein H, Greven J: Renal effects of mannitol in the early stage of glycerol-induced acute renal failure in the rat. *Nephron* 1979; 23:255

121. Paller MS, Sikora JJ: Hypothyroidism protects against free radical damage in ischemic renal failure. *Kidney Int* 1986; 29:1162

122. Cronin RE, Brown DM, Simonsen R: Protection by thyroxine in nephrotoxic acute renal failure. *Am J Physiol* 1986; 251:F408

123. Andrews PM, Bates SB: Dietary protein prior to renal ischemia dramatically affects postischemic kidney function. *Kidney Int* 1986; 30:299

124. Wait RB, White G, Davis JH: Beneficial effects of verapamil on postischemic renal failure. *Surgery* 1983; 94:276

125. Goldfarb D, Iaina A, Serban I, et al: Beneficial effect of verapamil in ischemic acute renal failure in the rat. *Proc Soc Exp Biol Med* 1983; 172:389

126. Osswald H, Nabakowski G, Hermes H: Adenosine as a possible mediator of metabolic control of glomerular filtration rate. *Int J Biochem* 1980; 12:263

127. Gerkens JF, Heidemann HT, Jackson EK: Effect of aminophylline on amphotericin B nephrotoxicity in the dog. *J Pharmacol Exp Ther* 1982; 224:609

128. Bidani AK, Churchill PC: Aminophylline ameliorates glycerol-induced acute renal failure in rats. *Can J Physiol Pharmacol* 1983; 61:567

129. Bowmer CJ, Collis MG, Yates MS: Effect of the adenosine antagonist 8-phenyltheophylline on glycerol-induced acute renal failure in the rat. *Br J Pharmacol* 1986; 88:205

130. Ono I, Ohura T, Azami K, et al: Anticoagulation therapy for renal insufficiency after burns. *Burns* 1984; 11:104

131. Zachee P, Lins RL, DeBroe ME: Serum amylase and lipase values in acute renal failure. *Clin Chem* 1985; 31:1237

132. Katz AI, Emmanouel DS: Metabolism of polypeptide hormones by the normal kidney and in uremia. *Nephron* 1978; 22:69

133. Luft FC: Acute renal failure: Contemporary management. *Indiana Medicine* 1985; 78:672

134. Bennet WM, Arnoff GR, Morrison G, et al: Drug prescribing in renal failure: Dosing guidelines for adults. *Am J Kidney Dis* 1983; 3:155

135. Nakayama M, Shinbo T, Nakamura K, et al: Experience of 26 acute renal failure cases. *Tokai J Exp Clin Med* 1982; 7:101

136. Tilney NL, Bailey GL, Morgan AP: Sequential system failure after rupture of abdominal aortic aneurysms: An unsolved problem in postoperative care. *Ann Surg* 1973; 10:117

137. Lien J, Chan V: Risk factors influencing survival in acute renal failure treated by hemodialysis. *Arch Intern Med* 1985; 145:2067

138. Cioffi WG: Probability of surviving postoperative acute renal failure: Development of a prognostic index. *Ann Surg* 1984; 200:205

139. Gornick CC Jr, Kjellstrand CM: Acute renal failure complicating aortic aneurysm surgery. *Nephron* 1983; 35:145

140. Mentzer SJ, Fryd DS, Kjellstrand CM: Why do patients with postsurgical acute tubular necrosis die? *Arch Surg* 1985; 120:907

141. Cameron JS: Acute renal failure in the intensive care unit today. *Intensive Care Med* 1986; 12:64

142. Rasmussen HH, Pitt EA, Ibels LS, et al: Prediction of outcome in acute renal failure by discriminant analysis of clinical variables. *Arch Intern Med* 1985; 145:2015

143. Bullock ML, Umen AJ, Finkelstein M, et al: The assessment of risk factors in 462 patients with acute renal failure. *Am J Kidney Dis* 1985; 5:97

144. Gillum DM, Dixon BS, Yanover MJ, et al: The role of intensive dialysis in acute renal failure. *Clin Nephrol* 1986; 25:249

145. Sawada Y, Momma S, Takamizawa A, et al: Survival from acute renal failure after severe burns. *Burns* 1984; 11:143

146. Abreo K, Moorthy AV, Osborne M: Changing patterns and outcome of acute renal failure requiring hemodialysis. *Arch Intern Med* 1986; 146:1338

147. Mackenzie TA, Zawada ET Jr, Stacy WK: Hemodialysis. Basic principles and practice. *Postgrad Med* 1985; 77:95

148. Huyghebaert M-F, Dhainaut J-F, Monsallier JF, et al: Bicarbonate hemodialysis of patients with acute renal failure and severe sepsis. *Crit Care Med* 1985; 13:840

149. Kohen JA, Whitley KY, Kjellstrand CM: Continuous arteriovenous hemofiltration: A comparison with hemodialysis in acute renal failure. *Trans Am Soc Artif Intern Organs* 1985; 31:169

150. Ronco C: Arterio-venous hemodiafiltration (A-V HDF): A possible way to increase urea removal during C.A.V.H. *Int J Artif Organs* 1985; 8:61

151. Kramer P, Seegers A, DeVivie R, et al: Therapeutic potential of hemofiltration. *Clin Nephrol* 1979; 11:145

152. Slive HL: Continuous arteriovenous hemofiltration. *JAMA* 1985; 253:1325

153. Silverstein ME: Treatment of severe fluid overload by ultrafiltration. *N Engl J Med* 1974; 291:747

154. Mault JR, Kresowik TF, Dechert RE, et al: Continuous arteriovenous hemofiltration: The answer to starvation in acute renal failure? *Trans Am Soc Artif Intern Organs* 1984; 30:203

155. Domoto DT: Two years clinical experience with continuous arteriovenous hemofiltration. *Trans Am Soc Artif Intern Organs* 1985; 31:581

156. Ronco C: Arteriovenous hemodiafiltration (AVHDF) combined with continuous arteriovenous hemofiltration (CADH). *Trans Am Soc Artif Intern Organs* 1985; 31:349

157. Miller RB, Tassistro CR: Peritoneal dialysis. *N Engl J Med* 1969; 281:945

158. Pomeranz A, Reichenberg Y, Schurr D, et al: Acute renal failure in a burn patient: The advantages of continuous peritoneal dialysis. *Burns* 1985; 11:367

159. Feinstein EI, Blumenkrantz MJ, Healy M, et al: Clinical and metabolic responses to parenteral nutrition in acute renal failure. A controlled double-blind study. *Medicine* 1981; 60:124

160. Teschner M, Heidland A: Nutrition in acute renal failure. *Blood Purification* 1985; 3:170

161. Teschan PE: Nutrition in renal failure. *Artif Organs* 1986; 10:301

162. Teschan PE: Acute renal failure versus nutrition: No free lunch in the ICU. *Trans Am Soc Artif Intern Organs* 1983; 29:764

163. Lazarus JM: Acute renal failure. *Intensive Care Med* 1986; 12:61

164. Ganda OMP, Aoki TT, Soeldner JS, et al: Hormone-fuel concentrations in anephric subjects. Effect of hemodialysis (with special reference to amino acids). *J Clin Invest* 1976; 57:1403

165. Blumenkrantz MJ, Gahl GM, Kopple JD, et al: Protein losses during peritoneal dialysis. *Kidney Int* 1981; 19:593

166. Thompson M: Use of essential amino acid/dextrose solutions in the nutritional management of patients with acute renal failure. *Drug Intell Clin Pharm* 1985; 19:106

167. Proietti R, Pelosi G, Santori R, et al: Nutrition in acute renal failure. *Resuscitation* 1983; 10:159

168. Kleinknecht D, Ganeval D, Gonzalez-Duque LA, et al: Furosemide in acute oliguric renal failure: A controlled trial. *Nephron* 1976; 17:51

169. Brown CB, Ogg CS, Cameron JS: High dose furosemide in acute renal failure: A controlled trial. *Clin Nephrol* 1981; 15:90

Chapter 12

Critical Care Technology: An Aid to Diagnosis

Philip D. Lumb, MB, BS

Outline

Educational Objectives

In this chapter the reader will learn:

1. to become familiar with new monitoring technologies which are applicable within the ICU and which do not require sophisticated transport or associated technology.

2. to determine the application of specific monitoring technologies to critical care medicine practice.

3. to discriminate between the costs, potential benefits, and drawbacks of various monitoring technologies.

4. to realize the indications and contraindications of new monitoring technology.

Introduction

In the late 1960s, a television phenomenon occurred which caused viewers "to boldly go" into uncharted galactic territory. The voyages of Starship Command's *Enterprise* and the adventures of her crew thrilled and amazed viewers of all ages. As importantly, the special effects created for the sets were envied and duplicated world-wide. In fact, an unsuccessful attempt was made to manufacture working models of the silently opening doors which led into the ship's various compartments, elevators, and onto the bridge. Despite the impressive recreations of extraterrestrial life and far-flung planets, for many viewers a prime achievement was the depiction of medical practice in the 23rd century. Even more amazing than the practices of Dr. McCoy and Nurse Chapel were the ideas underlying the equipment and techniques depicted in the series. For example, most fans will remember the medical "tricorder," a device which analyzed readings taken by the associated medical scanner. The tricorder recorded visually and audibly, and presented scientific or medical readings for rapid action. Also, "Trekkies" will recall the fact that McCoy's injections always were pressed through clothing and skin and took effect immediately.

However, probably the most lasting impression of the sick bay will be the medical diagnostic panel situated above the head of every bed. According to the description supplied by the producers, the device monitored temperature, brain activity, respiration, pulse, cell rate, and two blood chemistries. The panel could be programmed to function appropriately for different patients and species, and it monitored all of the patient functions without direct contact through the use of a scanning light beam. Finally, although McCoy sometimes disparaged the devices with which he was surrounded, he was portrayed as a physician capable of integrating the most modern technology with appropriate clinical skills. Perhaps the future of medical technology was predicted in the subsequent *Star Trek* motion pictures in which Chapel, now a physician, used a portable device to both sterilize and apply a plastic skin to Mr. Chekov's hand injury caused by electrical burns. In the final movie *(Star Trek IV, The Voyage Home),* the medical profession of the 20th century comes in for some tongue-in-cheek criticism when McCoy ridicules the treatment of end-stage renal failure and "rescues" Chekov from a neurosurgeon about to perform a craniotomy to relieve raised intracranial pressure due to a traumatic subdural hematoma.

More impressive than the inventiveness and perspicacity of the writers is the medical progress which has been made since the first *Star Trek* episode was aired. Although still working at the boundaries of medical possibility and dreams, many of the futuristic scenes appear strangely familiar when seen in reruns. Biologic dressings, noninvasive assessment capability of hemodynamic status and brain O_2 utilization, innovative drug delivery systems, and new body imaging techniques are all available in today's critical care units. Technology has paved the way to provide diagnostic and reassessment information in a new fashion. The clinician needs to learn how to control and direct the technology in order to benefit maximally from the massive amount of available raw information and integrate it into an overall patient care plan. This chapter will focus on the technology available to the clinician in the critical care unit rather than on devices which require complicated patient transport to specific, tailor-made facilities. Most of the information will focus on the devices which have been developed to ensure and assess adequate oxygen delivery ($\dot{D}o_2$), and this will include discussions of the following technologies: a) pulse oximetry; b) continuous invasive oximetry (arterial and venous); c) intravenous and noninvasive (transcutaneous) cardiac pacing techniques; d) noninvasive cardiac output determination; e) mechanical ventilatory support techniques and monitoring; f) near infrared O_2 sufficiency scope (niros-scope); and g) monitoring systems and integrated unit data processing.

Although important, the discussion will not detail changes in monitoring and diagnostic devices which are used outside the confines of the critical care unit and which may not be available to the majority of critical care practitioners. For example, although the technique of nuclear magnetic resonance imaging has received much attention in recent years, the likelihood that this will become an easily applied aid for the management of the critically ill is low. Also, the diagnostic and monitoring advances in the field of $\dot{D}o_2$ have been chosen for discussion because the alterations in this area of patient management have been associated with improved patient survival. Therefore, it is possible that improvements in the monitoring and management of $\dot{D}o_2$ will have a positive effect on patient outcome on a large scale.

Oxygen Delivery and Consumption

Oxygen transport is defined by the well described relationship between seven variables measured in most clinical environments. Initially, $\dot{D}o_2$ is seen as the product of cardiac output and arterial O_2 content (Cao_2). However, cardiac output is recognized as the product of heart rate (HR) times stroke volume (SV), and Cao_2 is the product of Hgb concentration times arterial oxygen saturation (Sao_2) times a constant plus the product of Po_2 in arterial blood times another constant. These relationships with clinical examples are detailed in Table 1. Because of the small contribution of O_2 dissolved in plasma to its overall transport by blood, this portion of the equation is often ignored to simplify calculations. Therefore, cardiac output and O_2 saturation (So_2) will be seen as the two most important variables which are likely to change rapidly during the course of a patient's illness.

TABLE 1: The seven variables of O_2 transport

Oxygen Transport	=	Cardiac output	$\times$	O_2 concentration (arterial)
(OT)	=	(CO)	$\times$	(Cao_2)
(Cao_2)	=	Hgb $\times$ 1.39	$\times$	Sao_2 = Pao_2 $\times$ .0031
(CO)	=	HR $\times$ SV		
(OT)	=	(HR $\times$ SV)	$\times$	([Hgb 1.39 $\times$ Sao_2] + [Pao_2 $\times$ .0031])

where 1.39 is the Hgb/O_2 binding constant and .0031 is the Bunsen O_2 solubility coefficient.

The evaluation of O_2 transport relies upon the determination of these seven variables. In order to determine the $\dot{D}o_2$ to a particular patient, a mixed venous O_2 sample must be analyzed in conjunction with the arterial specimen. Alteration of $\dot{D}o_2$ can be accomplished by careful manipulation of these variables with the clinical application of ventilatory and cardiac support systems. It is important to analyze any change in physiologic support with special reference to O_2 transport.

Obviously, further analysis must be performed to investigate alterations in SV which are not detailed in this discussion. Considerations of preload, afterload, and contractility will feature in these manipulations.

Adapted from: Kortz W, Lumb PD: The Seven Component Clinical Approach to All Types of Shock Based on Physiologic Considerations in Surgical Care: A Practical Guide. New York, Year Book Medical Publishers, 1984

Although delivery is important, the ability of tissues to utilize O_2 is associated with appropriate aerobic metabolism and the absence of acidosis. Ideally, the health of all tissue beds would be analyzed during the resuscitation and management of patients, but the practical aspects of this task, given the sophistication of available monitors, precludes this measurement. Therefore, the global assessment of O_2 utilization, which is obtained by comparing the amount of O_2 delivered to the tissues to the amount of O_2 returned to the lungs in venous blood prior to reoxygenation, is useful in assessing the response of patients to various therapeutic trials.

Theoretically, more normal $\dot{D}O_2$ and O_2 consumption values indicate improvement in a patient's condition and imply the appropriate selection of therapeutic options. The amount of returned O_2 is assessed by utilizing the same formulae and variables previously described with the substitution of mixed venous for arterial blood values. Mixed venous samples are obtained from the pulmonary artery and analysis may be either intermittent or continuous in nature. Utilization of these data is not new, but modern monitoring devices make the measurement easier and the responsiveness immediate. The assumption will be that therapeutic changes which are followed by an improvement in the $\dot{D}O_2$ to O_2 consumption ($\dot{V}O_2$) ratio (O_2 extraction [O_2 Extr] ratio) are beneficial and should be reinforced. Conversely, the deterioration of O_2 balance data indicate that the therapeutic course may not be optimal. The importance of these comments in the light of modern monitoring technology is that these changes can be followed continuously and on a real-time basis. This will provide clinicians the opportunity to modify therapeutic plans in a timely fashion with positive feedback. However, equally important to the management of critically ill patients is the accuracy with which the currently obtained values are reproduced, and the limits to which accuracy can and should be sought in a biologic system. For example, many publications in recent years have focused on the differences between values obtained for systolic and diastolic BP using indwelling arterial lines and routine auscultated measurements. To add to the confusion, differences are also noted between various arterial monitoring sites, and often the question is raised as to which value is "correct" and should be recorded and, more importantly, treated. Unfortunately, although a great deal of scientific argument can be brought to bear on answering this question, as much emotion as logic dictates the answer, and treatment appears to be based as much on superstition and clinical feel as on physiology. This phenomenon is equally evident in the monitoring of $\dot{D}O_2$ and utilization and in its interpretation, especially with respect to patient management. For too long the absolute partial pressure of oxygen in a patient's arterial blood sample has held pride of place in the eyes of the clinician and critical care nurse. Rather, it is far more important to evaluate the overall $\dot{D}O_2$ system, and initiate an investigation of aerobic metabolism. In fact, the likelihood exists that future management will be to modify a patient's physiologic state to approach optimal hemodynamic and O_2 transport values rather than to accept a return to normal values. In this context, the utilization of O_2 transport variables will prove more beneficial than reliance on more traditional monitoring and assessment aids. Therefore, the recently developed and available technologies in critical care medicine appear to be concentrating in an appropriate area of patient management which, hopefully, will improve outcome and decrease length of stay in the intensive care area.

Pulse Oximetry

Over the past several years, the pulse oximeter has become a widely accepted and used device in the operating room, and it is appearing more frequently in the intensive care environment. The ability to measure So_2 noninvasively stems from the research of Takuo Aoyagi, a Japanese physiological bioengineer, who was interested in using an ear oximeter to measure injected dye concentrations noninvasively during cardiac output determinations (1). The dye dilution curve obtained contained pulsatile variations which made calculation of cardiac output impossible. It was noted that the interfering pulse signal was detected at 900 nm while cardiogreen dye was sensed at 630 nm. In attempts to eliminate the variability of the curve, the pulse signal was electronically subtracted from the dye signal, but the cancellation was not complete, in retrospect due to the changes in So_2 occurring with the inflow of fresh arterial blood with each heart beat. Serendipity had placed appropriate absorption wavelengths together in the hands of an investigator who was able to recognize the potential for measuring So_2 noninvasively. Oxygenated and reduced Hgb have different absorption characteristics when exposed to red light at 660 nm and infrared light at 940 nm. As O_2 desaturates, red light transmission is decreased and infrared transmission is increased. Therefore, theoretically it became possible to measure blood So_2 by comparing the absorption spectra of the two different wavelengths when shone through a suitable tissue bed. The major barrier to calculating the So_2 of blood in living tissues has been to differentiate the absorption of light due to oxygenated and reduced Hgb and the absorption due to other tissue components through which the light shines. The advantage for pulse oximetry was the recognition that although each tissue component absorbs a portion of light at each of the wavelengths in question, this absorption is constant for a given site. The only variation is in the light absorption from the blood added during every cardiac cycle (2). This is the interference noted by Aoyagi but, when translated into a plethysmographic waveform at the red and infrared wavelengths, the relationship between the amplitude of the two pulsatile signals is linearly related to arterial saturation. Careful attention to probe position and effect of incident light and patient movement is necessary to provide an accurate reading, but if sufficient care is taken, the device works well and provides an extremely valuable aid to patient diagnosis and management (Fig. 1). Clinical judgment is notoriously unreliable when it comes to estimating Cao_2. The appearance of cyanosis depends upon the Hgb concentration and the observer, and often a patient is in extremis before desaturation is noted and appropriate remedial action is taken. However, the use of frequent arterial blood gas determinations is the hallmark of modern critical care medicine, and the necessity for continuous, noninvasive measurements could be questioned.

In fact, a debate between the utility of continuous versus intermittent measurements will be a focus of this discussion, and there is no compelling evidence at this point which establishes the validity of either position. In many advertisements, the implication is that if any measurement is valuable, then it must be more valuable if it is available continuously. Unfortunately, in no series has it been shown that clinicians are capable of responding in a continuous fashion to new data, but with the advent of increased use and sophistication of computer-assisted patient care programs, in the future continuous care may match the availability of the data.

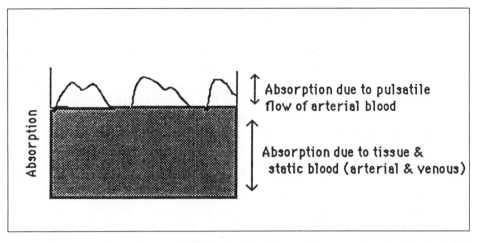

Fig. 1. Pulse oximetry and tissue light absorption. The problem associated with the development of a clinically useful device to measure So$_2$ was to differentiate between absorption by the tissues and absorption by oxygenated Hgb. The pulse oximeter overcomes this difficulty by measuring the saturation of blood added to the system with each heart beat. This corresponds to arterial O$_2$Hgb saturation. Adapted from: Petty TL: Clinical Pulse Oximetry Webb-Waring Lung Institute, Denver, CO (Sponsored by Ohmeda, Division BOC).

Another problem which affects the pulse oximeter is the lack of published data from critical care environments indicating the stability and reliability of the results obtained. In fact, in a recent case in our ICU in which a patient was being followed by pulse oximetry, a random arterial blood gas revealed an SaO$_2$ of 88% while the pulse oximeter was reading 96%. Further investigation showed a carboxyhemoglobin (HbCO) saturation of 10% and a methemoglobin (MetHb) saturation of 2.4%. The important feature of this illustration is that the patient's O$_2$ transport was markedly reduced, and the continuous monitoring was ineffective in providing an adequate warning. The pulse oximeter must be recognized for what it is, and unfortunately, the recent enthusiasm for this device may have provided physicians a false sense of security that the manufacturers never intended. Certainly, the product specification brochure from Ohmeda states that "Carboxyhemoglobin may erroneously increase readings. The level of increase is approximately equal to the amount of carboxyhemoglobin present" (3). In fact, this information is also incorrect, but it is far more sensible to overestimate the detrimental effect of the presence of HbCO on O$_2$ transport in this fashion than to minimize it and be left with a false sense of security as happened above. Also, it is important to realize that the presence of MetHb has little if any effect on the accuracy of pulse oximetry. Additionally, the various pulse oximeters available do not measure the same values and each may be calibrated in a different fashion from its competitor. For example, the device supplied by Nellcor deals with a concept called functional saturation described by the relationship O$_2$Hgb/O$_2$Hgb + RHb, while the device from Ohmeda claims to measure O$_2$Hgb or fractional saturation. In practice, this definition specification accounts for a 1% to 2% saturation difference between the two devices. When compared, the Nellcor product reads higher, while the Ohmeda machine comes closer to agreeing with laboratory values under some circumstances. To add to the confusion, the IL282 cooximeter (Instrumentation Laboratories Inc, Lexington, MA) used in many blood gas laboratories as the reference standard for O$_2$ transport measurements is also affected by presence of certain pigments in the blood, but because its results are derived from values obtained from absorption spectra analysis at four discrete wavelengths, reported values are more likely to be accurate.

Despite these disadvantages, these devices are finding their rightful place in the care of the critically ill. They will continue to gain in popularity and value as long as their faults are recognized as well as their obvious strengths, and users recognize their responsibility for appropriate interpretation and use of the data.

Continuous Invasive Oximetry (Arterial and Venous)

In the summer of 1969, Neil Armstrong took "One small step for man, but one large step for mankind." Undoubtedly, the lunar lander was equipped with the most sophisticated guidance system then available. As a matter of historical record, it is interesting to note that on landing, the automated guidance control was bringing the Eagle into an uncharted area filled with boulders and unsuitable for landing. Armstrong's skills and intuition played the most significant role in the mission and, with emergency fuel warning lights flashing, he disengaged the autopilot and landed, thereby establishing *Tranquility Base*. It is important to realize that no matter how sophisticated our modern technology becomes, it will be important always to have clinicians capable of interpreting the monitored data and integrating it into an overall patient care plan with some chance of success.

Therefore, with any new technology, not only will it be important to validate the science behind the measurement, but it will also be necessary to integrate the technology, once accepted, into clinical practice. Knowledge of physiologic abnormality by itself does not alter patient condition or affect outcome. Yet, integration of technology into clinical practice is often slow and based on bias rather than on easily proven morbidity and mortality statistics.

Utilization of mixed venous saturation data is not new. In the early 1970s the Extra Corporeal Membrane Oxygenator (ECMO) Project was established to study patients with severe respiratory failure and determine whether or not newer management techniques could alter mortality. Looking at the entry criteria for patients into the study in the light of our current practice, it appears clear that advances in patient management have been such that the sickest patients in that study would be considered routine today. One of the impacts of this study on routine patient care was the increased aggressiveness toward interventional therapy and the introduction of newer technologies into bedside management. Evaluation of $S\bar{v}O_2$ and its incorporation into the calculation of intrapulmonary shunt was advocated as a means of improving patient management. Increasingly aggressive approaches to patient care have been advocated recently, and it is likely that this trend will continue into the future. Over the past several years it has become possible to measure spectrophotometrically $S\bar{v}O_2$ continuously using a specially modified pulmonary artery catheter which contains two fiberoptic light bundles. Because, as detailed previously, oxyhemoglobin (HbO_2) and reduced Hgb absorb specific wavelength light differently, the absorption of the light transmitted through the catheter is directly proportional to the SO_2 of the blood in whatever vessel the catheter tip is placed. Therefore, using spectrophotometry, SaO_2 and $S\bar{v}O_2$ can be measured continuously. At this time, venous catheters have gained a wider reputation, and there is a large body of opinion which favors their use, although no definitive study exists which proves their efficacy, even though their accuracy is documented in a variety of situations.

The potential value to be obtained from monitoring $S\bar{v}O_2$ is in the belief that the obtained result may represent the end balance or adequacy of O_2 transport. In order to review O_2 transport, it is necessary to delineate the determinants of $S\bar{v}O_2$ and place the measurement in perspective. $S\bar{v}O_2$ is affected by the following four variables: a) Hgb concentration, b) cardiac output, c) $\dot{V}O_2$, and d) SaO_2. It is easily recognized that a change in any of these variables will result in an alteration in $S\bar{v}O_2$. Because of the interdependence of these variables, it is likely that $S\bar{v}O_2$ will change before the others, and continuous assessment may afford a greater precision in following a patient's condition and permit earlier treatment of perceived deficiencies in $\dot{D}O_2$. Adequacy of cardiac output becomes perceived not in the terms of a mechanical function, but rather in the context of the adequate support of aerobic metabolism as evidenced by lack of metabolic acidosis, with an appropriate $S\bar{v}O_2$ value indicating adequate venous O_2 reserves. This use is supported by the fact that partial pressure of O_2 is the driving pressure of O_2 into the tissues. On the arterial side of the circulation, all of us are familiar with the use of arterial blood gases to help adjust ventilatory support parameters. However, patients with a well maintained PaO_2 can exhibit inadequate $\dot{D}O_2$ in situations of anemia or low cardiac output. Also, in sepsis and many other critical situations, patients' O_2 requirements may increase out of proportion to the supply afforded by adequate pulmonary function. It is always important to remember that in terms of augmenting O_2 transport, the most important variables are Hgb concentration and cardiac output. Control of metabolic rate by sedation, muscle relaxation, and hypothermia is sometimes required to decrease $\dot{V}O_2$ to levels supportable by available cardiac output and SO_2. Utilization of $S\bar{v}O_2$ data can aid in the management of these patients by providing timely information on the progress of the patient and effectiveness of therapy.

As with all other medical measurements, however, the effective use of $S\bar{v}O_2$ data depends upon the clinicians' understanding of the technique and its limitations. Unlike the pulse oximeter previously described, continuous $S\bar{v}O_2$ determination is not affected to any significant degree by the presence of HbCO. The spectral reflectance of HbCO at the wavelengths used by the available systems does not interfere with the calculation of SO_2. In fact, the error is of the order of 14% HbCO causing a 1% reduction in the calculated saturation. Like the pulse oximeter, there will be a discrepancy noted between the result obtained from the IL 282 cooximeter and the reflectance $S\bar{v}O_2$ because of a difference in the definition of Hgb saturation. The cooximeter determines saturation by dividing the HbO_2 concentration by the total Hgb concentration, while the in vivo oximeters divide the HbO_2 concentration by the Hgb available for O_2 binding.

The situation for MetHb is a little more complicated. It has a larger impact on the calculation of HbO_2 saturation because of its spectral absorption characteristics which are closer to the wavelengths used in the in vivo oximeters. The problem is again one of definition, and because of the lower proportion of MetHb contamination of samples in clinical practice, it is of less significance than the possible errors which could result from a poor understanding of the problems associated with overestimating the actual saturation and making erroneous assumptions about the adequacy of O_2 transport. The primary advantage of measuring $S\bar{v}o_2$ continuously is not in receiving an indirect measurement of cardiac output which originally was promoted as the primary use of the technology, but rather in assessing the overall O_2 supply and demand relationship upon which metabolism is based. Normal metabolism is based on the premise that O_2 will be delivered to normally functioning tissue in adequate supply to support aerobic metabolism. In the usual setting, if cardiac output, Hgb concentration, or Sao_2 are inadequate, increased desaturation of the venous blood will be noted. In other words, the patient's metabolic rate controls O_2 Extr from the blood. Sometimes, especially in the critically ill, septic patients, $\dot{V}o_2$ appears to be driven by $\dot{D}o_2$ and increased O_2 Extr from the blood does not occur. In this group, $S\bar{v}o_2$ values are uniformly high, and although peripheral tissue death occurs, a lactic acidosis does not develop. Shoemaker and others have advocated maintaining a high $\dot{D}o_2$ in these patients in order to drive their metabolism to values which will be greater than those usually perceived as being necessary for survival under normal circumstances. Some interesting evidence is available which makes this an attractive argument, and it will be through the use of this type of technology that these advances will be possible. Additionally, clinicians increasingly will be forced to adjudicate over the development and acquisition of new technology and permit only those devices which can impact upon the quality of care rendered and the chances of survival. Beyond this, however, is the willingness of clinicians to pay attention to the data produced and processed by new monitors and to modify traditional management plans based on this new information. Certainly, adequate controlled clinical trials are lacking which provide strong support for the routine use of continuous oximetry.

Intravenous and Transcutaneous Cardiac Pacing Techniques

Although an obvious comment, cardiac output is the product of SV and HR. It is the single most important feature in the delivery of O_2 to the peripheral tissues, because in the absence of circulation, local metabolism is self-limited and futile. The traditional method of augmenting cardiac output in the ICU has been inotropic support which has, at times, produced unpredictable results which may be long-lived and resistant to corrective therapy. Electrical pacing has become a practical therapeutic reality over the past several years with the introduction of several different types of pacing pulmonary artery catheters, newer transvenous pacing probes, and transcutaneous and transesophageal pacing systems. For purposes of the ICU, the newest and possibly most serviceable of the pacing techniques are transcutaneous, utilizing specially designed, prejelled adhesive electrodes; and transvenous, via pacing wires located in specially modified pulmonary artery catheters.

Transcutaneous, noninvasive electric pacing is now recognized as an effective and safe technique. Earlier problems of excessive cutaneous nerve stimulation and discomfort have been reduced with more efficient electrodes. Minimal interference with diaphragmatic activity is encountered if the electrodes are placed appropriately. Available units have output currents variable up to 140 milliamperes with rates adjustable from 30 to 180 beat/min. Ready access emergency pacing is extremely valuable in the critical care setting in which unexpected circulatory arrest may follow anesthetic administration, surgery, angiography, and multiple other therapeutic and diagnostic procedures. Additional benefit may be obtained in situations where heart rate increase can be used to suppress an ectopic cardiac focus or improve $\dot{D}o_2$.

Transvenous pacing has become more efficient and certain over the past several years. The original pacing system based on a pulmonary artery catheter utilized conductive metal bands in rings around the catheter at special locations which, when stimulated by a pacing generator, would enable atrial, ventricular, or atrioventricular sequential pacing if the appropriate contact was made between the catheter and the myocardium. As can be imagined easily, although the technique proved to be lifesaving on numerous occasions, the regularity with which capture could be obtained was variable and dependent on operator skill and experience with the device. Additionally, pacing currents were quite high and long-term pacing was difficult. Recently, pacing pulmonary artery catheters have been developed which permit passage of a specially designed wire through one of the lumens which has an exit site in the cavity of the right ventricle. If appropriate location of the catheter is confirmed by observing the right ventricular pressure waveform prior to passage of the pacing wire, ventricular capture and pacing can be accomplished readily and reliably. In most cases, the pacing current requirement will be low and long-term pacing success rate is high. Although not yet released, another catheter which has a two-wire capacity and which enables independent or sequential pacing of the right atrium and/or ventricle has undergone clinical trials. When generally available, this catheter will provide extensive infusion, monitoring, and pacing capacity which will provide clinicians with enormous flexibility.

The addition of mixed venous oximetry capabilities to a pacing catheter has been accomplished within one of the ventricular pacing models. In this configuration, ventricular pacing is possible without losing the ability to monitor $S\bar{v}o_2$ continuously. Obviously, the clinician will never be satisfied completely, and further capability will be desired for each of the catheters. In the future, it is likely that general-purpose catheters will be produced which will have a variety of empty lumens into which specific purpose probes will be inserted and replaced as the requirement for patient monitoring changes. Electrodes capable of providing continuous readout of pH, sodium and potassium concentration, O_2 partial pressure and Sao_2, and lactate concentration have been discussed. The difficult task facing equipment manufacturers and clinicians is that monitoring capability currently outstrips medical knowledge. There is no agreement on the appropriate manner in which to manage many critical illnesses, and without agreement, the future of continuous monitoring will rest more in the realm of that which is possible rather than in the area of that which is either necessary or useful. In fact, it is interesting to speculate on the development of critical care technology and ask whether or not current management techniques are based on the information that became available through technical advances rather than on information which could have been more useful if it had been developed prospectively from physiologic "need to know." Certainly, $\dot{V}o_2$ data have been recognized as valuable for years, and the modern ICU handles these data in an efficient, accurate and timely fashion; it is likely that this trend will continue because of the practical and appropriate nature of this information to management of the critically ill of all etiologies.

Noninvasive Cardiac Output Determination

Rapid determination of cardiac output has become a mainstay of patient management. Until recently, the ICU has been dependent upon the use of invasive techniques to acquire this information. The gold standard for cardiac output determination has remained the direct Fick method, which relies on the determination of $\dot{V}_{O_2}$ to determine output. Following this, cardiac output determination by indocyanine green dye dilution and calculation of the area under the resultant dye curve became common in the ICU. However, both of these methods are cumbersome and do not lend themselves to multiple, repetitive measurement. Using indicator dilution theory, the next step was the development of thermal signals as the indicator, and the now familiar thermal dilution cardiac output computation was developed and became used routinely. Developments in equipment and theory have made the measurement easy to perform and highly reproducible, but the disadvantage of an invasive measurement remains. Therefore, over the past few years developments in echocardiographic and imaging techniques have enabled the study of cardiac function without the necessity for formal catheterization. Unfortunately, until recently these methods required the use of expensive and highly sophisticated, bulky equipment which scarcely served the needs of the crowded and busy critical care area. Two new methods for cardiac output determination have become available recently. One utilizes the concept that flow per unit area is equal to output. In this technique, a Doppler ultrasonic flow probe is placed in the suprasternal notch, and the sound signal is reflected off the moving column of blood as it is ejected from the left ventricle in a similar fashion to the sonar signals used to detect and size underwater objects. By assuming the area of the aortic root to be constant and based on the circumference of a circle, the velocity of the ejected blood and the cross sectional area of the aorta are readily calculated. From this, cardiac output can be determined. Unfortunately, the technique is not easy to perform, and the results are not consistent. On the other hand, the method has been used successfully, and it does provide a means for determining cardiac output noninvasively without the use of highly sophisticated equipment. Obviously, the data will be intermittent and subject to operator error. Also, recent criticism has focused on the fact that the algorithm for the aortic arch surface area is scarcely accurate for the condition which exists in conditions of changing afterload and cardiac output.

Another method has been described which uses the concept of transthoracic bioimpedance or the theory that the passage of an electrical current across the chest cavity will be impeded by the contained structures. In theory, all structures will remain constant over time, and the only variable will be the amount of blood ejected from the left ventricle with each systole. (This is similar to the concept underpinning the pulse oximeter technology described earlier.) Although the method suffers from several problems (difficult to use at high HRs, requires meticulous placement of electrodes, etc.), it is gaining acceptance because it provides a heretofore unobtainable measurement — continuous SV. In this context lies the value of the measurement. To date, the most sensitive indicator of myocardial ischemia is obtained by transesophageal echocardiography. In this technique, the underlying concept is that myocardial ischemia is first detected by changes in ventricular wall motion. These abnormalities are visible on the views of the heart obtained by echo, and they correlate well with experimental models of induced ischemia; in other words, it has been noted that the wall motion changes appear consistently before EKG or other changes such as increases in pulmonary artery occluded or diastolic pressures. It is possible that the continuous observation of SV could provide similar information if interpreted in light of constant myocardial demands and $\dot{D}_{O_2}$ requirements. The primary advantage of noninvasive cardiac output determination is that it provides the opportunity to monitor selected patients in a variety of clinical situations in which the knowledge of heart function is of primary importance. For example, recently a patient awaiting a heart transplantation required maintenance support on a variety of inotropic agents. In the early stages of his hospitalization, he was stabilized with the use of a pulmonary artery catheter and inotropic support adjusted to optimize myocardial function. For obvious reasons, the pulmonary artery catheter was discontinued and the patient was left on the same concentrations of inotropic support therapy which required maintenance in the closely monitored environment of the ICU. This situation persisted until noninvasive cardiac output determinations confirmed the fact that the patient tolerated reduced doses of inotropic support without $\dot{D}o_2$ deterioration. Indeed, the patient was weaned from inotropic support without complication and was able to remain in a step-down ICU until a successful transplant procedure was performed several days later. During his time under non-ICU observation, the clinical impression of adequate cardiac output was confirmed by noninvasive measurement continuously. An additional advantage of this technique may be the qualitative measurement of extravascular lung water which is interpreted from basal values obtained for impedance characteristics for the patient compared to standard, idealized normal data which have been collected over the life of the technique. Another area in which the technique has been reported to be of benefit has been in the Emergency Department during the early resuscitation of trauma victims. Certainly, the insertion of a pulmonary artery flotation catheter is not always possible or indicated in the management of these patients, but there is little doubt that management could be augmented by knowledge of cardiac output as early as possible. Further work needs to be performed to validate the technique in a variety of clinical situations, but undoubtedly the technique will gain accuracy, popularity, and acceptance in the intensive care areas and perhaps even more widely in the operating room and postanesthetic recovery area. The active therapeutic intervention in cardiac function abnormalities perceived as early as possible will probably be the hallmark of future hemodynamic progress in critical care management.

Mechanical Ventilatory Support Techniques and Monitoring

Over the past few years, it has been interesting to follow the changes which have taken place in the philosophy of mechanical ventilatory support. In the 1950s, large tidal volumes and intermediate ventilatory rates were used to ensure patient comfort. Unwanted mechanical hyperventilation was overcome with the addition of deadspace tubing added to the breathing circuit, and sedation and paralysis were used commonly. Weaning was a process of intermittent trials of breathing off the ventilator, and early tracheostomy was a common occurrence. In the late 1960s and years following, the concept of supporting a patient's breathing while receiving mechanical ventilation was popularized, and the use of assist/control and intermittent mandatory ventilatory (IMV) techniques became commonplace. In addition, the support of functional residual capacity (FRC) as a goal of mechanical ventilation became accepted, and the use of PEEP to support this endpoint was established. Early development of these ideas was confounded by an exceptionally confusing "alphabet soup" of ventilatory terms, and the confusion was heightened by a difference in definition of end-expiratory pressure applied during spontaneous breathing (continuous positive airways pressure [CPAP]) and that applied with mechanical ventilation —

PEEP. Even worse was the fact that CPAP was more commonly utilized in pediatric patients because the technique of utilizing spontaneous respiratory effort with support of FRC was established in infant respiratory distress syndrome patients treated with nasal prong CPAP. Unfortunately, this became interpreted and misunderstood that PEEP was for adults, and CPAP was a pediatric technique. Subsequent debate over extremely high levels of PEEP and the values of IMV vs. assist/control vs. controlled mechanical ventilation (CMV) occupied much of the literature. However, despite the perceived benefits of the various techniques and much investigative research and patient care, mortality from respiratory failure remained high. Because of the perceived disadvantages of positive-pressure ventilation on cardiac function, great anticipation heralded the introduction of a new ventilatory technique which promised less disruption of circulatory stability — high-frequency positive-pressure ventilation, or jet ventilation. A definite advantage was the markedly reduced positive intrathoracic pressure required to support ventilation, and the advantages in management of head-injured patients and patients with pulmonary barotrauma were obvious. Unfortunately, after a rapid start with a great deal of interest and early acceptance of the technique and support equipment, the promise of a significant improvement in morbidity and mortality statistics in respiratory failure was not forthcoming. In part, the lack of progress with these techniques may have been the perceived radical nature of the therapy and the lack of recognized logic which supported the concept. Certainly, some impressive results were and continue to be published, and it is possible that this concept will remain strong in specific areas, such as the management of bronchopleural fistulas in which a rapidly cycling, low-pressure technique is extremely valuable. However, routine application in the ICU is unlikely.

Current mechanical ventilatory philosophy supports the use of FRC supporting techniques and reduction in the patient's work of breathing. Over the past several years, interest has focused on the expiratory side of the ventilatory process, and heretofore unexplained failures in separating patients from mechanical support have been clarified. Initially, CPAP modes were felt to be extremely useful because they not only preserved FRC by maintaining alveoli open with continuous pressure, but also inspiratory work of breathing was decreased. Unfortunately, a hidden cost in increased expiratory work of breathing was not appreciated until recently. Basically, man is designed for passive expiration. As the chest wall is expanded, elastic elements are stretched and the chest wall becomes unstable in an expanded state. At the termination of active inspiration, passive exhalation is the norm with a resumption of the previously existing lung volume. If there is an obstruction to exhalation, work of breathing increases markedly, and the patient experiences a feeling of dyspnea. This increased work of breathing can be monitored by measuring the total $\dot{V}o_2$. If the $P\bar{v}o_2$ is monitored continuously, significant changes will be seen if ventilator patterns are chosen which place an increased load on expiration. Unfortunately, expiratory pressure valves are so designed that as higher gas flows pass through them, increased resistance to flow becomes pronounced. In the early attempts to eliminate the inspiratory component to ventilatory work, continuous flow through the circuit certainly diminished inspiratory work, but it also increased resistance to expiration by placing an increased flow load on the expiratory valve. In this manner, a hidden and unexpected expiratory cost of breathing prolonged patient separation from mechanical support and was difficult to

235

reduce because of the available technology. Recently, pressure-support ventilation (PSV) has become available, and this technique is proving valuable in the management of difficult to wean patients. Unfortunately, although clinically promising, it is difficult to document advantages for one mechanical ventilatory support mode over another, and clinical intuition is frequently the determining factor in deciding how to manage the problem patient. The advantage for PSV is that inspiration is augmented by a positive pressure which rises to a predetermined, physician-set peak pressure, usually well below the patient's peak ventilator inflation pressure. During exhalation, the machine's circuit is pressurized to the preset PEEP without a continuous flow component. Therefore, a lower flow rate is placed on the exhalation valve which now works against the patient's own exhaled flow rate without the additional CPAP flow. This reduces the resistance to exhalation caused by exhalation valve inefficiency and minimizes the O_2 cost of breathing. In this manner, a different interaction between machine and patient is possible which provides support more efficiently than previously. It is important to remember that as the patient's inspiratory effort increases, a higher degree of pressure support will be necessary to match the flow rate across the larynx so that the patient does not experience inspiratory dyspnea. Experience continues to grow with this technique, and it is likely to increase in popularity.

 .other support technique which has been introduced recently is augmented r..nute ventilation. In this mode, the patient-ventilator interaction is primarily one of a monitored T-tube until the patient's minute ventilation falls below a preset minimum. At this point, the ventilator assists the patient with breaths of preset tidal volume. The spontaneously initiated and ventilator breaths can be added to any of the other previously described modes such as PSV, PEEP, and IMV, and it is possible that this technique will decrease the time of patient separation from the machine because it diminishes the necessity for active participation on the part of the critical care team. Additionally, the patient will progress at his own rate rather than the arbitrary speed dictated by clinicians. Often, hypercarbia is vigorously and inappropriately treated, especially in the immediate postoperative period. Experience has shown that if left alone, the patient will breathe appropriately for the narcotic load administered during the anesthetic, and extubation will be accomplished without difficulty. Another advantage to this approach is that postoperative fluid shifts will have less effect on a patient's progress because the overall amount of mechanical ventilation is likely to be reduced. Certainly, patient comfort is improved and the asynchrony between patient and machine is less evident than with other support techniques.

Recent advances in mechanical ventilatory support have been more than cosmetic alterations, although little change has been seen in overall morbidity and mortality statistics. More frequently, practitioners are attempting to ventilate patients with physiologic endpoints as goals rather than attempting to control blood gases within narrow limits which may not be appropriate for the clinical condition. Attention is paid to a patient's preoperative condition, and it is not appropriate to attempt to improve these normal values during the weaning process. This concept is traditionally more rigorously obeyed in medical ICUs, and only recently have similar considerations become more widespread in surgical units. In part, this may be due to the increasing age of the surgical population. Certainly, over the last decade the patients undergoing significant elective procedures are older and in many cases more frail than in the past. For this reason, these patients require a more invasive and diligent approach to their care if success is to follow. In this group, strict attention to details of $\dot{D}o_2$ and $\dot{V}o_2$ will help optimize cardiovascular and ventilatory support modes. In this context, John Downs and his co-workers have been using the concept of "dual oximetry" to determine an on-line shunt calculation which they feel helps physicians optimize ventilatory and circulatory support with minimal delay. On the surface, the concept appears valid because the whole purpose of mechanical ventilatory support should be to maximize lung function. This ideal should be met at the point of minimal shunt and maximal compliance following the earlier work of Fairlie and Suter. However, over years of experience, this concept has not been borne out. The corollary to this approach was one supported by Civetta in the mid 1970s in which the suggestion was made to manipulate whichever variables were necessary to maintain an intrapulmonary shunt fraction of 15% or less. Indeed, high levels of PEEP were employed often to accomplish this goal, and mortality was reduced in only one of many studies performed in an attempt to validate the concept. It is possible that the newer methods of determining Sao_2 and $S\bar{v}o_2$ may be more appropriate than direct blood gas analysis because of the speed of response, but overenthusiasm will need to be curbed because critical care medicine cannot afford to enthusiastically endorse any new technologic advance without the benefit of appropriate clinical results validation. However, there is little doubt that utilization of these technologies permits the clinician to achieve rapidly a set of ventilator parameters which appear to give the patient the best chance of success, especially in those instances in which initiation of support is complicated by an unstable hemodynamic state, and in which maintenance of spontaneous ventilatory effort is desirable.

In summary, the initiation of mechanical ventilation cannot be discussed in isolation. Positive-pressure ventilation alters the normal intrathoracic pressure relationships, and therefore, hemodynamic function. It would seem logical that any monitoring techniques which give early feedback on the interactions between the circulatory and respiratory systems should benefit patient care. However, the widespread application of these devices will await the results of careful, prospective controlled studies. It is to be hoped that the results will be as promising as the expectation.

Niros-Scope

To this point, although multiple methods to estimate O_2 transport have been discussed, all of the measurements have been reflections rather than direct measurements of the activity occurring at the cellular level. Obviously, in a variety of clinical conditions such as the high output state associated with systemic sepsis, these indirect measurements will overestimate the health of certain organ systems. A new noninvasive, near-infrared monitoring device has been developed which measures the absorbance characteristics of the enzyme which catalyzes the major portion of oxygen utilization — cytochrome c oxidase or, as abbreviated, cyt $aa3$. Cyt $aa3$ is the terminal member of the respiratory chain and catalyzes the use of O_2 for the provision of high-energy phosphates by oxidative phosphorylation. Because man is an aerobic animal and cellular function is dependent on oxidative metabolism, this enzyme system is probably the most direct indicator of individual organ sufficiency. To date, the Niros-Scope (Near Infrared Oxygen Sufficiency Scope) has been used to follow the redox state of brain and skeletal muscle tissue. Reports from the anesthetic literature suggest that the device may have excellent potential as an adjunct to CNS monitoring, and it is hoped that further availability of the monitor in a clinical setting will prove its efficacy. Unfortunately, at the present time the monitor is capable only of following the trend in a patient's oxidized cyt $aa3$ once a baseline set of values has been obtained. Therefore, in anesthesia the baseline is easily obtained in the awake state, and further change is referenced to the patient's individual normal state. However, in the critical care unit, baseline values may be abnormal when first obtained, and it will be important to have a wide body of experience with this device to determine acceptable values representing adequate function of various cellular areas such as the brain, liver, kidney and peripheral musculature. Additionally, although not yet reported, possibilities for intrauterine fetal monitoring must be considered.

The theoretic and practical applications of the Niros-Scope are described in detail elsewhere in this textbook.

Monitoring Systems and Integrated Unit Data Processing

The look of the ICU has not changed greatly over the past several years, and indeed the techniques used and responsibilities of the various members of the health care team have not developed as fast as might have been anticipated. In part, this phenomenon has been due to the large amount of time spent by nursing staff in the simple collection of data, and the integration of this information into a workable data base. Although multiple data acquisition and handling methods have been proposed to support the nursing effort and free the nurse from much of the charting responsibilities which have become necessary to the routine of the ICU, no single method has gained acceptance uniformly. At present, the answer to this challenge to critical care nursing practice and patient care may hold one of the keys to improved morbidity and mortality statistics. In most busy units, nursing availability is diminishing and nursing manpower studies do not show a reversal of this trend. In fact, the likelihood is that the future will bring even lower staff-to-patient ratios, and the manner of critical patient management will have to change in an appropriate manner without compromising care. One of the ways in which this redeployment of effort may be accomplished is in the automated entry of data into the patient's record and the concomitant diminution of the nurse's role as a secretary. Additionally, this will increase the information available at the bedside which will become more of a data collection point than a passive charting station. This increased capability will make the nurse more independent in carrying out appropriate therapeutic interventions, and delays in initiation of indicated treatment should decrease. New monitor capabilities and displays will help the nurse organize data so that physicians on rounds will have a more interactive discussion about each patient, and hopefully more complete plans will be made in a timely fashion.

The concept of the automated physiologic profile is not new, and in many units this has become a routine method of patient care. However, it is important to realize that in a number of ICUs this concept is neither understood nor practiced. In part, this is due to poor or outdated equipment which, coupled with the current nursing manpower shortage, has made gathering routine hemodynamic data difficult and often incompatible with the available nurse/patient ratio. Certainly, data acquisition can be accomplished with varying degrees of automation, but usually any lack of sophistication has been overcome by a variety of dedi-

238

cated personnel whose duty it has been to be monitor or computer watchers. As research systems became commonplace, these tasks fell to nursing, and the care given to each patient began to suffer because of the increased demands placed on the nurse's time. Requirements for preparation of individual care plans, quality assurance mandated surveillance responsibilities, and change of shift reports have taken up much of the time. In fact, the critical care unit has become an area of documentation rather than of care. This is a trend which must be reversed by available technology.

However, certain problems need to be addressed before the wide variety of available data can be entered into the patient record. In all respects, the acquisition must be predetermined by the physician and nursing staff of the individual units concerned, and it must be remembered that it is unlikely that a system that works well in one institution will duplicate its success in another. Also, the personality and special function of specialized units must be remembered when the system is designed. It is unlikely that the needs of a coronary care unit will be met by the system placed into a busy trauma or surgical unit. The problems are different, and therefore, the solutions will also differ. Obviously, there will be similarities, and a multidisciplinary critical care committee will benefit most hospitals as a repository of ideas and an arena in which critical decisions can be made with maximum information. Some of the simple decisions to be made will involve the types of data which will be transferred directly into the data base and at what sampling frequency. Most automated systems can store far more information than can be used, and in many situations a lack of selectivity leads to confusion and data paralysis, i.e., the results are available and the correct therapy may be indicated, but the data display may preclude easy access to the appropriate alternative.

Therefore, the concept of user friendliness takes on a new meaning in this context. No longer is it adequate for a computer-driven system to prescribe the prerogatives of a unit; rather, the unit will impose its personality and specific requirements on the system. Nursing care plans will become a reflection of the needs of specific patient groups, and physicians will receive the information necessary to treat specific abnormalities rather than the whole range of raw information collected. Data collection, organization, and manipulation must become a transparent process which becomes second nature to the caregivers. If the setup and calibration of ICU monitors, and the initial entry of a patient into the data base requires a lot of time which otherwise could be spent providing care, nursing staff will ignore the technology appropriately. On the other hand, if the staff can appreciate a patient benefit early in the initiation of a new system, the likelihood is that the interaction between machine and unit will be appropriate. The ideal situation is one in which nursing is involved in the design and purchase of any data base and monitoring system. In this manner, a realistic appreciation of nursing requirements will be obtained, and all staff members will have a vested interest in making the system work.

A major potential benefit of this type of ICU system is the potential for medical organization and display of relevant information. Unfortunately, medical decisions in the ICU are often hindered by the ability of the physicians to have an organized presentation of relevant information in an appropriate time period. Too frequently the information is jumbled, and in many instances a great deal of time is spent reviewing normal information.

In fact, unless a great deal of care is taken to avoid the pitfall of complacency, the recitation of normal information may lull the practitioner into a false sense of security, and an abnormal data point may be overlooked in the rush. Although the critical care unit should not become a nonclinical area, more frequently than not, subtle changes in the information derived from special investigations may warn clinicians of impending problems. For example, a recent admission to our surgical ICU was a 77-yr-old female who had suffered a massive GI hemorrhage and associated colon perforation. Surgical control was accomplished with a left hemicolectomy, and the abdomen was irrigated copiously and drained appropriately. In the emergency department prior to surgery, the patient had complained of crushing substernal chest pain, and intraoperative pulmonary artery pressures revealed high filling pressures with a depressed cardiac output and wide arterial-to-venous O_2 content difference. Postoperative isoenzyme determinations were positive for myocardial infarction, and the patient had a prolonged ICU course complicated by severe pulmonary dysfunction, renal and cardiac insufficiency, hematologic abnormalities, and sepsis. Prognosis in this group of patients is poor, and yet all critical care practitioners have treated similar problems with success. It is possible that the monitoring capacities now available will enable a greater degree of success in the management of these problems than in the past by providing timely, physiologically important information which alters treatment. At present, this is an unrealized wish. However, as this patient went on to make a good recovery, so future patients will with increasing frequency. In part, this must come from the rapid interpretation of measurements obtained invasively, and appropriate and timely therapeutic interventions based upon these data. In this particular patient, a major problem was in balancing the undeniable need for increased $\dot{D}o_2$ with the fact of a recent myocardial infarction and the desire to minimize myocardial work. It is possible that the use of continuous, dual oximetry methods enabled the care team to make rational decisions regarding ventilator support, inotropic and vasodilator therapy, and nutritional formulae. It was also interesting to watch how $S\bar{v}o_2$ changes correspond to antibiotic administration.

The ICU is becoming more of a clinical laboratory than ever before. Appropriate data handling and integration into patient care may hold one of the future keys to reduced morbidity and mortality. Certainly, individual unit analysis of available data and comparison among other ICUs, both local and national, may aid in interpretation and future therapy. It is not appropriate to throw much of the information away for lack of the ability to store it and manipulate it. Nursing staff can not be expected to solve the problem by improvements in charting, and patient care requirements will demand more nursing time, not less.

Summary

Patient care in the modern critical care unit is nurse, physician, and monitor-intensive. Acquisition and organization of data from a variety of sources have become major challenges. Not only is it important to guarantee the accuracy of data entered into the chart, but also, appropriate manipulation and display of the information is mandatory if timely therapeutic decisions are to be made. Unfortunately, information common to all critical illness is undefined, and it will be necessary to analyze data in a prospective, comparative fashion to define this required body of knowledge. In turn, this will require a more accurate and "friendly" means of entering information into a data base which will not require a large amount of nursing effort and which will be free of observer bias and documentation error. The amount of information available to the critical care practitioner has increased greatly over the past several years, and the technologic support of critical care medicine has made many therapeutic and diagnostic advances possible. However, the tendency for small successes to breed traditions is well documented in the field, and management controversies will continue to smoulder until adequate data are available for analysis and interpretation. For example, the use of steroids in critical illness has been a mainstay of therapy in a large number of situations. Certainly, there has been a wide variety of opinion on this issue, and recently, the results of two large series were released which may alter practice in future. However, I am sure all practitioners recognize the fact that steroid use will continue to be a heavily debated topic, and that one publication is unlikely to alter established therapeutic regimens.

This discussion has focused on some of the newer devices which are available to the ICU staff for assessing adequacy of O_2 transport and managing deficiencies if they occur. The important feature of many of these technologies is that they provide information noninvasively, rapidly, and in a format which is compatible with management of patients in a variety of environments. No longer are bulky, slow machines a requirement. Rather, the newer trends are more like the futuristic devices alluded to earlier in the *Star Trek* series. As our technology grows, so will the information provided. It will be important for future advances in critical care technology to reflect physiologic requirements of patient management rather than the capabilities of the equipment manufacturers. In this fashion, critical care technology will continue to be state of the art and responsive to the practitioner.

References

1. Severinghaus J, Honda Y: History of blood gas analysis. VII. Pulse oximetry. *J Clin Monit* 1987; 3:135

2. Petty TL: Clinical Pulse Oximetry. Webb-Waring Lung Institute, Denver, CO, 1986 (Sponsored by Ohmeda, Division of BOC)

3. Ohmeda: Biox 3700 Pulse Oximeter. Operating/Maintenance Manual, Boulder, CO, Revision H, 1985, p 28

Selected References

Oxygen Transport

Bryan-Brown CW, Ayres S (Eds): New Horizons: Oxygen Transport and Utilization. Fullerton, CA, Society of Critical Care Medicine, 1987

Shoemaker WC: Pathophysiology, monitoring, outcome prediction, and therapy of shock states. *In:* Critical Care Clinics. Systemic Responses to Anesthesia and Surgery. Waxman K (Ed). Philadelphia, WB Saunders and Co, 1987, p 307

Snyder JV, Pinsky MR (Eds): Oxygen Transport in the Critically Ill. New York, Year Book Medical Publishers, 1987

These three references support the concept that the determination and manipulation of $\dot{D}o_2$ is of primary importance in the management of critically ill patients. It is exciting to think that this interest is a continuation of the physiologic observations that have been made over the years and which have been forgotten in the more obvious and easier management modes in the ICU. All of these references are exceptionally well written and referenced, and the critical care practitioner is encouraged to obtain them.

Pulse Oximetry

In addition to references 1, 2, and 3 above, the following articles discuss some newer applications for and drawbacks of pulse oximetry.

Mihm FG, Halperin BD: Noninvasive detection of profound arterial desaturations using a pulse oximetry device. *Anesthesiology* 1985; 62:85

Partridge BL: Use of pulse oximetry as a noninvasive indicator of intravascular volume status. *J Clin Monit* 1987; 3:263

Raemer DB, Warren DL, Morris R, et al: Hypoxemia during ambulatory gynecologic surgery as evaluated by the pulse oximeter. *J Clin Monit* 1987; 3:244

Sidi A, Rush W, Gravenstein N, et al: Pulse oximetry fails to accurately detect low levels of arterial hemoglobin oxygen saturation in dogs. *J Clin Monit* 1987; 3:257

Yelderman M, New W: Evaluation of pulse oximetry. *Anesthesiology* 1983; 59:349

Continuous Invasive Oximetry

Baele PL, McMichan JC, Marsh HM, et al. Continuous monitoring of mixed venous oxygen saturation in critically ill patients. *Anesth Analg* 1982; 61:513

Boutros AR, Lee C: Value of continuous monitoring of mixed venous blood oxygen saturation in the management of critically ill patients. *Crit Care Med* 1986; 14:132

Gutierrez G, Pohil RJ: Oxygen consumption is linearly related to O_2 supply in critically ill patients. *J Crit Care* 1986; 1:45

Lumb PD: Monitoring Beyond the Wedge: Theories, Applications and Controversies of Continuous $S\bar{v}O_2$ Monitoring. Abstracts of the Intensive Care Symposium of the College of Medicine of King Saud University, King Saud University Press, 1407 A.H. (12-13 April,1987)

McMichan JC, Baele PL, Wignes MW: Insertion of pulmonary artery catheters — A comparison of fiberoptic and nonfiberoptic catheters. *Crit Care Med* 1984; 12:S17

Norwood JH, Nelson LD: Continuous monitoring of mixed venous oxygen saturation during aortofemoral bypass grafting. *Am Surg* 1986; 52:114

Orlando R: Continuous mixed venous oximetry in critically ill surgical patients: High-tech cost effectiveness. *Arch Surg* 1986; 121:470

Whire KM: Completing the hemodynamic picture: $S\bar{v}O_2$. *Heart Lung* 1986; 14:272

Cardiac Pacing Techniques

Lumb PD: Atrioventricular sequential pacing with a pulmonary artery catheter: A comparison with epicardial wires. Abstr. 9th Annual Meeting of the Society of Cardiovascular Anesthesiologists, Palm Desert, CA, May 10-13, 1987

Instruction manual for the Zoll Noninvasive Temporary Pacemaker. Cambridge, MA, ZMI Corporation, 1987

Noninvasive Cardiac Output Determination

Huntsman LL, Stewart DK, Barnes SR, et al: Noninvasive Doppler determination of cardiac output in man: Clinical validation. *Circulation* 1983; 67:593

Levy BI, Payen DM, Tedgui A, et al: Noninvasive ultrasonic cardiac output measurement in intensive care unit. *Ultrasound Med Biol* 1985; 11:841

Loeppky JA, Hoekenga DE, Greene ER, et al: Comparison of noninvasive pulsed Doppler and Fick measurements of stroke volume in cardiac patients. *Am Heart J* 1984; 107:339

Mancini GBJ, Costello D, Bhargava V, et al: The isovolemic index: A new noninvasive approach to the assessment of left ventricular function in man. *Am J Cardiol* 1982; 50:1401

Nishimura RA, Callahan MJ, Schaff HV, et al: Noninvasive measurement of cardiac output by continuous-wave Doppler echocardiography: Initial experience and review of the literature. *Mayo Clin Proc* 1984; 59:484

Sramek BB: Why Should Cardiac Output be Measured/Monitored? Customer Information Bulletin # 0005. Irvine, CA, BoMed Medical Manufacturing, Ltd, March 20, 1986

Near-Infrared Oxygen Sufficiency Scope

Jobsis-VanderVliet FF, Fox E, Sugioka K: Monitoring of cerebral oxygenation and cytochrome *aa3* redox state. *Intern Anes Clin* 1987; 25:209

These references will amplify the individual monitoring sections and provide background information on which individual physicians will be able to base acquisition decisions. Technological capacity is in advance of clinical management in many areas, and the clinician must understand the available equipment fully in order to maximize its use and improve patient care.

General

Extracorporeal Support for Respiratory Insufficiency. A Collaborative Study in Response to RFP-NHLBI-73-20. Bethesda, MD, National Heart, Blood and Lung Institute, 1979

Protocol for Extracorporeal Support and Respiratory Insufficiency. Bethesda, MD, National Heart, Lung and Blood Institute, 1974

Gattinoni L, Pesenti A, Mascheroni D, et al: Low-frequency positive-pressure ventilation with extracorporeal CO_2 removal in severe acute respiratory failure. *JAMA* 1986; 256:881

NIH Consensus Development Conference on Critical Care Medicine. *Crit Care Med* 1983; 11:466

These references will give a great deal of insight into the progress which has been made in the management of patients with acute lung injuries. Also, the frustration of the early investigators can be implied from some of the results and the recognition of current inability to manage the next generation of acute lung injuries. It is interesting to think that a return to a modified ECMO may hold a great deal of promise as demonstrated by Gattinoni et al.

Chapter 13

The Hepatorenal Syndrome

Guido O. Perez MD, and Eugene R. Schiff, MD

Outline

Educational Objectives

In this chapter the reader will learn:

1. the pathogenesis of functional renal failure in patients with liver disease.

2. to properly evaluate patients with renal failure and liver disease.

3. to attempt to maximize efforts to reverse the hepatorenal syndrome among that select group of patients where this is possible.

Introduction

The hepatorenal syndrome (HRS) is defined as the development of progressive acute renal failure in a patient with advanced liver disease, unexplained by other known causes of renal dysfunction (1, 2). It is generally believed that the HRS is a functional disorder characterized by renal hypoperfusion with preferential renal cortical ischemia. This cortical vasoconstriction may be triggered by decreased "effective" blood volume, but the putative effectors that mediate these changes remain incompletely defined.

The HRS can be prevented and prompt attention should be paid to contributory factors such as bleeding, sepsis, vomiting, excessive diuresis or paracentesis, and nephrotoxic agents that may precipitate acute renal failure. Among the latter, particular care should be taken to avoid inhibitors of prostaglandin synthesis (nonsteroidal anti-inflammatory drugs) and antibiotics such as aminoglycosides and demeclocycline, especially in patients with decreased renal function. Finally, profuse diarrhea induced by excessive lactulose or other agents may induce extracellular fluid volume contraction and precipitate the HRS.

Clinical Approach

As recently emphasized in the literature (3), the serum creatinine concentration is not a reliable index of renal function in patients with decompensated cirrhosis. Many patients exhibit markedly reduced creatinine or inulin clearances in the presence of a normal or near-normal serum creatinine concentration. This may relate to decreased lean body mass and to other unidentified factors. Likewise, the BUN may also underestimate the degree of renal functional impairment. Thus, it is recommended that the clearance of creatinine or one of the commercially available radiopharmaceuticals be used to assess the renal function in these patients.

Conditions in which hepatic and renal dysfunction result from simultaneous injury to both organs (pseudo-hepatorenal syndrome) should be excluded. They include sepsis (leptospirosis, Gram-negative sepsis), circulatory problems (shock, heat stroke, end-stage congestive heart failure), genetic disorders (polycystic kidneys, Wilson's disease, sickle cell anemia), coagulopathies (DIC), toxins (carbon tetrachloride, amanita phalloides), and systemic vasculitis (lupus, polyarteritis). Chronic glomerular disease in the form of IgA nephritis or as a result of hepatitis B infection may also occur in patients with chronic liver disease.

It should be kept in mind that patients with obstructive jaundice, sepsis, or GI bleeding may be prone to acute intrinsic renal failure (ATN) and that extracellular fluid volume depletion leading to pre-renal azotemia is very common in cirrhosis. Because ATN and pre-renal azotemia are so prevalent in this population, and are reversible, measurement of urinary sodium concentration or fractional sodium excretion (F_{ENa}) and examination of the urinary sediment should be performed during the initial evaluation. In oliguric ATN, the F_{ENa} is greater than 2% and urinary osmolality (Uosm) is similar to that of plasma (Fig. 1, Table 1). Nevertheless, ATN cannot always be separated from HRS or from pre-renal failure using the urinary diagnostic indices. In addition, in some patients ATN develops following the onset of pre-renal azotemia or HRS. Thus, patients with HRS may exhibit active urinary sediments with numerous renal tubular epithelial cells suggestive of ATN (4).

A greater difficulty may be encountered in separating the HRS from prerenal azotemia because the urinary indices (Uosm, F_{ENa}) are similar in both (Fig. 1, Table 1). Measurement of CVP or pulmonary capillary wedge pressure (WP) and a carefully conducted trial of volume expansion is indicated in this situation. A CVP or WP of >8 to 10 mm Hg and a lack of response to volume expansion are suggestive of HRS. Unfortunately, some patients exhibit a WP in the range of

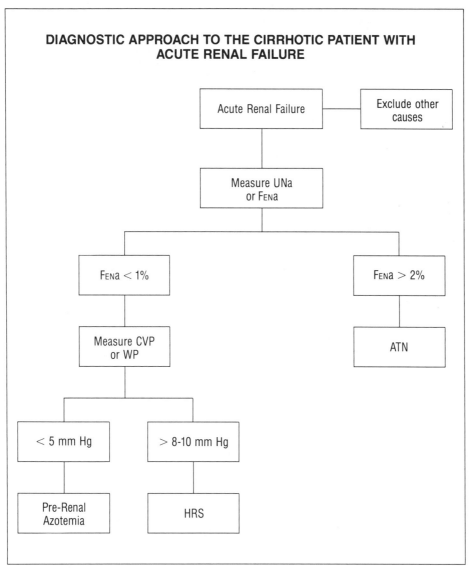

DIAGNOSTIC APPROACH TO THE CIRRHOTIC PATIENT WITH ACUTE RENAL FAILURE

Acute Renal Failure — Exclude other causes

Measure UNa or F_{ENa}

$F_{ENa} < 1\%$

$F_{ENa} > 2\%$

Measure CVP or WP

ATN

< 5 mm Hg

> 8-10 mm Hg

Pre-Renal Azotemia

HRS

Fig. 1. The main diagnostic considerations are pre-renal azotemia, acute tubular necrosis and the hepatorenal syndrome (HRS). The fractional excretion of sodium (F_{ENa}) or the urinary sodium concentration in a spot urine, and the pulmonary capillary wedge pressures (WP) or the central venous pressure (CVP) may help to distinguish among these diagnostic possibilities.

only 5 to 10 mm Hg, which fails to increase substantially in response to volume expansion. This may be related to increased venous capacitance and to rapid movement of fluid out of the intravascular compartment. The renal function response to volume expansion may also be inconclusive in these patients.

In order to illustrate the application of the above-mentioned approach to patients with suspected HRS, we present here the data recently obtained in several patients. Of note, in the only study of the HRS in which hemodynamic measurements were reported (5) the diagnostic criteria were not rigidly defined. We believe that the clinical diagnosis of HRS should be made on the basis of

Table 1. Urinary findings in the differential diagnosis of the hepatorenal syndrome

	Pre-renal Azotemia	Hepatorenal Syndrome	Acute Renal Failure (ATN)
Urine Sodium Concentration (mEq/L)	< 10	< 10	> 30
F_{ENa} (%)	< 1	< 1	> 2
Urine to Plasma Creatinine Ratio	> 30:1	> 30:1	< 20:1
Urine to Plasma Osmolality Ratio	> 1	> 1	1
Urine Sediment	Normal	Cellular Debris	Casts, Cellular Debris

a) clinical or biopsy diagnosis of cirrhosis or hepatic failure; b) acute azotemia usually associated with oliguria; c) urinary sodium concentration of less than 10 mEq/L or F_{ENa} less than 1%; d) CVP or WP greater than 8 to 10 mm Hg; and e) partial or no response to colloid volume expansion.

Because our patients fulfilled these criteria, they were transferred to the intensive care unit for close monitoring. Cardiac output ranged from 5.3 to 14 L/min and peripheral vascular resistance from 442 to 1441 dyne·sec/cm⁵ (Table 2). Volume expansion was performed with 5% albumin given at 50 ml/h for at least 24 h. Two patients experienced a partial response with an increase in urine

Table 2. Initial renal function and hemodynamics in patients with HRS

	Patient						
	1	2	3	4	5	6	7
Serum Creatinine (mg/dl)	6.8	2.8	4.0	2.6	4.5	5.2	2.9
Urine Flow (ml/min)	5.0	5.0	40.0	30.0	10.0	5.0	10.0
UNa (mEq/L)	<10	<10	<10	12	<10	<10	<10
Uosm (mOsm/kg)	370	340	70	-	-	-	400
Mean BP (mm Hg)	83	91	90	80	70	90	76
CVP (mm Hg)	21	9	8	12	11	8	10
WP (mm Hg)	14	14	8	14	12	16	13
PAP (mm Hg)	45/23	26/12	30/20	39/17	28/15	35/20	30/18
CO (L/min)	5.8	12.4	9.5	14.0	10.7	7.8	5.3
PVR (dyne·sec/cm⁵)	1412	498	902	652	442	970	996

UNa = urine sodium concentration, Uosm = urine osmolality, CVP = central venous pressure, WP = pulmonary capillary wedge pressure, PAP = pulmonary artery pressure, CO = cardiac output, PVR = pulmonary vascular resistance.

output and stabilization in serum creatinine concentration. One of these patients (No. 4) remained azotemic for about one month and then improved progressively so that 6 months after admission the serum creatinine concentration was 1.4 mg/dl. The remaining five patients failed to respond to volume expansion and expired soon after the studies were performed.

Pathophysiology

There is a strong evidence that the renal failure in HRS is functional in nature. The documentation of normal sodium reabsorption and intact urinary concentrating ability suggests tubular functional integrity. Several studies utilizing varied techniques have demonstrated a substantial reduction in renal perfusion with marked cortical ischemia in this condition. Moreover, the abnormality appears to be reversible as evidenced by the return of renal function once the kidneys are transplanted into a normal host.

The mechanism(s) associated with the renal hypoperfusion in HRS has not been elucidated. Most studies suggest enhanced synthesis of vasoactive humoral factor(s) capable of causing intense renal vasoconstriction and/or decreased production of endogenous vasodilatory agent(s). The abnormalities may arise in response to decreased effective plasma volume and as a result of the inability of the liver to produce, metabolize, or inactivate endogenous substances.

Vasoconstrictive Mechanisms That May Participate in the HRS

Endotoxins

It has been proposed that endotoxemia may contribute to the pathogenesis of HRS (6). Endotoxin has profound effects on renal function that could result in some of the renal abnormalities in the HRS. Nevertheless, a correlation between endotoxemia and the HRS has not been confirmed by all investigators (7, 8).

Sympathetic Nervous System

Several studies have shown increased adrenergic activity in cirrhosis. Presumably, the enhanced sympathetic tone is due to decreased effective plasma volume and may lead to renal vasoconstriction. A relationship between changes in renal function and plasma catecholamine levels has not been shown by all investigators, however (9). In addition, there is no conclusive evidence that false neurotransmitters play a role in the pathogenesis of HRS.

Renin-Angiotensin System

Plasma renin activity is frequently elevated in decompensated cirrhosis with or without the hepatorenal syndrome (10, 11). In light of the clinical and experimental evidence that angiotensin plays an important role in the control of renal circulation, it has been suggested that the enhanced activity of the renin-angiotensin system in cirrhosis contributes to the pathogenesis of the HRS.

Thromboxanes

The studies of Zipser et al. (12) showed enhanced urinary thromboxane B_2 activity in the urine of patients with HRS. Unfortunately, administration of a thromboxane synthetase inhibitor to patients with the HRS did not result in reversal of the progressive impairment of renal function (13).

Deficient Vasodilatory Mechanisms That May Contribute to the Pathogenesis of HRS

Prostaglandins

The possibility that a decrease in the renal synthesis of vasodilatory prostaglandins contributes to the pathogenesis of HRS has been raised in several studies (14, 15). Specifically, it has been shown that administration of prostaglandin synthetase inhibitors to these patients may result in marked decrements in renal function and precipitation of the HRS. Nevertheless, intrarenal infusion of PGE in the HRS did not improve natriuresis or renal function (16).

Kallikrein-Kinin System

Bradykinin and other kinins may participate in the modulation of renal blood flow. Patients with HRS may exhibit very low prekallikrein levels (17), raising the possibility that decreased vasodilatory kinin formation may contribute to the renal vasoconstriction associated with HRS.

Atrial Natriuretic Factor

Atrial natriuretic factor (ANF) induces glomerular vasodilation and its deficiency could explain some of the renal functional abnormalities of HRS. Recent studies, however, suggest that ANF levels are normal to elevated in patients with decompensated cirrhosis (18). Nevertheless, it has been suggested that defective release of ANF in response to volume expansion might play a role (12).

Glomerulopressin

The liver may produce a hormone (glomerulopressin) that is involved in the regulation of glomerular function (19, 20). It has been proposed (21) that the diseased liver may not be able to synthesize this substance and that the abnormality may contribute to the pathogenesis of HRS.

Treatment

Supportive measures include provision of adequate nutrients and vitamins, correcting fluid and electrolyte abnormalities, and avoiding hepatotoxic and nephrotoxic agents.

Correction of Decreased Effective Plasma Volume

Once all correctable causes of acute renal failure are excluded, an attempt should be made to increase the effective plasma volume, even in patients with normal or near-normal CVP or WP, by intravenous infusion of colloid. The latter may be performed with albumin or by reinfusion of ascites. The use of fresh frozen plasma as a source of renin substrate has also been advocated (22). Unfortunately, these measures only result in transient improvement in renal function.

Head-out water immersion is known to augment central blood volume (23) and it has been suggested that it could be used for the treatment of HRS (24). Although systematic evaluation of this procedure has not been carried out, patients could only reasonably be immersed for short periods of time and only in specialized medical facilities.

Because ascites may have a negative influence on cardiac function, paracentesis has been advocated not only for the removal of ascites but also to improve renal perfusion (25). The procedure, if attempted, should be coupled with intravenous colloid infusion in view of the decreases in creatinine clearance associated with paracentesis.

Another way to improve a contracted plasma volume is to decrease vascular capacitance. Several vasoconstrictive agents such as metaraminol, norepinephrine, and phenylephrine have been used. Generally, these agents fail to increase the reduced systemic vascular resistance and do not induce a sustained improvement in renal function.

Correction of Renal Cortical Vasoconstriction

In light of the striking renal cortical ischemia that has been documented in patients with HRS, it is not altogether surprising that there have been numerous attempts to reverse this renal hemodynamic abnormality pharmacologically. Diverse agents including furosemide, dopamine, phentolamine, beta-blockers, captopril, saralasin, thromboxane inhibitors, and antibiotics (to decrease the production of endotoxin) have been utilized in an attempt to decrease cortical vasoconstriction. These manipulations generally have not resulted in sustained beneficial effects.

Hemodialysis and Ultrafiltration

Several investigators have reported that peritoneal dialysis and hemodialysis are ineffective in the management of HRS (26, 27). Although most of the published literature indeed suggests a dismal prognosis for patients who are dialyzed, such reports have dealt almost exclusively with patients with chronic end-stage liver disease. Our experience and that of others (28) suggests that in carefully selected patients, i.e., patients with hepatic dysfunction in whom there is reason to believe that the underlying liver disease may reverse (making long-term survival and even spontaneous recovery of renal function possible), dialytic therapy is indicated. Thus, sporadic case reports describe prolonged survival and improvement in renal function in selected patients with acute, or acute superimposed on chronic liver disease treated by dialysis alone (29, 30) or combined with other modalities (31, 32).

Dialysis may also play a role in the treatment of acute renal failure in patients with severe end-stage liver disease awaiting hepatic transplantation. Aside from complicating the medical management, the development of acute renal failure in this setting is associated with considerable morbidity and mortality not improved by dialysis. Nevertheless, in one study dialytic therapy was helpful in the life support of patients awaiting liver transplantation, and four of seven patients with HRS experienced recovery of renal function 1 to 5 weeks after successful hepatic replacement (33).

Because many patients with HRS are in hepatic coma, dialysis with a large pore-size polyacrylonitrile membrane may have a beneficial effect (34-38). Although in most studies there has been some neurologic improvement, survival was not improved. The available studies suggest that removal of toxic middle-sized molecules with this membrane may be responsible for the improvement in mental status. Charcoal hemoperfusion with or without prostacyclin infusion, as well as other therapeutic modalities for hepatic coma such as exchange transfusion, have been utilized in combination with dialysis for the treatment of combined hepatic and renal failure (32, 39).

Peritoneovenous Shunt

In 1974, LeVeen and associates (40) introduced the peritoneovenous shunt (PVS) for the treatment of refractory ascites. Subsequently, these authors reported five long-term survivals in nine patients whose HRS was treated with PVS. Other reports that followed (41-52) (Table 3) claimed long-term survival rates of approximately 40%. Nevertheless, careful scrutiny of the reported cases reveals that diagnosis of HRS was frequently inadequately documented, and that many of the original cases were included in subsequent series. Clear-cut beneficial results in patients with carefully established HRS were reported by Schroeder et al (44). Four of their five cases treated in this manner experienced long-term survival; nevertheless, all of their patients exhibited creatinine clearances greater than 50 ml/min prior to shunting, suggesting that they were treated at a very early stage of HRS. Of interest, there were no long-term survivors in ten patients with well established criteria for HRS recently reported by Smith et al (49).

Table 3. The peritoneovenous shunt in the treatment of hepatorenal syndrome

Author	No. Patients	Long-term Survival*	Comments
1. LeVeen et al (1976)	9	5	First report
2. Grossberg et al (1978)	11	4	May include 3 patients reported by Wapnick et al
3. Fullen (1979)	2	1	One patient bled 3 days post op
4. Schroeder et al (1979)	5	4	Baseline CcR 50 ml/min
5. Kinney et al (1979)	7	3	Cases may overlap with series 2
6. Greig et al (1980)	5	3	_____
7. Schwartz et al (1980)	5	2	Includes case reported by Pladson and Parrish
8. Bernhoft et al (1982)	9	3	One patient alive at 24 mo
9. Smith et al (1984)	10	0	Inhospital mortality
10. Kearns et al (1985)	1	1	Survival 13 mo
11. Stanley et al (1985)	14	7	Survival not different from controls
12. Daskalopoulos et al (1985)	11	3	_____
13. Linas et al (1986)	10	1	Patient survived 210 days
14. Cade et al (1987)	6	6	_____
	105	43	

Prospective randomized studies: 11, 12 and 13. Rigorous criteria for HRS only found in series 4, 9, 11, 12, and 13.
* Greater than 2 months.

Only three prospective randomized studies of the role of the PVS in the treatment of HRS have been performed (50-52). Linas et al. (50) prospectively compared the effects of the PVS shunt (n = 10) or medical therapy (n = 10) on renal function and mortality in 20 patients who had HRS associated with alcoholic liver disease. After 48 to 72 h, body weight and serum creatinine were increased with medical therapy and decreased (from 3.6 ± 0.4 to 3.0 ± 0.5, p <0.05) in patients with the shunt. Despite improvement of renal function, only one patient with PVS had a prolonged survival (210 days). In the remainder, survival was 13.0 ± 2.2 days compared to 4.1 ± 0.6 days with medical therapy.

The preliminary results of the Veterans Administration Cooperative study (51) showed that although there were seven long-term survivors in a group of 14 patients treated with PVS, the results were not statistically significant when compared to those of a group of 19 patients undergoing medical therapy. The mean half life of patients treated with the shunt did not differ significantly from that of controls. Of note, the group of patients with HRS was carefully selected, and patients with severe complications of chronic liver disease were excluded. Another study (52) suggested that PVS does not alter the survival in patients with HRS, but appears to prevent further progression of renal impairment.

From the above information, it can be concluded that the role of the PVS in the treatment of HRS has not been established. Although some patients exhibit an improvement in renal function, further controlled studies, with larger number of patients, are necessary to assess the effect of the PVS on long-term survival, quality of life, and the incidence of complications.

Portacaval Shunt

Schroeder et al. (44) reported encouraging results in patients with the HRS syndrome treated with side-to-side portacaval shunts. Unfortunately, the results have not been confirmed by others. In addition, the procedure itself is attended by substantial morbidity and mortality. This procedure should be regarded as experimental, and not established therapy.

Hepatic Transplantation

This is the ultimate modality of therapy that results in correction not only of the HRS (33, 53, 54), but also many of the metabolic complications of advanced liver disease. Obviously, the procedure is complicated, expensive, and performed a limited number of centers around the world. Thus, transplantation does not currently constitute a practical, cost-effective approach to managing these patients.

In summary, we recommend the following schema for the evaluation and management of acute renal failure in cirrhosis (Fig. 1). The three important diagnostic considerations are pre-renal azotemia, acute tubular necrosis, and the hepatorenal syndrome. The FE_{Na} or the urinary sodium concentration in a spot urine, and the WP or CVP may help to distinguish among these diagnostic possibilities. There is, however, considerable overlap between the three categories, and patients often present with more than one diagnosis. For example, patients with HRS often exhibit acute tubular necrosis; HRS and pre-renal failure often coexist. In fact, the response to colloid infusion is the only feature that may help differentiate the latter two conditions.

Treatment should be aimed initially to correct decreased plasma volume, discontinuing nephrotoxic agents, and optimizing nutrition and liver function.

Attempts to decrease cortical vasoconstriction with pharmacological agents have not been successful. Intensive hemodialysis and/or hemoperfusion is indicated for the management of HRS complicating acute (reversible) liver injury. In patients with advanced liver failure who are candidates for hepatic transplantation, dialysis may maintain the patient until a suitable liver donor is found. Otherwise, good-risk patients may be treated by the PVS. The role of paracentesis combined with colloid infusion in the management of HRS needs further study.

References

1. Papper S: Hepatorenal syndrome. *In:* The Kidney in Liver Disease, Second Edition. Epstein M (Ed). New York, Elsevier Biomedical, 1983, pp 86-106

2. Epstein M: Hepatorenal syndrome. *In:* Gastroenterology, Fourth Edition. Berk JE (Ed). Philadelphia, WB Saunders Co, 1985, pp 3138-3149

3. Papadakis MA, Arieff AI: Unpredictability of clinical evaluation of renal function in cirrhosis. Prospective study. *Am J Med* 1987; 82:945

4. Mandal AK, Lansing M, Fahmy A: Acute tubular necrosis in hepatorenal syndrome: An electron microscopic study. *Am J Kidney Dis* 1982; 2:363

5. Tristani FE, Cohn JN: Systemic and renal hemodynamics in oliguric hepatic failure. Effect of volume expansion *J Clin Invest* 1967; 46:1894

6. Liehr H, Jacob AI: Endotoxin and renal failure in liver disease. *In:* The Kidney in Liver Disease, Second Edition. Epstein M (Ed). New York, Elsevier, 1983, p 535

7. Clemente C, Bosch J, Rodes J, et al: Functional renal failure and haemorrhagic gastritis associated with endotoxaemia in cirrhosis. *Gut* 1977; 18:556

8. Gatta A, Milani L, Merkel C, et al: Lack of correlation between endotoxemia and renal hypoperfusion in cirrhotics without overt renal failure. *Eur J Clin Invest* 1982; 12:417

9. Epstein M, Larios O, Johnson G: Effects of water immersion on plasma catecholamines in decompensated cirrhosis. Implications for deranged sodium and water homeostasis. *Miner Electrolyte Metab* 1985; 11:25

10. Hollenberg NK: Renin, angiotensin and the kidney: Assessment by pharmacological interruption of the renin-angiotensin system. *In:* The Kidney in Liver Disease, Second Edition. Epstein M (Ed). New York, Elsevier, 1983, p 395

11. Schroeder ET, Eich RH, Smulyan H, et al: Plasma renin level in hepatic cirrhosis. *Am J Med* 1970; 49:186

12. Zipser RD, Radvan GH, Kronborg KJ, et al: Urinary thromboxane B2 and prostaglandin E2 in the hepatorenal syndrome: Evidence for increased vasoconstrictor and decreased vasodilator factors. *Gastroenterology* 1983; 84:697

13. Zipser RD, Kronborg I, Rector W, et al: Therapeutic trial of thromboxane synthesis inhibition in the hepatorenal syndrome. *Gastroenterology* 1984; 87:1228

14. Boyer TD, Zia P, Reynolds TB: Effect of indomethacin and prostaglandin A1 on renal function and plasma renin activity in alcoholic liver disease. *Gastroenterology* 1979; 77:215

15. Zipser RD, Hoefs JC, Speckart PF, et al: Prostaglandins: Modulators of renal function and pressor resistance in chronic liver disease. *J Clin Endocrinol Metab* 1979; 48:895

16. Zusman RM, Axelrod L, Tolkoff-Rubin N: The treatment of the hepatorenal syndrome with intrarenal administration of prostaglandin E. *Prostaglandins* 1977; 13:819

17. O'Connor DT, Stone RA: The renal kallikrein-kinin system: Description and relationship to liver disease. *In:* I The Kidney in Liver Disease, Second Edition. Epstein M (Ed). New York, Elsevier, 1983, p 469

18. Davidson EW, Dunn MJ: Pathogenesis of the hepatorenal syndrome. *Ann Rev Med* 1987; 38:361

19. Uranga J, Fuenzalida R, Rappaport AL, et al: Effect of glucagon and glomerulopressin on the renal function of the dog. *Horm Metab Res* 1979; 11:275

20. Uranga J, Fuenzalida R: Effect of glomerulopressin and a rabbit glomerulopressin and a rabbit glomerulopressin-like substance in the rat. *Horm Metab Res* 1979; 7:180

21. Coratelli P, Passavanti G, Munno I, et al: New trends in hepatorenal syndrome. *Kidney Int* 1985; 28:S-143

22. Cade R, Wagemaker H, Vogel S, et al: Hepatorenal syndrome. Studies of the effect of vascular volume and intraperitoneal pressure on renal and hepatic function. *Am J Med* 1987; 82:427

23. Levinson R, Epstein M, Sackner MA, et al: Comparison of the effects of water immersion and saline infusion on central hemodynamics in man. *Clin Sci Mol Med* 1977; 52:343

24. Bichet DG, Grines BG, Schrier RW: Effect of head out water immersion on hepatorenal syndrome. *Am J Kidney Dis* 1984; 3:258

25. Simon DM, McCain J: Effects of therapeutic paracentesis on systemic and hepatic hemodynamics and on renal and hormonal function. *Hepatology* 1987; 7:423

26. Perez G, Oster JR, Epstein M: Role of dialysis and ultrafiltration in the treatment of the renal complications of liver disease. *In:* The Kidney in Liver Disease. Third Edition. Epstein M (Ed). Baltimore, Williams & Wilkins Co, (In Press)

27. Ring-Larsen H, Clausen E, Ranek L: Peritoneal dialysis in hyponatremia due to liver failure. *Scan J Gastroenterol* 1973; 8:33

28. Wilkinson SP, Weston MJ, Parsons V, et al: Dialysis in the treatment of renal failure in patients with liver disease. *Clin Nephrol* 1977; 8:287

29. Strand V, Mayor G, Ristow G, et al: Concomitant renal and hepatic failure treated by polyacrylonitrile membrane hemodialysis. *Int J Artif Organs* 1981; 4:136

30. Keller F, Wagner K, Lenz T, et al: Hemodialysis in "hepatorenal syndrome": Report on two cases. *Gut* 1985; 26:208

31. Kearns PJ, Polhemus RJ, Oakes D, et al: Hepatorenal syndrome managed with hemodialysis then reversed by peritoneovenous shunting. *J Clin Gastroenterol* 1985; 7:341

32. Landini S, Coli U, Lucatello S, et al: Plasma-exchange and dialysis. Combined treatment in acute renal insufficiency secondary to severe hepatopathies. *Minerva Nefrol* 1981; 28:179

33. Ellis D, Avner ED: Renal failure and dialysis therapy in children with hepatic failure in the perioperative period of orthotopic liver transplantation. *Clin Nephrol* 1986; 25:295

34. Opolon P, Rapin JR, Huguet C, et al: Hepatic failure coma (HFC) treated by polyacrylonitrile membrane (PAN) and hemodialysis (HD). *Trans Am Soc Artif Intern Organs* 1976; 22:701

35. Silk DBA, Williams R: Experiences in the treatment of fulminant hepatic failure by conservative therapy, charcoal hemoperfusion and polyacrylonitrite hemodialysis. *Int J Artif Organs* 1978; 1:29

36. Opolon P: Large pore hemodialysis in fulminant hepatic failure. *In:* Artificial Liver Support. Brunner G, Schmidt FW (Eds). Berlin, Springer Verlag, 1981, pp 141-146

37. Sakai K, Suzuki M, Hirashawa Y, et al: Artificial hepatic support device with polyacrylonitrile (PAN) membrane, with special reference to hemodiafiltration. *Nippon Rinsho* 1982; 40:890

38. Mathieu D, Gosselin B, Paris JC, et al: Hemofiltration continue dans le traitement de l'encephalopathie hepatique. *Nouv Press Med* 1982; 11:1921

39. Krumlovsky FA, Del Greco F, Niederman M: Prolonged hemoperfusion and hemodialysis in management of hepatic failure and hepatorenal syndrome. *Trans Am Soc Artif Intern Organs* 1978; 24:235

40. LeVeen HH, Christoudias G, Luft R, et al: Peritoneovenous shunting for ascites. *Ann Surg* 1974: 180:580

41. LeVeen HH, Wapnick S, Grosberg S: Further experience with peritoneovenous shunt for ascites. *Am Surg* 1976; 184:574

42. Grosberg SJ, Wapnick S: A retrospective comparison of functional renal failure in cirrhosis treated by conventional therapy or the peritoneovenous shunt (LeVeen). *Am J Med Sci* 1978; 276:287

43. Fullen WD: Hepatorenal syndrome: Reversal by peritoneovenous shunt. *Surgery* 1977; 82:337

44. Schroeder ET, Anderson GH, Smulyan H: Effects of a portacaval or peritoneovenous shunt on renin in the hepatorenal syndrome. *Kidney Int* 1979; 15:54

45. Kinney MJ, Schneider A, Wapnick S, et al: The hepatorenal syndrome and refractory ascites: successful therapy with the LeVeen-type peritonealvenous shunt and valve. *Nephron* 1979; 23:228

46. Greig PD, Blendis LM, Langer B: Renal and hemodynamic effects of the peritoneovenous shunt. II. Long-term effects. *Gastroenterology* 1981; 80:119

47. Schwartz ML, Vogel SB: Treatment of hepatorenal syndrome. *Am J Surg* 1980; 139:370

48. Bernhoft RA, Pellegrini CA, Way LW: Peritoneovenous shunting for refractory ascites. *Arch Surg* 1982; 117:631

49. Smith RE, Nostrant TT, Eckhauser FE, et al: Patient selection and survival after peritoneovenous shunting for nonmalignant ascites. *Am J Gastroenterol* 1984; 79:659

50. Linas SL, Schaefer JW, Moore EE, et al: Peritoneovenous shunt in the management of the hepatorenal syndrome. *Kidney Int* 1986; 30:736

51. Stanley MM and Members of VA Cooperative Study 142. Peritoneovenous shunting vs medical treatment of alcoholic cirrhotic ascites. Abstr. *Hepatology* 1985; 5:980

52. Daskalopoulos G, Jordan DR, Reynolds TB: Randomized trial of peritoneovenous shunt in the treatment of the hepatorenal syndrome. *Gastroenterology* 1985; 88:1655

53. Koppel MH, Coburn JW, Mims MM, et al: Transplantation of cadaveric kidneys from patients with hepatorenal syndrome. Evidence for the functional nature of renal failure in advanced liver disease. *N Engl J Med* 1969; 280:1367

54. Iwatsuki S, Popovtzer MM, Corman JL, et al: Recovery from "hepatorenal syndrome" after orthotopic liver transplantation. *N Engl J Med* 1973; 289:1155

Chapter 14

Circulatory Support

Lazar J. Greenfield, MD

Outline

Educational Objectives

In this chapter the reader will learn:

1. to understand the physiology of the sympathetic nervous system and the variety of adrenergic receptors which are affected by catecholamines. The reader will also learn about the pharmacology of the most commonly used sympathomimetic pharmacological agents and the circumstances in which they should be employed.

2. the management of specific shock states including cardiogenic, hypovolemic and septic shock with suggestions for appropriate drug therapy.

3. about the variety of mechanical devices currently used to assist the failing circulation, including counterpulsation by intra-aortic balloon and ventricular assist devices.

4. the mechanical approaches to a total artificial heart and the types of pumps currently being evaluated both in the laboratory setting and in selected patients.

Introduction

Clinical recognition of circulatory failure occurs in the setting of systemic hypotension; the usual sequence of treatment proceeds from concern for adequate circulatory volume to the effectiveness of the cardiac pump and finally to systemic vascular resistance. Each of these areas has been the subject of intensive investigational efforts. There have been recent major improvements in both pharmacological and mechanical support of the circulation, and these will be the focus of this review. Some areas of study, such as the opioid peptide system and prostaglandins which show very promising animal experimental results, have not reached the stage of clinical application and will not be included.

Catecholamines

Adrenergic Receptor Physiology

Adrenergic receptors are glycoproteins bound to the cell surface membrane and designated alpha and beta subtypes with a separate group of dopamine receptors. The $beta_1$-adrenergic receptors are found on myocardial cells and mediate cardiac sympathomimetic effects, producing both inotropy and chronotropy. $Beta_2$ receptors are located on vascular and bronchial smooth muscle cells, and produce bronchodilation and vasodilation of the pulmonary, mesenteric, and skeletal vascular beds. Visceral effects include increased hepatic glucose production, insulin release, and decreased granulocyte lysosomal release.

The $alpha_1$-receptors are found on vascular smooth muscle and mediate calcium-dependent vasoconstriction. The $alpha_2$-receptors are presynaptic as opposed to the $alpha_1$-postsynaptic locus; their stimulation produces decreased norepinephrine release and vasodilation. They also inhibit both insulin release and lipolysis.

The cerebral, coronary, mesenteric, and renal vascular beds also contain postsynaptic dopamine (d_1-receptors) which mediate vasodilation while the presynaptic d_2-receptors inhibit norepinephrine. All the adrenergic receptors are subject to varying sensitivity depending on the extent and length of exposure to either exogenous or endogenous catecholamines. For example, catecholamine depletion or the use of antagonists will increase the sensitivity ("up-regulation") (1) whereas increased exposure to catecholamines may produce "down-regulation" with decreased adrenergic receptor sensitivity (2).

Available Pharmacologic Agents

Epinephrine

Epinephrine is a potent inotropic agent which stimulates both alpha- and beta-adrenergic receptors in dose-related fashion. Lower-dose epinephrine enhances $beta_1$ effects, producing increased cardiac output by inotropic and chronotropic effects. Infusion at a rate of 0.1 to 0.4 μg/kg·min can increase systolic pressure without raising diastolic BP as a result of peripherally mediated vasodilation. There is, however, an increase in myocardial $\dot{V}O_2$ and increased myocardial irritability due to a decrease in the refractory period of the myocardium.

At higher doses there is predominant alpha activity causing intense vasoconstriction with decreases in renal blood flow and increases in both preload and afterload. Adding to these effects are renin and angiotensin released by beta stimulation of the juxtaglomerular apparatus (3). There is no direct cerebral vasoconstriction and the potential increase in cerebral blood flow adds to its usefulness in cardiopulmonary resuscitation. Its bronchodilator effect also makes it the drug of choice for treatment of acute asthma and anaphylaxis. Its primary value as an inotropic agent can be obtained without the intense vasoconstriction of norepinephrine (Table 1).

TABLE 1: Catecholamine effects on adrenergic receptors

Catecholamine	Receptor				
	Alpha$_1$	Alpha$_2$	Beta$_1$	Beta$_2$	DA
Epinephrine	+ + +	+ + +	+ + +	+ + +	0
Norepinephrine	+ + +	+ + +	+ + +	+	0
Isoproterenol	0	0	+ + +	+ + +	0
Dopamine[a]	0 to + + +	+	+ + to + + +	+ +	+ + +
Dobutamine	0 to +	0	+ + +	+	0

+ Relative degree of stimulation; 0, no stimulation.
[a] Variable dose-dependent effects. High doses produce predominant alpha-adrenergic effects.

From: Zaritsky A: Catecholamines and sympathomimetics. *In:* The Pharmacologic Approach to the Critically Ill Patient. Chernow B, Lake CR (Eds). Baltimore, Williams & Wilkins Co, 1983, p 483

Norepinephrine

The alpha$_1$ effects of norepinephrine constrict both veins and arteries, increasing both preload and afterload. The beta$_1$ stimulation increases myocardial contractility, resulting in increased O$_2$ demand; however, the net result is little change in cardiac output. There is usually an increase in coronary blood flow because of the increased pressure gradient between systemic pressure and left ventricular end-diastolic pressure. Visceral effects include a decrease in renal blood flow which may be angiotensin-II mediated (4), and both hepatic and splanchnic vasoconstriction (5). There is also increased pulmonary vascular resistance but no effect on cerebral blood vessels. The primary indication for norepinephrine is when other vasoconstrictors fail and when vasoconstriction is essential to elevate systemic BP.

Isoproterenol

Through its beta-adrenergic effects, isoproterenol is a potent cardiac stimulant with minimal alpha-adrenergic activity. Its vasodilator effects reduce preload, while its inotropic and chronotropic effects increase cardiac work out of proportion to coronary blood flow, resulting in a decrease in myocardial

261

efficiency. The preferential dilation of skeletal muscle vasculature may shunt blood away from splanchnic or renal areas. In addition to bronchodilation, there is a decrease in pulmonary vascular resistance and intrapulmonary shunt may be increased. Isoproterenol is indicated for hypotension associated with bradycardia and occasionally to improve cardiac contractility, but its major benefit is in children with status asthmaticus.

Dopamine

Dopamine is the endogenous precursor of norepinephrine and produces differing effects dependent upon the rate of administration. With doses of 0.5 to 2 μg/kg·min, there is an increase in renal blood flow and glomerular filtration rate with enhanced sodium excretion (6). With infusion rates of 2 to 5 μg/kg·min, there is a beta-adrenergic inotropic effect without significant increase in heart rate or peripheral resistance (7). At infusion rates in excess of 5 μg/kg·min, there is some endogenous release of norepinephrine and at rates above 10 μg/kg·min, there is alpha-adrenergic vasoconstriction including the renal vascular bed (8). With infusion rates above 20 μg/kg·min, dopamine becomes a potent vasoconstrictor increasing preload, afterload, and myocardial wall tension. With its unique low-dose effect of selective renal vasodilatation, dopamine is indicated to improve renal blood flow and urine output. It also serves as an effective inotropic agent without significant vasoconstriction until higher doses are achieved.

Dobutamine

Dobutamine is a selective beta$_1$-agonist capable of increasing cardiac contractility with very little alpha-adrenergic effect. It has less chronotropic effect than isoproterenol but augments S-A node activity and increases A-V node conduction (9). At an infusion rate of 10 μg/kg·min, dobutamine improves cardiac output while decreasing myocardial $\dot{V}o_2$. Although it has no specific effect on the renal circulation, it can increase urine output on the basis of an increase in cardiac output. It is indicated primarily in cardiogenic shock, congestive heart failure, and in septic shock when cardiac output is insufficient (10).

Specific Shock Management

Cardiogenic Shock

When the volume of muscle damaged as the result of an acute myocardial infarction is sufficient to produce cardiogenic shock, there is a very high mortality rate. The remaining myocardium remains in jeopardy because of increased wall tension, O_2 demand, and decreased coronary perfusion. Additional mechanical problems such as a ventricular septal defect or papillary muscle rupture may require mechanical circulatory support (as will be described in the next section). The principles of management of cardiogenic shock include the utilization of inotropic support and peripheral vasodilation in preference to vasoconstriction. Dopamine in doses which emphasize its beta effects can increase the cardiac output, but it may increase the $\dot{V}o_2$; higher doses should be avoided to prevent the afterload effects of vasoconstriction. Dobutamine is particularly valuable in this situation because it produces an inotropic effect along with mild vasodilation and very little tachycardia. Epinephrine also serves as a potent inotrope at lower dosages, but it can increase $\dot{V}o_2$ and may cause tachycardia and arrhythmias. It should be considered when dobutamine is not effective, but higher dosage levels should be avoided. Isoproterenol is not indicated in this situation unless there is an associated bradycardia and norepinephrine should be avoided because of its vasoconstrictor afterload effects (Table 1).

Hypovolemic Shock

The physiological response to significant volume loss is a strong adrenergic response which produces peripheral vasoconstriction and increased heart rate to compensate for decreased stroke volume and impaired O_2 delivery. If circulating volume is not restored, compensatory mechanisms fail and there is loss of vasoconstriction with hypotension and systemic shock. The principle of management in this situation is to replace volume as rapidly as necessary to correct the hypovolemia. Although catecholamine administration may be used as a temporizing measure until volume replacement can be initiated, it will further impair perfusion and may complicate the hemodynamic assessment of adequacy of volume repletion. Only if there is secondary myocardial dysfunction after adequate volume resuscitation should catecholamine inotropic support be considered.

Septic Shock

The early stage of septic shock, which has been characterized as "hyperdynamic," is associated with vasodilation and increased cardiac output. There are increases in both epinephrine and norepinephrine in plasma that do not correlate with systemic BP (11). The principles of management are to control the septic focus, if possible by drainage of any infected material, to administer appropriate antibiotics, and to provide circulatory support usually by optimizing circulating volume. Lower-dose dopamine can be helpful in maintaining an adequate urine output. In later stages of septic shock, more inotropic support will be required and may be combined with a vasodilator, although it is doubtful that there is any alteration in outcome.

The role of corticosteroids remains controversial, although well controlled animal studies reported by Hinshaw et al. (12,13), using live organism infusion, have demonstrated significant improvement in survival when antibiotics are combined with steroid administration, especially if the steroids are begun within 30 min of an *E. coli* infusion. The rationale for the use of steroid therapy is based on its ability to stabilize lysosomal membranes, prevent platelet aggregation, prevent the complement/white blood cell interaction, increase cardiac output, improve organ perfusion, normalize insulin levels, and preserve cellular mitochondria. Despite these potential beneficial effects, clinical studies performed in a prospective randomized fashion have yielded conflicting results. The 8-yr prospective study reported by Schumer in 1976 (14) showed a 10% mortality in patients treated with antibiotics, steroids, and other supportive measures, while there was a 38% mortality without steroids. In 1984, however, Sprung et al. (15) published the results of a smaller 3-yr prospective study of 59 patients with septic shock and found no difference in outcome, although there was a suggestion of increased superinfection with the use of dexamethasone. Since experimental studies document the maximal beneficial effect of steroids when administered early after the onset of sepsis, and since it is so difficult to determine at the bedside exactly when sepsis begins, the issue of a potential beneficial effect from steroid administration remains an attractive but unconfirmed adjunct to management.

Mechanical Support

The total artificial heart received worldwide attention when the first implantation occurred in 1982 in Utah. Using an external energy source and controller, this application was the result of major improvements in long-term mechanical circulatory support systems for the entire cardiac output. The stimulus and precedent for this can be traced to circumstances when patients undergoing cardiac surgery could not be weaned from cardiopulmonary bypass by either pharmacological or intra-aortic balloon support. A variety of ventricular assist devices was developed for short-term use until there was recovery of intrinsic myocardial function. In the absence of recovery, the remaining alternative was cardiac transplantation. This section will review briefly the variety of mechanical systems available to support the circulation.

Counterpulsation

The intra-aortic balloon pump (IABP) is the most widely used device for prolonged circulatory support. The original concept of counterpulsation, as proposed by Harken in 1958 (16), suggested that blood could be removed from the body via the femoral artery during ventricular systole and then rapidly reinfused during diastole to augment coronary perfusion pressure. This approach, however, required bilateral femoral arteriotomies and led to excessive hemolysis. In 1962, Moulopoulos et al. (17) suggested the use of an intra-aortic balloon to accomplish the same purpose as external counterpulsation. The concept was based on rapid inflation of the balloon during diastole to augment coronary perfusion and then rapid deflation during systole to decrease left ventricular afterload. The first successful clinical application of this technique was reported in 1968 (18).

The conventional approach to operative insertion of the intra-aortic balloon device required a second surgical procedure to repair the artery; there was a high incidence of complications, averaging 20% in most clinical series (19). In 1979 a technique for percutaneous insertion was developed using the modified Seldinger technique through a 12-Fr sheath (20) (Fig. 1). The remaining problem of compromised blood flow to the extremity distal to the point of insertion of the balloon should be minimized by the development of a new 10.5-Fr balloon device which will allow more blood flow distally (21). The most frequent indication for use of the intra-aortic balloon pump is for circulatory support in patients with postoperative left ventricular failure; it is widely used for unstable angina refractory to medical treatment or recurrent angina following an acute myocardial infarction. With increasing experience, the indications have widened to include prophylactic management of patients with mild to moderate hemodynamic compromise and some noncardiac situations, although the results in the management of noncardiogenic shock have not been encouraging. In one series of 149 successful balloon insertions (21), 74 patients had a surgical indication for insertion; 45 of these patients died, for a mortality rate of 61%. Of the 75 patients who had a medical indication for insertion, 59 eventually underwent a cardiac surgical procedure and only six of these patients died, for a mortality rate of 10%. Although the use of IABP is generally measured in days, its use chronically has been reported for periods of 2 to 5 months (22).

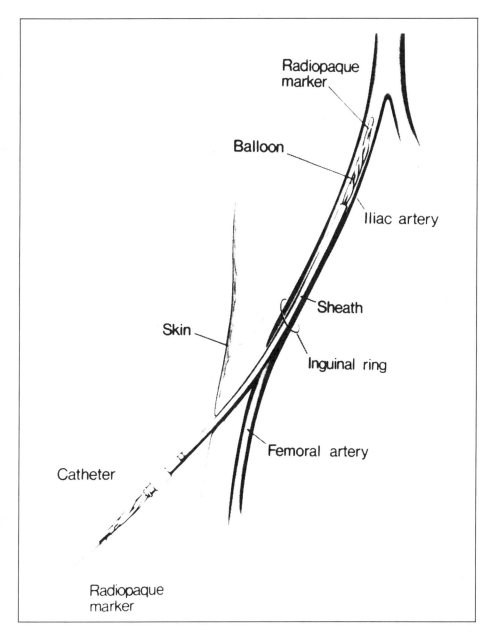

Fig. 1. The intra-aortic balloon can be inserted percutaneously and positioned in the descending thoracic aorta for effective counterpulsation. Reproduced with permission from Bregman and Kaskel (21).

Ventricular Assist Devices

The principle of paracorporeal ventricular assist devices is based on the utilization of a parallel bypass circuit which can reduce pressure work during systole, thereby decreasing myocardial $\dot{V}o_2$. The left ventricular assist device (LVAD) is designed to provide sufficient flow to maintain adequate systemic

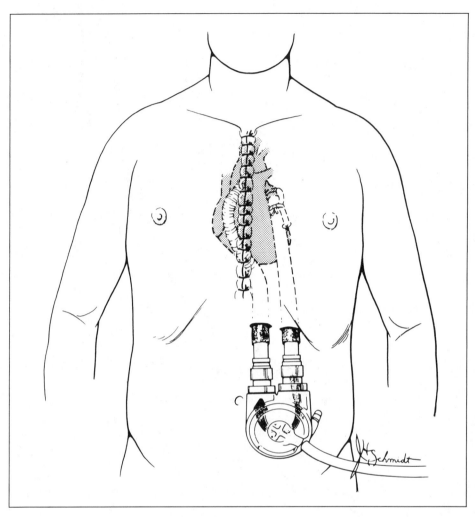

Fig. 2. The Pennsylvania State University sac-type LAVD is a parallel circuit shunting blood from the left atrium to the ascending aorta. The cannulae exit the body below the costal margin. A right ventricular device can also be used to shunt blood from the right atrium to the pulmonary artery. Reproduced with permission from Richenbacher et al (24).

perfusion and coronary blood flow, which allows metabolic recovery of injured myocardium. A right ventricular assist device can be used alone or in conjunction with an LVAD to decompress the right heart and maintain flow through the pulmonary vasculature. The first clinical report of a left heart assist device was in 1963 by Liotta et al (23). Since then, additional experience has been obtained using pneumatic pumps for both left and right heart support for ventricular failure following cardiac surgery (24). Their experience consisted of 17 patients who could not be weaned from cardiopulmonary bypass following a cardiac procedure; eight patients were long-term survivors. The device used was the Pennsylvania State University sac-type LVAD which shunted blood from the left atrium to the ascending aorta (Fig. 2). The pump is driven pneumatically and functions either in a synchronous mode through the electrocardiogram signal or in a fixed rate asynchronous mode. The hemodynamic criteria for insertion include a left atrial mean pressure in excess of 25 mm Hg, systolic aortic pressure < 90 mm Hg, and cardiac index < 1.8 L/min·m². Systemic anticoagulation was not used, although 5% low-molecular-weight dextran was administered to reduce platelet adhesiveness. Weaning from the LVAD was accomplished by discontinuing pumping for periods of up to 60 sec to evaluate the patient's ventricular function. The rate of pumping was then progressively decreased to 30 beat/min and the pump removed by reoperation.

A nonpulsatile ventricular assist device using a centrifugal pump has been reported by Pennington et al. (25) and employed in 16 patients. In 15 of them, additional pulsatility was provided by an IABP. Variations in cannula access included inserting the withdrawal catheter through the left ventricular apex, retrograde across the aortic valve into the left ventricle, or directly into the left atrium. The infusion cannula was placed directly into the ascending aorta through a prosthetic graft or directly into the aorta. Although these patients were not initially heparinized, the development of thromboembolism in two patients led to a policy of using heparin to maintain the activated partial thromboplastin time at twice normal beginning 36 to 48 h postoperatively. The most frequent complication was bleeding; all but two patients required reoperation. Although seven patients had improved ventricular function, only four were successfully weaned and there were two long-term survivors out of 16 who had the pump inserted.

An electrically powered implantable LVAD has been reported by Portner et al (26). The system uses a novel belt skin transformer for transmission of primary power across the intact skin. Implant durations of up to 6 months have been achieved but clinical studies have not been reported. More extensive clinical experience with a simplified LVAD has been reported by Rose et al. (27) using an external roller pump as well as the IABP. Heparin administration was continued postoperatively and reoperation was required for pump removal. There were 13 long-term survivors out of 35 in whom the device was used.

Total Artificial Heart

Artificial hearts maintain separate pulmonary and systemic circulations and have either pneumatic or electric power sources. The most common pneumatic pulsatile devices use compressed air to move a flexible pumping diaphragm with or without a pressure plate support. These devices are reliable, are of simple design, and have a wide range of pumping capabilities. To achieve a totally implantable system, however, the disposal of exhausted air or gases limits the pneumatic pump; efforts have been made to develop small electric motors with mechanical linkages behind pusher plates. In addition to the mechanical requirements, separate control of the drive system for each ventricle is required to adjust for shunted blood and differences in afterload between the left and right circulations.

The pneumatic artificial heart, with a flexible pumping diaphragm, has the ability to accommodate a change in stroke volume according to filling pressure with no change in driving pressure, heart rate, or amount of vacuum applied during the diastolic phase. This Starling-like response allows for a range in cardiac output with minimal adjustments of the external control systems (28). Studies in calves and sheep in dedicated laboratories around the world have confirmed the durability of the device (Jarvik-7) to maintain the animals during growth and exercise for periods in excess of 200 days. Since the original implantation in man in 1982, additional clinical experience has demonstrated the ability of the total artificial heart to reverse pulmonary edema, sustain normal organ function, and improve renal performance. Neither thrombus formation within the artificial heart nor infection from percutaneous leads has presented serious problems. Examination of the pumping components of the artificial heart after removal has shown no evidence of wear or damage (28).

Future Directions

There are two electric motor-driven systems currently under development at Pennsylvania State University (29). One system uses a low-speed/high-torque motor to rotate a triple-track drum cam that converts rotary motion into rectilinear motion (Fig. 3). The other uses a higher-speed/lower-torque motor to rotate a roller-screw mechanism that also converts rotary to rectilinear motion. Both units drive pusher plates which alternately compress and retract a diaphragm to achieve systole and diastole. The cam-drive system has undergone successful long-term implantation in calves, and has demonstrated both reliability and portability when a battery pack is attached to the animal (29). When a transcutaneous energy system is developed, an external battery pack and primary coil will be used to activate a secondary coil to achieve a totally implantable artificial heart in man.

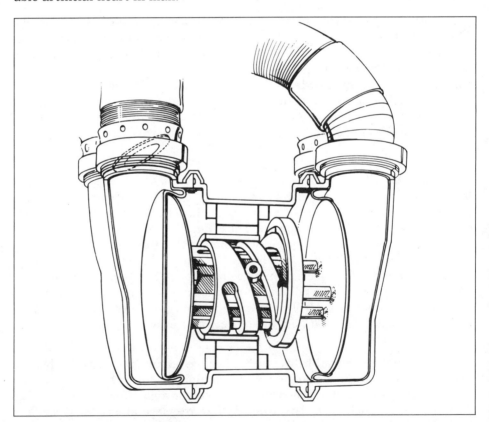

Fig. 3. In the cam-drive artificial heart, the triple-track drive cam is driven by a DC brushless motor. The motor rotates in one direction for systole, then stops and counter-rotates for diastole. Reproduced with permission from Rosenberg et al (29).

References

1. Boudoulas H, Louis RP, Kates RE, et al: Hypersensitivity to adrenergic stimulation after propranolol withdrawal in normal subjects. *Ann Intern Med* 1977; 87:433

2. Tohmeh JF, Cryer PE: Biophasic adrenergic modulation of beta-adrenergic receptors in man. *J Clin Invest* 1980; 65:836

3. Vander AJ: Effect of catecholamines and the renal nerves on renin secretion in anesthetized dogs. *Am J Physiol* 1965; 209:659

4. Bomzon L, Rosendorff E: Renovascular resistance and noradrenaline. *Am J Physiol* 1975; 229:1649

5. Greenway CV, Stark RD: Hepatic vascular bed. *Physiol Rev* 1971; 51:23

6. Goldberg LI: Cardiovascular and renal actions of dopamine: Potential clinical applications. *Pharmacol Rev* 1972; 24:1

7. Goldberg LI: Dopamine-clinical uses of an endogenous catecholamine. *N Engl J Med* 1974; 291:707

8. Goldberg LI, Hsieh Y, Resnekov L: Newer catecholamines for treatment of heart failure and shock: An update on dopamine and a first look at dobutamine. *Prog Cardiovasc Dis* 1977; 19:327

9. Loeb HS, Sinno MZ, Saudye A, et al: Electrophysiologic properties of dobutamine. *Circ Shock* 1974; 1:217

10. Jardin F, Sportiche M, Bazil M, et al: Dobutamine: A hemodynamic evaluation in septic shock. *Crit Care Med* 1981; 9:329

11. Sugarman HJ, Newsome HH, Greenfield LJ: Hemodynamics, oxygen consumption and serum catecholamine changes in progressive lethal peritonitis in the dog. *Surg Gynecol Obstet* 1982; 154:8

12. Hinshaw LB, Archer LT, Beller-Todd BK, et al: Survival of primates in lethal septic shock following delayed treatment with steroid. *Circ Shock* 1981; 8:291

13. Hinshaw LB, Beller-Todd BK, Archer LT, et al: Effectiveness of steroid/antibiotic treatment in primates administered LD[100] *E. coli. Ann Surg* 1981; 194:51

14. Schumer W: Steroids in the treatment of clinical septic shock. *Ann Surg* 1976; 184:333

15. Sprung CL, Caralis PV, Marciel EH, et al: The effects of high-dose corticosteroids in patients with septic shock: A prospective, controlled study. *N Engl J Med* 1984; 311:1137

16. Harken DE: Counterpulsation. Presentation at the International College of Cardiology meeting. Brussels, Belgium, 1958

17. Moulopoulos SE, Topaz S, Kolff WF: Diastolic balloon pumping (with carbon dioxide) in the aorta-mechanical assist to the failing circulation. *Am Heart J* 1962; 63:669

18. Kantrowitz A, Tjonneland F, Freed PS, et al: Initial clinical experience with intra-aortic balloon pumping in cardiogenic shock. *JAMA* 1968; 203:135

19. LaFemine AA, Kosowshi B, Madoff I, et al: Results and complications of intra-aortic balloon pumping in surgical and medical patients. *Am J Cardiol* 1977; 40:416

20. Bregman D, Casarella WJ: Percutaneous intra-aortic balloon pumping: Initial clinical experience. *Ann Thorac Surg* 1980; 29:153

21. Bregman D, Kaskel P: Clinical experience with percutaneous intra-aortic balloon pumping. *In:* Assisted Circulation 2. Unger F (Ed). New York, Springer-Verlag, l984, p 13

22. Gaul G, Blazek G, Deutsch M, et al: Chronic use of an intra-aortic balloon pump in congestive cardiomyopathy. *In:* Assisted Circulation 2. Unger F (Ed). New York, Springer-Verlag, 1984, p 28

23. Liotta D, Hall CW, Walter SH, et al: Prolonged assisted circulation during and after cardiac or aortic surgery. Prolonged partial left ventricular bypass by means of intracorporeal circulation. *Am J Cardiol* 1963; 12:399

24. Richenbacher WE, Wisman CB, Rosenberg G, et al: Ventricular assistance: Clinical experience at the Pennsylvania State University. *In:* Assisted Circulation 2. Unger F (Ed). New York, Springer-Verlag, 1984, p 70

25. Pennington DG, Merjavy JP, Codd JE, et al: Temporary mechanical support of patients with profound ventricular failure. *In:* Assisted Circulation 2. Unger F (Ed). New York, Springer-Verlag, 1984, p 85

26. Portner PM, Oyer PE, Jassawalla JS, et al: A totally implantable ventricular assist device for end-stage heart disease. *In:* Assisted Circulation 2. Unger F (Ed). New York, Springer-Verlag, 1984, p 115

27. Rose DM, Cunningham JN Jr, Spencer FC: New York University experience with a roller-pump-type left ventricular assist device. *In:* Assisted Circulation 2. Unger F (Ed). New York, Springer-Verlag, 1984, p 153

28. Olsen DB, Murray KD: The total artificial heart. *In:* Assisted Circulation 2. Unger F (Ed). New York, Springer-Verlag, 1984, p 197

29. Rosenberg G, Pierce WS, Landis DL: Progress in the development of the Pennsylvania State University motor-driven artificial heart. *In:* Assisted Circulation 2. Unger F (Ed). New York, Springer-Verlag, 1984, p 270

Self-Assessment Questions

1. Myocardial inotropic and chronotropic effects are mediated through:
   A. $alpha_1$-receptors
   B. $alpha_2$-receptors
   C. $beta_1$-receptors
   D. $beta_2$-receptors
   E. dopamine receptors

2. Dopamine d_1-receptors are found in all of the following vascular beds except:
   A. cerebral
   B. coronary

C. mesenteric
D. musculoskeletal
E. renal

3. The drug of choice in the management of anaphylactic shock is:
   A. dopamine
   B. dobutamine
   C. norepinephrine
   D. epinephrine
   E. isoproterenol

4. The drug of choice in the management of cardiogenic shock is:
   A. dopamine
   B. dobutamine
   C. norepinephrine
   D. epinephrine
   E. isoproterenol

5. Which of the following devices is most suitable for an implantable total artificial heart:
   A. pneumatic pump
   B. LVAD
   C. electrical pump
   D. intra-aortic balloon
   E. none of the above

Self-Assessment Answers

1. C. Beta$_1$ receptors are found on myocardial cells and mediate cardiac sympathomimetic effects including inotropy and chronotropy

2. D. The postsynaptic dopamine d$_1$-receptors are found in cerebral, coronary, mesenteric, and renal vascular beds.

3. D. Because of its bronchodilator effect, epinephrine is the drug of choice for the treatment of anaphylactic shock.

4. B. Dobutamine is particularly valuable in the management of cardiogenic shock because it produces an inotropic effect along with mild vasodilation and very little tachycardia.

5. C. Electric motor-driven pumps provide the best available drive system for an implantable total artificial heart since the pneumatic pump requires a means for discharge of vented air or gas.

Chapter 15

Magnetic Resonance Imaging in Critically Ill Patients

Robert H. Posteraro, MD, and Carl E. Ravin, MD

Outline

Educational Objectives

In this chapter the reader will learn:

1. the basic physical principles involved in magnetic resonance imaging.

2. the differences between permanent, resistive, and superconducting magnet systems.

3. the types of diagnosis in which magnetic resonance imaging may be helpful in the critically ill patient.

4. the risks and limitations involved when working with patients in a strong magnetic field.

Introduction

Magnetic resonance imaging (MRI) has been hailed as a revolutionary technique which will ultimately have as profound an impact on diagnostic medical imaging as did the initial discovery of x-rays. Unlike radiography, which exposes the patient to potentially harmful ionizing radiation in order to produce an image, MRI exposes the patient to nonionizing electromagnetic radiation in the form of magnetic fields and radiofrequency (RF) emissions. The images produced, while similar to computed tomographic images in appearance, are not derived from differences in attenuation of an x-ray beam by organs in the body, but rather, are based upon the chemical characteristics of the tissues imaged and, in the case of flowing blood or cerebrospinal fluid, the velocity and characteristics of flow. In the critically ill patient, MRI offers the potential of several

273

unique improvements in diagnosis and, therefore, treatment. First, because flowing blood is readily distinguishable from surrounding soft tissues, there is no need to use iodine-based contrast agents to opacify the blood vessels. Second, because the images reflect the chemical composition of the tissues, it is possible that disease progression or response to treatment may be assessed earlier and more accurately than with conventional radiographic techniques.

Principles of Magnetic Resonance Imaging

Basic Physics

All atoms are composed of a central nucleus surrounded by one or more electrons. The nucleus of an atom consists of protons, which are positively charged particles and (with the exception of the lightest isotope of hydrogen) neutrons, which have no charge. Protons and neutrons, because they are found in the nucleus of atoms, are collectively referred to as nucleons. Nuclei which have an odd number of protons and/or neutrons possess a property known as magnetic moment. These magnetic moments behave like tiny bar magnets, having a north pole and a south pole. In the absence of any outside influence, the magnetic moments of the nuclei will be pointing in random directions. If a strong external magnetic field is applied, the magnetic moments will align themselves parallel to the direction of that field. Unlike ordinary bar magnets which would all align themselves pointing in the same direction when placed in a magnetic field, the nuclear magnetic moments will orient themselves with some pointing in the direction of the field (parallel) and others pointing in the opposite direction (antiparallel). This distribution of parallel and antiparallel magnetic moments is not an equal distribution. Slightly more than half of the magnetic moments line up in the parallel orientation. This slight advantage produces a net magnetic vector pointing in the direction of the externally applied magnetic field. If we could now look at one of the nuclei in the presence of the strong external field, we would see that its magnetic moment is not rigidly fixed in the direction of the field but, rather, is slowly revolving around the axis of that field. Its motion is similar to that of a spinning toy top which has been tipped slightly. This type of motion is called precession. The rate at which the nuclear magnetic moment moves in precession around the axis of the magnetic field is determined by the strength of the externally applied field and another quantity referred to as the magnetogyric (gyromagnetic) ratio, which is determined by the composition of the atomic nucleus. The rate or frequency of the precession is given by the Larmor equation:

$$\omega_0 = \gamma B_0$$

which states that the frequency of precession (ω_0) is equal to the magnetogyric ratio (γ) times the strength of the externally applied magnetic field (B_0). The strength of a magnetic field is measured in units of either gauss (G) or tesla (T), (one tesla = 10,000 gauss). As a point of reference, the strength of the earth's magnetic field is approximately 0.00005 T. For nuclei of hydrogen atoms in a 1.5-T magnetic field, the frequency of precession is 63.9 MHz. If the precessing nuclei are exposed to a second magnetic field oriented perpendicular to the B_0 field, the effect of the newly applied field will be to draw the direction of the magnetic moments away from the axis of the static field. How do we introduce a second magnetic field perpendicular to the static field? It is known that electromagnetic radiations (for example, radio waves) consist of an electric field and a magnetic field oriented perpendicular to each other. Whenever a radio signal is transmitted, an electric field and a magnetic field are radiated simultaneously. In the MR imager, the second magnetic field is produced by transmitting an RF signal into the patient in such a way that the direction of the magnetic field generated by the RF signal is perpendicular to the axis of the static field. In order for the magnetic moments of the nuclei to respond to this field, the RF signal must be generated at a frequency equal to that given by the Larmor equation (63.9 MHz for hydrogen nuclei in a 1.5-T magnetic field). The longer the second field is applied, the farther the axis of the nuclear spins will be pulled away from their original direction. If the second field is applied for a long enough time, the magnetic moments will end up rotating in a plane perpendicular to the axis of the static magnetic field. Due to the presence of the second magnetic field, the magnetic moments all come to point in the same direction as they precess in this plane; that is, they are "coherent," and form a net magnetic vector. As this net magnetic vector moves in precession it emits an RF signal. The magnitude of this signal is measured in the perpendicular plane. If, at this point, the second magnetic field is removed, the nuclei will once again be subject only to the influence of the static magnetic field and will return to their original equilibrium condition, precessing and pointing along the axis of the static field. As the nuclei return to their equilibrium position, the strength of their RF signal in the perpendicular plane decreases. However, the nuclei do not return to this condition all at once. They return to equilibrium in a logarithmic fashion over time with a time constant defined as T1. The value of T1 is a function of temperature, pH, the strength of the external field, and the chemical nature of the individual nuclei. Nuclei with long T1 values return to the equilibrium state more slowly than those with short T1 values. The different appearances of different tissues on MR images is due, in part, to differences in T1 values between the nuclei of atoms which make up those tissues.

Let us return to the situation where we had applied a second magnetic field perpendicular to the static field. The magnetic moments of the nuclei were drawn away from the direction of the static magnetic field and are spinning in a plane perpendicular to the axis of the static field. Because of the effect of the second field, the magnetic moments of the individual nuclei are pointing in the same direction as they rotate and emit an RF signal which can be measured. When the second magnetic field is removed, the individual nuclear magnetic moments begin to lose coherence. Some begin to precess at a slightly faster rate than the average and some begin to precess at a slightly slower rate. The reason for this alteration is that each magnetic moment is influenced by the local magnetic fields produced by the molecules around it. Some of these local fields increase the effect of the external field, causing some nuclei to spin at a faster rate. Others decrease the effect of the external field, causing some nuclei to spin at a slower rate. The effect of this loss of coherence is that after a short time the individual nuclear magnetic moments are pointing in random directions within the plane perpendicular to the axis of the static magnetic field. Once the individual magnetic moments are randomly oriented, there is no net magnetic vector; thus, no RF signal can be measured. The time it takes for the magnetic moments to lose coherence is described by a time constant T2. Different atoms of the same element located in different chemical environments lose coherence at different rates and, therefore, have different T2 time constants. These differences also contribute to the various appearances of tissues on an MR image.

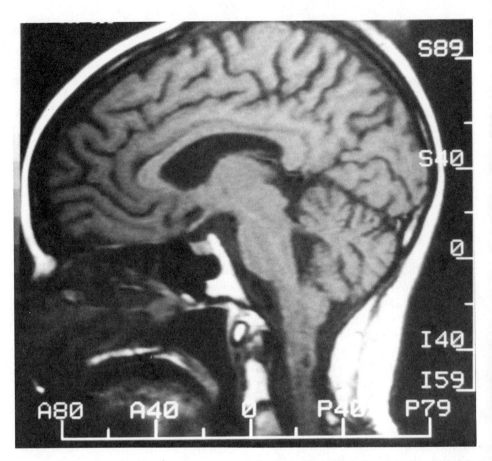

Fig. 1. Midline sagittal MR image of the brain. Note the high resolution especially of the cerebellum and brain stem. These are areas which are very difficult to evaluate on CT images.

By exposing the patient to additional magnetic fields of varying strength and direction during the course of the imaging process, selected slices of the patient's body can be imaged in any desired plane of orientation. Unlike reformatted CT images, which are produced by reconstructing data from axial images and therefore suffer a loss of resolution, MR images are obtained directly in the desired plane of interest. Sagittal and coronal images have as fine a resolution as images taken in the axial direction (Fig. 1). Depending on the imaging parameters used for scanning, flowing blood may be made to appear black or white on images (Figs. 2 and 3). This attribute of MRI allows us to see blood in the heart and great vessels without the use of intravenous contrast (Fig. 4).

The advantages of MRI are: a) there is no ionizing radiation used and, so far, there have been no reported ill effects produced solely by the magnetic field strengths and RF signals used in the clinical setting; b) no iodine-based contrast needs to be used to visualize blood flow or cerebrospinal fluid; and c) images may be directly acquired in any plane desired.

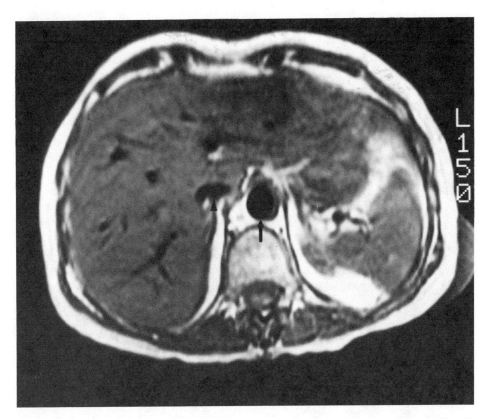

Fig. 2. Axial MR image of the upper abdomen. Flowing blood produces no signal; thus, the aorta (arrow), *inferior vena cava* (arrowhead), *and hepatic vessels appear black.*

Types of Magnetic Resonance Scanners

There are three categories of MR units which are defined by the type of magnet used to generate the static magnetic field: permanent, resistive, and superconducting.

The permanent magnet is similar to the bar or horseshoe magnets with which we are all familiar, although for clinical use the magnet must be larger. This magnet is usually built on site from magnetized ceramic blocks. It can produce a magnetic field strength of about 0.3 T.

The resistive magnet is, in essence, an electromagnet. It can produce a magnetic field of approximately 0.7 T.

The superconducting magnet is a resistive magnet whose electrical wiring has been cooled to a temperature of 4° above absolute zero. At that temperature the electrical resistance in the wires drops to zero, allowing more current to flow through the wires and thus producing a stronger magnetic field. This magnet is able to produce a magnetic field of 1.5 to 2.0 T.

There are advantages and disadvantages associated with each type of system. Permanent magnets require no power or cooling and are therefore the least expensive to operate. They do require a constant temperature environment, and

277

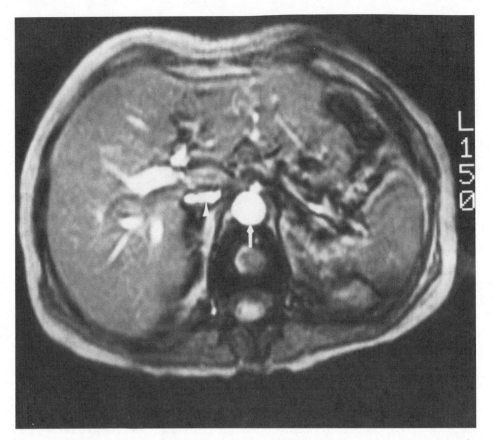

Fig. 3. Axial MR image of the upper abdomen. Using different imaging parameters, the flowing blood produces a strong signal. The aorta (arrow), inferior vena cava (arrowhead), and hepatic vessels appear white.

are very heavy, weighing from 12,000 to 200,000 pounds. Resistive magnets require a constant supply of electricity to maintain the magnetic field. The magnet must also be cooled because of the heat generated by the electric current in the wires. Superconducting magnets are the most expensive to operate. They require liquid helium and liquid nitrogen to keep the wires of the magnet at superconducting temperatures.

The magnetic field produced by the magnet is not confined to the physical volume of the magnet's structure. The field extends out for a distance from the magnet. How far out the field extends depends on the construction of the magnet and its strength. Shielding of the magnet must be provided in order to reduce the effects which the magnetic field would have on nearby metallic or magnetic devices, and also to reduce the effect which these devices would have on the magnetic field. Permanent magnets are, for the most part, self-shielding. The fringe field does not extend very far outside the magnet. The resistive and superconducting magnets must have external shielding. This requires additional space around the magnet in which metallic objects are prohibited. This limits access to the patient by ancillary personnel, or delays access to the patient while personnel remove metallic objects from their pockets. Electronic devices, magnetic tapes, and computer disks must be kept even farther away from the mag-

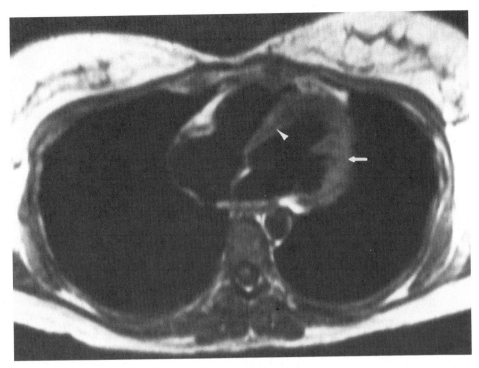

Fig. 4. Axial MR image of the heart. The flowing blood produces no signal. The cardiac chambers appear black. The myocardial wall (arrow) *and interventricular septum* (arrowhead) *are well demarcated.*

net. Electronic devices may malfunction and magnetic tapes or computer disks may be erased by the magnetic field. In general, it is easier to work around the permanent magnet systems, but for improved diagnostic capability, the 1.5-T superconducting systems are preferred.

Uses of Magnetic Resonance Imaging in the Critically Ill

Myocardial Infarction

MRI has been shown to be effective in the identification of acute myocardial infarction. Patients with acute myocardial infarction as diagnosed by ECG have been imaged as early as 2 days following the onset of infarction (1). Infarcted myocardial tissue exhibits longer T1 relaxation times as compared with normal myocardium. In another study (2), areas of infarction demonstrated increased T2 relaxation times and increased signal intensity on the MR images. Foci of chronic infarction showed decreased signal intensity and thinning of the myocardial wall. In eight patients with acute myocardial infarction who underwent both MRI and left ventriculography, increased signal intensity was seen in those segments of the cardiac wall which had appeared akinetic or hypokinetic on the left ventriculogram (3). Gated cardiac MR studies have been shown to be reliable for measuring left ventricular function. Measurements of left ventricular wall thickness and left ventricular wall motion from gated cardiac MR images have proven comparable to measurements obtained from x-ray ventriculography (4). MRI has also been used to calculate left ventricular ejection fraction, and has been found to have good correlation with ventriculography (5).

Pulmonary Embolism

A number of case reports and experimental studies have been reported showing that MRI can identify the presence of pulmonary emboli (6, 7). These reports make use of the fact that, using the appropriate imaging techniques, flowing blood will produce no MR signal. The pulmonary emboli were seen as areas of increased signal intensity in the pulmonary arteries. This finding, however, is nonspecific and could as easily have been produced by tumor, hilar adenopathy, or slowly flowing blood. At this time, MRI is not specific for diagnosing central pulmonary emboli and is not considered effective for identifying peripheral emboli.

Acute Head Injury

Due to the speed and ease of monitoring and supporting critically ill patients, CT is still considered a better modality for diagnosing acute head injuries. MRI, on the other hand, has been shown to be more sensitive in identifying small hypothalamic and brainstem infarcts and small areas of contusion (8). For this reason, MRI may prove to be of great value for determining the prognosis of patients who have suffered head injury.

Transplantation

MRI has been used to evaluate the status of transplanted kidneys. In cases of acute and/or chronic rejection, the MR images showed a decrease in the renal corticomedullary differentiation and a decrease in the renal parenchymal vascularity (9). These findings are not specific, however, and may be seen in cases of acute tubular necrosis as well. Additional work is being done using nuclear magnetic resonance spectroscopy, in addition to imaging, in order to try to differentiate transplant rejection from acute tubular necrosis.

Musculoskeletal Injury

Although plain films and CT scans are better for identifying fractures, MRI is more sensitive for evaluating disorders of ligaments, cartilage, and bone marrow. While conditions affecting these structures are often not life-threatening, MRI may play a role in evaluating the extent of musculoskeletal injury in the stabilized multiple-trauma patient. Internal derangements of joints can be diagnosed without resorting to arthrography or surgical exploration (Fig. 5).

Risks

Thus far, this exciting technology has seen only limited application in the evaluation of critically ill patients because the critically ill patient presents some difficult MRI problems. The first of these is examination time. Most body scans take 45 min to 1.5 h to perform. Cardiac MR scans require cardiac gating and, therefore, require longer times. Patients with irregular heart rhythms are, by the nature of the gated study, not good candidates for cardiac imaging.

The length of the magnet bore is approximately 6 ft and the diameter of the bore is approximately 22 inches. Approximately 5% of healthy people experience acute claustrophobia when placed in this long narrow tube. In an already anxious patient, this sensation may be intensified.

The presence of the magnetic and RF fields has been shown to adversely affect electronic monitoring and life-support apparatus. T wave abnormalities

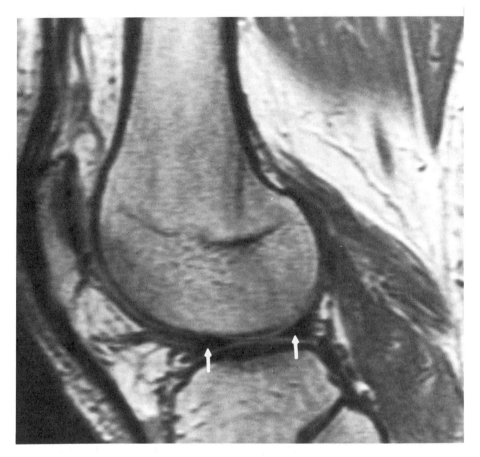

Fig. 5. Sagittal MR image of the knee. The anterior and posterior horns of the lateral meniscus (arrows) *are seen as well defined black triangles. Meniscal tears and ligament ruptures may be easily diagnosed by MR imaging.*

have been seen on ECGs of patients in static magnetic fields up to 0.3 T (10). Pacemakers have been shown to malfunction during MR scanning. The reed switches on the pacemakers closed under the influence of a 0.15-T magnetic field. This caused the pacemakers to assume an asynchronous mode of pacing. During imaging, two of the four pacemakers tested developed rapid pacing rates, probably in response to the rapidly changing RF fields (11). In another study (12), four pacemakers were tested in a 0.5-T imaging system. All functioned normally in the static magnetic field, but all malfunctioned during imaging. Three of the four experienced total inhibition of atrial and ventricular output. In the fourth, ventricular backup pacing was activated at high RF pulse repetition rates. The MR scanner was also able to trigger atrial output at rates up to 800/min.

Intravenous drip regulators have been found to vary in their response to MR scanners (13). When placed within 3 feet of the magnet bore, one regulator failed to function completely (0 drip rate). Another operated but with inaccurate flow rates and a third operated normally.

The need to provide ventilatory support to critically ill patients undergoing MRI has been addressed by a number of authors. Gas cylinders which are ferromagnetic must be kept away from the magnet at all times lest they become projectiles into the bore of the magnet. Similarly, ventilators which are constructed of ferromagnetic material may not be brought too close to the magnet. Those which rely on ferromagnetic or electrical components for their operation may become nonfunctional if placed within the magnetic field. Dunn et al. (14) described a commercially available ventilator which is pneumatically driven, fluid controlled, and has no electrical components. The distance of the ventilator to the patient in an MR scanner required approximately 8 ft of ventilator tubing. This resulted in increased CO_2 retention during ventilation. In order to compensate for this, the tidal volume needed to be increased approximately 20%.

Monitoring of a patient's vital functions also requires an ingenious approach. The customary electronic monitoring devices must be located remotely and connected to the patient via nonelectronic pathways. Fiberoptic telemetry links (10, 15), rubber bellows to monitor respirations, and nylon tubing connectors have all been used for monitoring during MR scanning. If the patient requires the personal attention of physicians, nurses, or other ancillary staff, these people must not bring ferromagnetic objects with them into the scan room. Laryngoscopes, scissors, and even ball-point pens may be attracted into the magnet with great force and become, in essence, projectiles hurtling toward the patient. This risk should not be minimized. A few examples may help to demonstrate the magnitude of this effect. A laryngoscope (batteries included) suspended by a string at the portal of a 0.5-T MR scanner will be attracted to the magnet with a force of 3.54 newtons, causing the string to be deviated 55 degrees from the vertical. A pair of scissors similarly placed will be attracted by a force of 4.453 newtons, sufficient to deviate the supporting string 86 degrees from the vertical (10). A letter to the editor of the *New England Journal of Medicine* (16) reported a case in which a 0.5-T magnet was being installed. A technician was in the bore of the magnet directing a forklift to approach him. When the extension tines of the forklift (each 2 meters long and weighing 50 kg) came within 30 cm of the magnet, they shot into the bore. The technician was hit with such a force that he was propelled 6 meters across the chamber into a wall. He was knocked unconscious, suffered fractures of the right forearm and right femur, and had several lacerations. He was treated in the hospital for 18 days and was discharged.

Hospital personnel are not the only ones who may pose a hazard to the patient in MR scanners. The patient may bring with him his own potential projectiles. A number of surgical hemostatic and aneurysm clips have been found to be ferromagnetic (17). Nonsteel (silver or titanium) clips, suture wires, and hip prostheses are nonmagnetic and pose no hazard. Stainless steel clips may or may not be ferromagnetic and it is the rare patient, indeed, who would know into which category his surgical clips fell. Metallic objects such as shrapnel or iron filings may be lodged in the body, and like surgical clips, could be potential internal projectiles if the patient were placed in proximity to the MR magnet. For these reasons, many institutions will refuse to scan patients with surgical clips, a history of embedded metallic foreign bodies, or a history of having worked around metal filings. The use of metal detectors or magnetometers has been advocated for screening patients prior to MR scanning. Some of these devices can distinguish ferromagnetic from nonferromagnetic objects (18).

Nonferromagnetic wheelchairs and stretchers should be standard equipment in the MR area. One group (19) experimented with a nonferromagnetic crash cart stocked with nonferromagnetic supplies but chose, instead, to use a standard crash cart located outside the scanning area. Their decision was based on the premise that a nonstandard cart and nonstandard equipment would be unfamiliar to personnel in the hospital and might increase the risk of error during a code. Also, people who responded to a code might carry metallic objects into the scan room resulting in a "missile effect." Therefore, they decided that the best course of action was to train the MR personnel in CPR, to get the patient out of the scanner rapidly, and to proceed with the code away from the scan room.

Summary

Clearly, one can see, there are a number of uses for MRI in critically ill patients. With more experience and development of newer techniques such as magnetic resonance spectroscopy, and the ability to image atoms such as phosphorus and sodium, MRI will become even more useful. However, at the present time there are significant difficulties which limit the use of MRI in the critically ill patient. As newer scanning techniques are developed which decrease the time needed for a scan, as we become more accustomed to working in strong magnetic fields, and as more equipment is developed which is capable of operating safely in the magnetic environment, MRI will become more widely used in the diagnosis of critical care patients.

References

1. Been M, Smith MA, Ridgeway JP, et al: Characterisation of acute myocardial infarction by gated magnetic resonance imaging. *Lancet* 1985; ii:348

2. Tscholakoff D, Higgins CB: Gated magnetic resonance imaging for assessment of cardiac function and myocardial infarction. *Radiol Clin North Am* 1985; 23:449

3. Johnston DL, Thompson RC, Liu P, et al: Magnetic resonance imaging during acute myocardial infarction. *Am J Cardiol* 1986; 57:1059

4. Underwood SR, Rees RSO, Savage PE, et al: Assessment of regional left ventricular function by magnetic resonance. *Br Heart J* 1986; 56:334

5. Stratemeier EJ, Thompson R, Brady TJ, et al: Ejection fraction determination by MR imaging: Comparison with left ventricular angiography. *Radiology* 1986; 158:775

6. Thickman D, Kressel HY, Axel L: Demonstration of pulmonary embolism by magnetic resonance imaging. *AJR* 1984; 142:921

7. Moore EH, Gamsu G, Webb WR, et al: Pulmonary embolus: Detection and follow up using magnetic resonance. *Radiology* 1984; 153:471

8. Zimmerman RA, Bilaniuk LT, Hackney DB, et al: Head injury: Early results of comparing CT and high field MR. *AJR* 1986; 147:1215

9. Baumgartner BR, Nelson RC, Ball TI, et al: MR imaging of renal transplants. *AJR* 1986; 147:949

10. Nixon C, Hirsch NP, Ormerod IEC, et al: Nuclear magnetic resonance, its implications for the anesthetist. *Anesthesia* 1986; 41:131

11. Holmes DR, Hayes DL, Gray JE, et al: The effects of magnetic resonance imaging on implantable pulse generators. *PACE* 1986; 9:360

12. Erlebacher JA, Cahill PT, Pannizzo F, et al: Effect of magnetic resonance imaging on DDD pacemakers. *Am J Cardiol* 1986; 57:437

13. Engler MB, Engler MM: The hazards of magnetic resonance imaging. *Am J Nurs* 1986; 86:650

14. Dunn V, Coffman CE, McGowan JE, et al: Mechanical ventilation during magnetic resonance imaging. *Magn Reson Imaging* 1985; 3:169

15. Legendre JP, Misner R, Forester GV, et al: A simple fiber optic monitor of cardiac and respiratory activity for biomedical magnetic resonance applications. *Magnetic Resonance in Medicine* 1986; 3:953

16. Fowler JR, terPenning B, Syverud SA, et al: Magnetic field hazard. *N Engl J Med* 1986; 314:1517

17. Barrafato D, Henkelman RM: Magnetic resonance imaging and surgical clips. *Can J Surg* 1984; 27:509

18. Finn EJ, Di Chiro G, Brooks RA, et al: Ferromagnetic materials in patients: Detection before MR imaging. *Radiology* 1985; 156:139

19. Weinreb JC, Maravilla KR, Peshock R, et al: Magnetic resonance imaging: Improving patient tolerance and safety. *AJR* 1984; 143:1285

Chapter 16

Tissue Oxygen Monitoring

Thomas L. Whitsett, MD, FACP

Outline

Educational Objectives

In this chapter the reader will learn:

1. to understand the factors that influence tissue oxygenation.

2. that tissue Po_2 is independent of arterial Po_2 under low-flow conditions and correlates well with Pao_2 during hyperperfusion.

3. to use these techniques to assess microvascular flow in a variety of clinical and investigative conditions.

Introduction

The monitoring of Po_2 in blood and other tissues became a reality in 1956 when Dr. Leland C. Clark, Jr. developed the electrode that carries his name (1). He desired a relatively simple method to continuously monitor the O_2 tension in venous and arterial blood circulating in the heart-lung machines (2). Realizing further possibilities with this technology, Huch et al. (3) and Eberhardt et al. (4), working independently, reported on the application of the Clark electrode for measurement of transcutaneous Po_2 ($Ptco_2$). The original expectation was that $Ptco_2$ measurements would closely correspond to arterial Pao_2 values. This promise was often realized in infants and was frequently utilized in the intensive care setting. Initially, the lack of correlation was disappointing and poorly understood. It was subsequently realized that low-flow conditions obviously limit tissue oxygenation (5). There was special concern in adults whose $Ptco_2$ values were approximately 80% of the Pao_2 values. This, too, was better understood with the realization that skin thickness increased with age while capillary density decreased, both resulting in lower $Ptco_2$ values.

Currently, much has been accomplished regarding O_2 monitoring systems. The Clark electrode was modified to measure conjunctival Po_2 ($Pcjo_2$). Electrode systems are available for measuring continuous Pao_2 from an arterial catheter. $Ptco_2$ has also been measured by mass spectrometry and gas chromatography (6). However, this more expensive and less functional technology has given way to applications of the Clark electrode and oximetry. A symposium was presented on $Ptco_2$ and $Ptcco_2$ measurements that reviews many important aspects (7). This chapter: a) briefly reviews some of the theoretical aspects that underlie measuring tissue Po_2, b) describes methodological aspects, and c) discusses some of the more common uses. Brief comments are made regarding oximetry and its uses. Table 1 is a representative list of numerous applications for monitoring tissue oxygenation. This list continues to grow as the technology and familiarity with its capabilities expands.

TABLE 1. Partial listing of uses for oxygen monitoring systems

TRANSCUTANEOUS

Shock Syndrome	(8)	Liver & Gastric Perfusion	(23)
Peripheral Vascular Disease	(9,10,11)	Intraoperative Apnea	(24,25)
During Exercise Testing	(12)	During Extubation	(26)
Congenital Heart Disease	(13,14,15)	Inoperative Vascular Disease	(27)
Limb Lesions in Diabetics	(16,17)	Major Trauma	(28)
PEEP Titration	(18)	Healing of Amputation Sites	(29,30)
During Asthma	(19)	Conscious Oral Surgery	(31)
Critically Ill Newborns	(20,21)	Skin Flaps	(32,33)
Bowel Viability	(22)		

CONJUNCTIVAL

Cardiopulmonary Resuscitation	(34)
Monitoring Hemorrhage	(35,36)
Carotid Surgery	(37)
During Patient Transport	(38)

Instrumentation

The Clark Electrode

A modern-day electrode is illustrated in Figure 1. This system employs the principle that a small voltage applied to a cathode produces an electric current that passes to an anode. As each O_2 molecule is reduced at the cathode, four electrons will pass through the circuit, thus altering the flow of electricity that is monitored by an ampmeter.

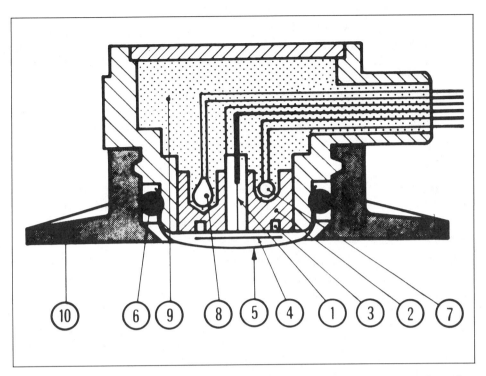

Fig. 1. Cut-away view of electrode: 1) *platinum cathode;* 2) *silver anode;* 3) *electrolyte chamber;* 4) *cuprophane spacer;* 5) *polypropylene membrane;* 6) *O ring;* 7) *heating element;* 8) *NTC resistor;* 9) *epoxy resin;* 10) *retaining ring.*

It is important for the platinum-wire cathode to be of a sufficiently small dimension to avoid a level of O_2 consumption ($\dot{V}o_2$) that would exceed availability under low-Po_2 conditions. The replaceable membrane that covers the electrode permits O_2 molecules to diffuse through to the platinum wire. The material and its thickness are important to provide an optimum rate of diffusion from the skin surface to the electrode. The most commonly used material is polypropylene, with a thickness of 25 mm. Membranes that are too thin can increase "diffusion error" and underestimate Po_2. Questions have been raised regarding halothane causing a falsely high $Ptco_2$ value when used with a polypropylene membrane, but not with a Teflon membrane. This appears to be a problem discovered in vitro when higher-than-standard concentrations of anesthetic were used; it was not a problem during standard anesthesia (39). The heating element is a critical part of this system and will be discussed later.

Calibration, preferably at 2 points, especially when low values are to be measured, is rather easy with most instruments. The zero point may be established by use of nitrogen gas or a "zeroing solution," while higher levels are determined by calibrating with room air. When moving the electrode every 4 h to avoid burns, or under certain conditions when it is desirable to measure $Ptco_2$ in more than one site, room-air calibrations should be checked between measurements.

To obtain a measurement, the skin is shaved and cleaned with alcohol to remove any oil. The electrode is attached to the skin surface with a double-stick O ring or an adaptor. The electrode temperature is set at 44 to 45°C. There is a warm-up time of 5 to 20 min to establish diffusion equilibrium, but subsequently there is minimal lag time. Although it clearly does not have the instantaneous response of oximetry, results can be taken from a digital read-out or a strip-chart recorder if a permanent or continuous record is desired. This electrode has been modified to fit beneath the eyelid and permit measurement of $Pjco_2$ (40). It does not require heating since the problems with the skin do not have to be overcome. Interestingly, it also has similar findings as skin in regard to decreases with advancing age (41). Although this is relatively new instrumentation, it is improving and its usefulness is evolving (Table 1).

Oximetry

Oximetry is the term applied to the instrument that was developed in 1942 to noninvasively measure the O_2 saturation of arterial blood. While it is not the intent of this presentation to critically review the topic, as this has recently been accomplished (42), general comments are presented.

This technique is ideal for continuous measurement of arterial O_2 saturation and has correlation coefficients of 0.97 under conditions of general use (43). The principle of operation concerns the difference in light absorption between oxygenated and reduced Hgb. A light source of appropriate wavelength is transmitted through the skin, e.g., ear lobe, finger, or toe. A sensor detects the amount of light absorbed, which is related to the concentration of oxyhemoglobin (Hbo_2). The analog waveform reflects the pulsatile nature of flow and can be used to monitor the adequacy of capillary flow as well as heart rate and rhythm.

While the technique has become the mainstay for monitoring Hbo_2 saturation, it is influenced by carboxyhemoglobin (Hbco), skin pigments (bilirubin) and circulating dyes (indocyanine green). Of course, this is not a sensitive technique for assessing tissue O_2 delivery since that is also determined by cardiac output, Hgb concentration, and the O_2 affinity of Hgb.

Theoretical Considerations

Much work has been done to understand the various factors that influence skin surface Po_2 and its measurement with the Clark electrode. There are excellent reviews by Lubbers (44) and Tremper and Waxman (45) which summarize in considerable detail both the physical and physiological factors that are important for proper application of this technique.

The structure, $\dot{V}o_2$ and blood supply of the skin are important factors that influence $Ptco_2$ measurements (Fig. 2). The epidermis is metabolically active and has a $\dot{V}o_2$ of 0.28 ml/100 g·min at 37°C and 0.37 ml/100 g·min at a temperature of 44°C while the stratum corneum or the "dead layer" is inactive (46). The epidermis is relatively thin at birth, becomes thicker at puberty, and thinner again by reduction in the size of papillae around the fifth to sixth decade (47). Also, the epidermis is thicker in men and on the palms and soles. Thickness of the skin is a major variable in the ability of $Ptco_2$ to reflect Pao_2.

The blood supply of the epidermis involves a series of hairpin-shaped capillary loops (48). The dome of the capillaries are in close contact with the basal cells of the epidermis (Fig. 2). Capillary density varies from one region of the body to another; in newborns, the capillaries are more dense than in adults. This is another factor that explains a lower $Ptco_2$ compared to Pao_2 in adults.

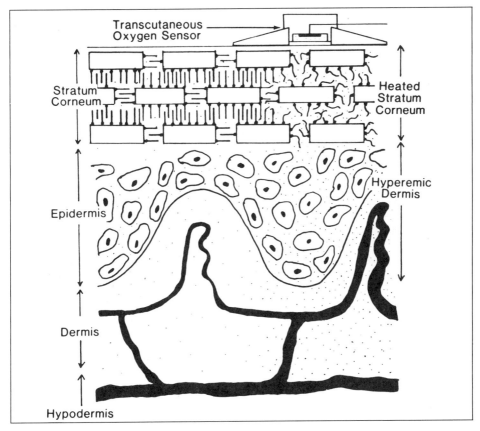

Fig. 2. Schematic cross section of the electrode and skin: stratum corneum, epidermis, dermis, and hypodermis. This irregular structure of the stratum corneum beneath the electrode represents the melted lipid. The dots represent O_2. Reproduced from Tremper et al. (45) with permission.

The capillary loop at the base of the epidermis is situated in close parallel proximity to the arterial and collecting venule. This results in a counter-current mechanism that permits an O_2 "shunt diffusion" to take place between the arterial and venous capillary limbs (49). At normal skin temperature and during low cutaneous blood flow (even with elevated skin temperature), the surface Po_2 is virtually zero as a result of shunt diffusion. As capillary blood flow increases, shunt diffusion decreases. This explains the so-called arteriolization of the capillaries, i.e., a level of capillary blood flow that provides a Po_2 in the dome of the capillary comparable to Pao_2.

The relationship of blood flow to the venous O_2 concentration is important, since adequate flow is necessary to avoid shunt diffusion. This relationship was termed "circulatory hyperbola" by Lubbers (44) (Fig. 3). Clearly, it is necessary to operate in region 3 to negate the effect of flow on capillary O_2 concentration. Under low-flow conditions (region 1), there is a proportional drop in capillary O_2; small changes in flow produce dramatic effects on O_2. This explains how $Ptco_2$ measurements can reflect tissue perfusion while Pao_2 is unchanged. Attempts at adequately increasing capillary flow to approach region 3 by pharmacologic means has not been successfully accomplished, since values were in the range of 30 to 40 ml/100 g·min. From Figure 3 it can be seen that skin blood flow must be in the range of 80-plus ml/100 g·min to be on the portion of the curve that is flow-independent. The application of heat produces vasodilation by a non-neuronal mechanism. At room temperature, only 75% of the capillaries are perfused with blood. By heating the skin, the maximum flow occurs around 45°C (50) (Fig. 4). Interestingly, the $Ptco_2$ values are not influenced by heat as is argon diffusion. Argon diffusion reflects skin permeability and is directly related to temperature. The improved skin O_2 permeability with heating is due to changes in the lipid content of the stratum corneum from a solid to liquid phase (51). This permits gases to diffuse through the skin several hundred times faster. Heating the skin by means of the electrode has another effect unrelated to cutaneous blood flow and O_2 diffusion. Increasing temperature shifts the O_2 dissociation curve to the right. Thus, for a given O_2 concentration there is an increase in Po_2; therefore, with locally applied heat the $Ptco_2$ increases accordingly. The magnitude of the shift is relatively small and should not produce $Ptco_2$ values above those of Pao_2.

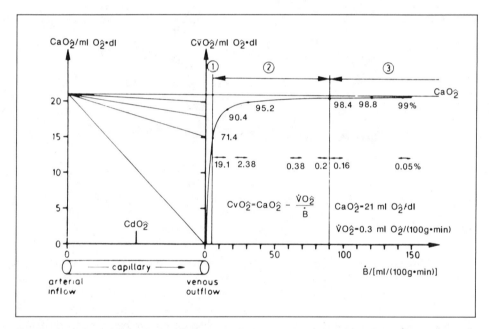

Fig. 3. Circulatory hyperbole for the overall O_2 supply of the skin. The arterial O_2 concentration (Cao_2) decreases linearly along the capillary to the venous O_2 concentration ($C\bar{v}o_2$) (left side). With a constant $Cao_2 = 21$ ml/dl and $\dot{V}o_2 = 0.3$ ml/100 g·min, the flow (B) is calculated according to the equations on the right side. $C\bar{v}o_2$ depends on B in a hyperbolic way. The numbers at the dots of the curve describe the percental approach to Cao_2. There are three different regions: 1) $C\bar{v}o_2$ changes very much with flow, 2) distinct changes of $C\bar{v}o_2$ with flow changes, and 3) $C\bar{v}o_2$ is almost independent of flow. The lines with two arrows correspond to a flow change of 10 ml/100 g·min and the numbers to the concomitant percental change of $C\bar{v}o_2$. $CdO_2 = O_2$ concentration at the dome of the capillary loop. Reproduced from Lubbers (44) with permission.

The effect of gas and heat exchange on different layers of the skin was reviewed (52). The outer layer of the epidermis (stratum-corneum) does not consume O_2; O_2 transport is by diffusion. Any factor that increases the thickness of this dead material will reduce the $Ptco_2$. The inner layer contains metabolically active cells and while O_2 transport is by diffusion, these cells consume O_2. Dry skin has an increased O_2 diffusion resistance; to modify that, the skin is moistened at the site of electrode attachment. Also, $Ptco_2$ values have been used to reflect the state of hydration and the adequacy of fluid replacement (53). Heat also decreases O_2 solubility while it increases skin $\dot{V}o_2$. However, these contrasting effects are known; when $Ptco_2$ measurements are made at skin temperatures around 44°C, these factors are minimized.

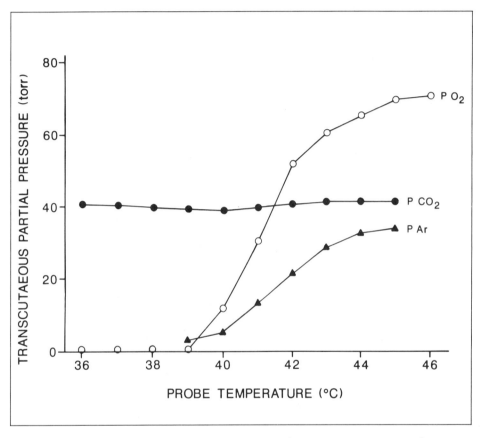

Fig. 4. The influence of skin probe temperature on the transcutaneous partial pressure measurement of three gases: ○ = $Ptco_2$ using a PVC membrane; ● = tcP Ar using PVC membrane; ▲ = $Ptco_2$ using an oriented polypropylene membrane. PtcAr = argon. Modified from Al-Siaidy and Hill (50) with permission.

Clinical Use of Oxygen Monitoring Systems

During the 14 yr since this technique became generally available, there have been many reports of varied uses. Much of this was reviewed with particular emphasis in areas involving pediatric patients (54). While early use focused on $Ptco_2$ as a technique that would reflect Pao_2 values, it was subsequently learned that the $Ptco_2$ measuring devices also reflect tissue perfusion, and definite use was established in areas that might otherwise interfere with Pao_2 correlation (Table 2). However, there was a real need for a noninvasive method to monitor the state of blood oxygenation with a minimum of distracting factors. Measurement

TABLE 2. Factors associated with altered $Ptco_2$ and Pao_2 correlations

Thickened & Keratotic Skin	Hypothermia
Edema	Severe Anemia
Shock	Severe Acidosis
Vascular Disease	Tolazoline in Infants

of Hbo_2 saturation by oximetry has moved into that role and has replaced $Ptco_2$ as a means of assessing moment-to-moment changes in blood oxygenation.

Neonatal

The newborn infant is particularly well suited for $Ptco_2$ measurements since the skin is rather thin, has a low O_2 diffusion resistance, and there is naturally a high density of skin capillary loops. Avoiding repeated arterial punctures that cause crying and possibly reduce Pao_2 is of obvious benefit. Correlation of $Ptco_2$ with Pao_2 is especially good, particularly when the various factors listed in Table 2 are excluded. In numerous studies involving over 3,000 comparisons, the correlation coefficient was greater than 0.9 (54). Values of 0.98 were obtained when appropriate conditions were recognized and excluded.

Obstetrics

While maternal and newborn oxygenation monitoring is in common clinical use, fetal measurements are much more complicated; there still remains considerable investigative work to resolve many of its special problems. Fetal $Ptco_2$ measurements can be performed with a standard Clark electrode but special instrumentation is necessary for sterile attachment of the electrode to the scalp (55). Electrodes may be attached after rupture of the membranes and with at least a 2 to 3-cm cervical dilation; monitoring may be accomplished over a 12-h period. The inability to closely observe the site of electrode attachment and recognize edema or pressure on the electrode is a methodological problem that can interfere with obtaining precise and reliable results.

Data are not available correlating fetal scalp $Ptco_2$ with Pao_2 in humans, but have been obtained in fetal lambs with excellent agreement (56). Comparisons were made between human fetal scalp capillary blood and $Ptco_2$ values (57). These measurements were, on the average, 17 torr with good correlation. Other experiences have recognized a reliably large number of false-positive results, that is, values less than 12 torr in individuals without evidence of fetal distress. Obviously, these problems need further clarification before its use can be generally recommended.

Anesthesiology

Since there is normally a 10% to 20% difference in adult $Ptco_2$ and Pao_2, and the anesthesiologist needs to know the state of oxygenation, measurement of $Ptco_2$ has not been generally accepted (58). Table 1 lists a variety of uses in anesthesiology. The conjunctival electrodes have been used with a better Pao_2 correlation. Measurement of blood oxygenation by oximetry, as already discussed, is widely used to provide quick and relatively inexpensive moment-to-moment determinations.

Surgery

PtcO$_2$ has been employed in a variety of situations, as listed in Table 1. While there are similar criticisms as noted for anesthesiology, there are still circumstances of definite value. Intraoperative monitoring of extremity PtcO$_2$ values in patients undergoing revascularization is a good example of utilizing this technique's ability to assess adequacy of tissue perfusion (27). This technique can also be used to follow individuals in the postoperative state to recognize early circulatory failure that may require reoperation. A particularly innovative use concerns the assessment of bowel viability at the time of operation (22). Conjunctival O$_2$ was shown to correlate well with cerebral blood flow, and was proven useful during carotid artery surgery (37), although this was questioned (38). Cutaneous monitoring of O$_2$ and CO$_2$ during conscious sedation for oral surgery revealed a 36% incidence of significant hypoxia that was not recognized by clinical appearance (31). Usefulness has also been demonstrated in skin-flap viability assessment (32, 33).

Vascular Disease

PtcO$_2$ measurements have found considerable use in patients with peripheral vascular disease (9-11, 16, 17, 27, 29, 30). This is a result of the ability of PtcO$_2$ to reflect tissue perfusion and not just PaO$_2$. The use of measurements on the leg and particularly the dorsum of the foot may have merit, but interpretation may be difficult since control values measured from the subclavian or deltoid area are sometimes surprisingly low. This is likely related to a variety of factors, e.g., the patient's age, presence of obstructive lung disease, dehydration, and cigarette smoking. To distinguish between local and systemic effects, the limb/chest PtcO$_2$ ratio was used and termed the regional perfusion index (RPI) (9). This has helped in quantifying deficits in tissue perfusion, and corrected for fluctuations in O$_2$ delivery and changes in circulatory status. However, without some maneuver there still remains excessive overlap when comparing individuals with claudication, ischemic rest pain, and nonhealing lesions (30, 59).

Patients with diabetes mellitus and peripheral vascular disease are a particularly challenging group when medialsclerosis causes the cuff pressure to greatly exceed intra-arterial pressure and thus, falsely elevate ankle or segmental pressures determined by Doppler. PtcO$_2$ measurements have been used successfully in this setting (15), particularly when RPI is determined with the leg elevated as well as supine (17) (Fig. 5). While worsening of ischemia is not surprising when the legs are elevated, it is interesting to note that PtcO$_2$ is increased in ischemic legs that are placed in the dependent position. This is a possible explanation for the relief of pain in individuals with resting ischemia when they sit or stand.

There is an additional maneuver that is helpful in categorizing patients with vascular disease, and which is especially helpful in assessing their response to therapy (60). This was termed the transcutaneous O$_2$ recovery half-time. PtcO$_2$ values, or preferably, RPI values are obtained at rest and following 4 min of arterial occlusion by a thigh pneumatic compression cuff. Transcutaneous O$_2$ recovery half-time is the time required for the RPI to return to 50% of the control value. In normals, this occurs by 1.5 min. Patients with peripheral vascular disease require longer times depending upon the degree of disease (Fig. 6).

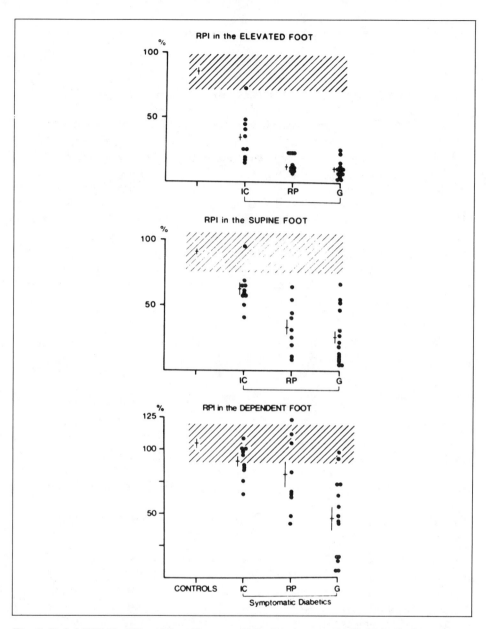

Fig. 5. Pedal RPI (foot $Ptco_2$/chest $Ptco_2$ × 100) of symptomatic diabetic limbs as measured in the elevated, supine, and dependent positions. The hatched areas represent 95% confidence limits of RPI in normal limbs. IC = intermittent claudication; RP = rest pain; G = gangrene. Reproduced from Hauser et al. (17) with permission.

Experimental Applications

The importance of an adequate concentration of tissue O_2 is uncontested, and its measurement is a continuing challenge. A variety of techniques are available and the resulting information has clearly demonstrated that tissues are inhomogenously oxygenated (61). While a bell-shaped distribution of tissue O_2 normally exists, under pathologic conditions it is disrupted with a clustering of values toward the lower range of Po_2 (Fig. 7). Such a finding could result from

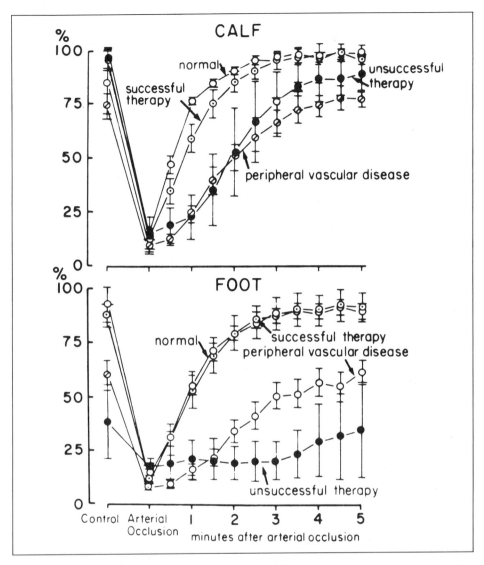

Fig. 6. *Effect of temporary arterial occlusion on calf and foot* $Ptco_2$ *values, expressed as percentage of simultaneously recorded chest* $Ptco_2$, *in normal volunteers, in patients with PVD, in patients who had successful and unsuccessful therapy. Values are mean ± SEM. Reproduced from Kram et al. (60) with permission.*

inadequate cardiac output, excessive hypotension, arterial occlusive disease, and microvascular disease with arteriolar and capillary narrowing. When using $Ptco_2$ as a reflection of tissue perfusion, it is important to recall that resting blood flow in these conditions may not be associated with ischemia, but with increased O_2 demand in the face of fixed or limited blood supply; tissue hypoxia and cellular dysfunction then ensue. Given this reality, the choice of a monitoring technique depends upon whether one is interested in summing microvascular units with a surface electrode (as in a skin-flap graft) or assess disrupted patterns of perfusion (as seen in shock) that would be reflected by smaller multi-wire electrodes that obtain numerous samples.

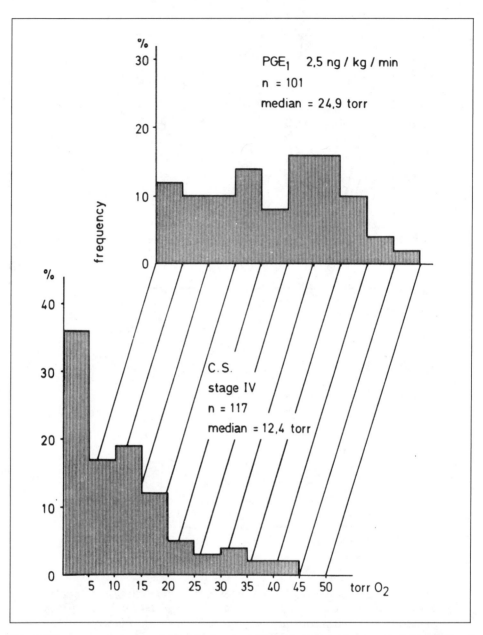

Fig. 7. Histogram of a patient before (bottom) and during (top) an intra-arterial infusion of prostaglandin E_1 (2.5 ng/kg·min). Median Po_2 is doubled and changes are noted in the distribution type of the histogram. Reproduced from Lund et al. (61) with permission.

Surface Electrode

The Clark or surface electrode has been applied successfully to the surface of a variety of organs, permitting better understanding of tissue oxygenation. Using a miniaturized electrode, this technique was applied to the intraoperative assessment of net tissue oxygenation associated with a variety of vascular procedures (23). It was applied to brain, liver, gallbladder, stomach, jejunum, ileum, colon, and kidney. This means of assessing organ perfusion and O_2 transport can

296

also be applied to experimental circumstances for monitoring tissue O_2 during induced shock or other forms of experimental intervention.

Needle Electrode

Measuring tissue PO_2 at deeper levels has been somewhat successful with a needle electrode (62). While the needle electrodes that are commercially available may have some utility, there is considerable movement artifact and drift that occurs in many tissues because the electrode size (22-ga) is disruptive. Special skills are required to make needles that are small enough (2 to 4 μm in diameter) and yet properly insulated. Also, a micromanipulator is necessary to move the electrode through 10 mm of tissue over a 5 to 10-min period. This provides a good sample of the microvasculature to assess homogeneity of tissue perfusion. These electrodes have been used in humans with peripheral vascular disease demonstrating the benefits of ancrod, a defibrinating agent (62), and pentoxifylline, a rheologically active drug (63).

Multiwire Electrode

The surface electrode was modified to provide a means of assessing inhomogenous oxygenation. Multiple (8 to 16) platinum wires, 15 μm in diameter, are enclosed in a single assembly. Each electrode measures O_2 in a 20 to 25-micron radius which permits assessment between capillaries. Multiple sites are sampled and a histogram is generated (64). This technique is commercially available and has been applied to skeletal muscle (by a skin incision) in patients with peripheral vascular disease to measure PO_2 response to dextran 40 and prostaglandin E_1, (65) (Fig. 7). It has also been applied in renal transplantation (66) and on the liver during portacaval anastomosis (67).

While the multiwire system provides valuable information concerning disrupted microvascular oxygenation, the technology is somewhat complex and relatively expensive. However, it is not difficult to use once exposure of the tissue for placement of the electrode has been achieved. It appears that this method is ideally suited for evaluating the microvascular response to pharmacologic agents and other forms of experimental intervention.

References

1. Clark LC Jr: Monitor and control of blood and tissue oxygen tensions. *Trans Am Soc Artif Intern Organs* 1956; 2:41

2. Clark LC Jr: Measurement of oxygen tension: A historical perspective. *Crit Care Med* 1981; 9:690

3. Huch A, Huch R, Menzer K, et al: Eine schnelle, betizte proberlachenelek trode zer kontinuier lichen uberwach ung des Po_2 beim menschjen. Electro denautbautbau Und-eigen Schaften. Stuttgart: Proc Medizin-Technik, May, 1972

4. Eberhard P, Mint W, Hammacher K: Perkutane messung des sauerstatpartialdruckes. Methodick und Anwendungen. Stuttgart: Proc Medizin-Technik, May, 1972

5. Tremper KK, Waxman K, Shoemaker WC: Effects of hypoxia and shock on transcutaneous Po_2 values in dogs. *Crit Care Med* 1979; 7:526

6. Delpy DT, Parkwood D, Reynolds EOR, et al: Transcutaneous blood gas analysis by mass spectrometry and gas chromatography. *In*: Continuous Transcutaneous Blood Gas Monitoring. Original Article Series - Birth Defects. The National Foundation March of Dimes. Volume 15. Huch A, Huch R, Lucey JF (Eds). New York, Alan R Liss, 1979, pp 91-101

7. Shoemaker WC, Vidyasagar D (Eds): Physiological and clinical significance of $Ptco_2$ measurements. A symposium on transcutaneous Po_2 and Pco_2 measurements. *Crit Care Med* 1981; 9:689

8. Tremper KK, Shoemaker WC: Transcutaneous oxygen monitoring of critically ill adults, with and without low flow shock. *Crit Care Med* 1981; 9:706

9. Hauser CJ, Shoemaker WC: Use of a transcutaneous Po_2 regional perfusion index to quantify tissue perfusion in peripheral vascular disease. *Ann Surg* 1983; 197:337

10. Hauser CJ, Appel PL, Shoemaker WC: Pathophysiologic classification of peripheral vascular disease by positional changes in regional transcutaneous oxygen tension. *Surgery* 1983; 95:689

11. Kram HB, Appel PL, White RA, et al: Assessment of peripheral vascular disease by postocclusive transcutaneous oxygen recovery time. *J Vasc Surg* 1984; 1:628

12. Gidding SS, Rosenthal A, Moorehead C: Follow-up evaluation of transcutaneous Po_2 monitoring before and after adult exercise testing. *Respiratory Care* 1981; 26:963

13. Gidding SS, Rosenthal A, Moorehead C: Transcutaneous oxygen monitoring. Its use in the treatment of outpatients with congenital heart disease. *Am J Dis Child* 1985; 139:288

14. Heinonen K, Hakulinen A: Transcutaneous Po_2 recording using two sensors in a neonate with preductal coarction of the aorta. *Crit Care Med* 1986; 14:298

15. Hauser CJ, Klein SR, Mehringer CM, et al: Superiority of transcutaneous oximetry in noninvasive vascular diagnosis in patients with diabetes. *Arch Surg* 1984; 119:690

16. Wyes CR, Matsen F, Simmons CW, et al: Transcutaneous oxygen tension measurements on limbs of diabetic and nondiabetic patients with peripheral vascular disease. *Surgery* 1984; 95:339

17. Hauser CJ, Klein SR, Mehringer CM, et al: Assessment of perfusion in the diabetic foot by regional transcutaneous oximetry. *Diabetes* 1984; 33:527

18. Tremper KK, Waxman K, Shoemaker WC: Use of transcutaneous oxygen sensors to titrate PEEP. *Ann Surg* 1981; 193:206

19. Wennergren G, Engstrom E, Bjure J: Transcutaneous oxygen and carbon dioxide levels and a clinical symptom scale for monitoring the acute asthmatic state in infants and young children. *Acta Paediatr Scand* 1986; 75:465

20. Peabody JL, Emery JR: Noninvasive monitoring of blood gases in the newborn. *Clin Perinatol* 1985; 12:147

21. Kilbride HW, Merenstein GB: Continuous transcutaneous oxygen monitoring in acutely ill preterm infants. *Crit Care Med* 1984; 12:121

22. Locke R, Hauser CJ, Shoemaker WC: The use of surface oximetry to assess bowel viability. *Arch Surg* 1984; 119:1252

23. Kram HB, Shoemaker WC: Method for intraoperative assessment of organ perfusion and viability using a miniature oxygen sensor. *Am J Surg* 1984; 148:404

24. Hauser CJ, Harley DP: Transcutaneous gas tension monitoring in the management of intraoperative apnea. *Crit Care Med* 1983; 11:830

25. Mikatti NE: Arterial and transcutaneous oxygen tension measurement during hypotensive anaesthesia. *Ann R Coll Surg Engl* 1982; 64:328

26. Tahvanainen J, Nikki P: The significance of hypoxemia with low inspired O_2 fraction before extubation. *Crit Care Med* 1983; 11:708

27. Kram HB, Shoemaker WC: Use of transcutaneous O_2 monitoring in the intraoperative management of severe peripheral vascular disease. *Crit Care Med* 1983; 11:482

28. Kram HB, Shoemaker WC: Diagnosis of major peripheral arterial trauma by transcutaneous oxygen monitoring. *Am J Surg* 1984; 147:776

29. Burgess EM, Marsen FA, Wyss CR, et al: Segmental transcutaneous measurements of Po_2 in patients requiring below-the-knee amputation for peripheral vascular insufficiency. *J Bone Joint Sur* 1982; 64-A:382

30. Franzeck UK, Talke P, Bernstein EF, et al: Transcutaneous Po_2 measurements in health and peripheral arterial occlusive disease. *Surgery* 1982; 91:156

31. Kraut RA, Colonel DC: Continuous transcutaneous O_2 and CO_2 monitoring during conscious sedation for oral surgery. *J Oral Surg* 1985; 43:489

32. Archauer BM, Black KS, Litke DK: Transcutaneous Po_2 in flaps: A new method of survival prediction. *Plast Reconstr Surg* 1980; 65:738

33. Sloan GM, Reinisch JF: Flap physiology and the prediction of flap viability. *Hand Clinics* 1985; 1:609

34. Abraham E, Smith M, Silver L: Conjunctival and transcutaneous oxygen monitoring during cardiac arrest and cardiopulmonary resuscitation. *Crit Care Med* 1984; 12:419

35. Abraham E, Smith M: Conjunctival oxygen tension monitoring during hemorrhage. *Crit Care Med* 1985; 13:353

36. Abraham E, Oye RK, Smith M: Detection of blood volume deficits through conjunctival oxygen tension monitoring. *Crit Care Med* 1984; 12:931

37. Shoemaker WC, Lawner PB: Method for continuous conjunctival oxygen monitoring during carotid artery surgery. *Crit Care Med* 1983; 11:946

38. Abraham E, Lee G, Morgan M: Conjunctival oxygen tension monitoring during helicopter transport of critically ill patients. *Crit Care Med* 1983; 11:946

39. Samra KS: Halothane interference with transcutaneous oxygen monitoring: In vivo and in vitro. *Crit Care Med* 1983; 11:612

40. Fink S, Ray CW, McCartney S, et al: Oxygen transport and utilization in hyperoxia and hypoxia: Relation of conjunctival and transcutaneous oxygen tensions to hemodynamic and oxygen transport variables. *Crit Care Med* 1984; 12:943

41. Isenberg SJ, Green BF: Changes in conjunctival oxygen tension and temperature with advancing age. *Crit Care Med* 1985; 13:683

42. Chapman KR, Rebuck AS: Oximetry. *In*: Noninvasive Respiratory Monitoring. Nochomovitz ML, Cherniack NS (Eds). New York, Churchill Livingstone, 1986, pp 203-221

43. Saunders NA, Powles ACP, Rebuck AS: Ear oximetry: Accuracy and practicability in the assessment of arterial oxygenation. *Am Rev Respir Dis* 1976; 113:745

44. Lubbers DW: Theoretical basis of the transcutaneous blood gas measurements. *Crit Care Med* 1981; 9:721

45. Tremper KK, Waxman KS: Transcutaneous monitoring of respiratory gases. *In*: Noninvasive Respiratory Monitoring. Nochomovitz ML, Chernaiack NS (Eds). New York, Churchill Livingstone, 1986, pp 1-28

46. Severinghaus JW, Stafford M, Thunstrom AM: Estimation of skin metabolism and blood flow with $Ptco_2$ and $Ptcco_2$ electrodes by cuff occlusion of the circulation. *Acta Anaesthesiol Scand* 1978; 68:9

47. Southwood WFW: The thickness of the skin. *Plast Reconstr Surg* 1956; 15:423

48. Ellis RA: Vascular patterns of the skin. *In*: Advances in Biology of Skin. Volume II. Blood Vessels and Circulation. Montagna W, Ellis RA (Eds). New York, Pergamon Press, 1961, pp 20-37

49. Grossman U, Huber J, Fricke R, et al: A new model for simulating oxygen pressure field of skin. *In*: Oxygen Transport to Tissue. Kovach AGB, Dora E, Kessler M, et al (Eds). Budapest, Pergamon Press, 1981, pp 319-320

50. Al-Siaidy W, Hill DW: The importance of an elevated skin temperature in transcutaneous oxygen tension measurement. *In*: Continuous Transcutaneous Blood Gas Monitoring. Original Article Series - Birth Defects. The National Foundation March of Dimes. Huch A, Huch R, Lucey JF (Eds). New York, Alan R Liss, 1979, pp 223-233

51. Van Duzee BJ: Thermal analysis of human stratum corneum. *J Invest Dermatol* 1975; 65:404

52. Huch R, Huch A, Lubbers DW: Gas and heat exchange in the different layers of skin. *In*: Transcutaneous Po_2. Huch R, Huch A, Lubbers DW (Eds). New York, Theime-Stratton, Inc, 1981, pp 20-41

53. Yonfa AE: Use of TC-Po_2 as an aid in fluid and blood administration. *Anaesthesiol Rev* 1983; 10:33

54. Huch R, Huch A, Lubbers DW: Applications in clinical medicine and physiologic research. *In*: Transcutaneous Po_2. New York, Thieme-Stratton, Inc, 1981, pp 118-151

55. Huch R, Huch A, Lubbers DW: Characteristics of electrode construction significant for measurement on the skin. *In*: Transcutaneous Po_2. New York, Thieme-Stratton, Inc, 1981, pp 82-94

56. Mueller-Heuback E, Seiler D, Huch R, et al: Use of the $Ptco_2$ Electrode in the animal fetus. *In*: Continuous Transcutaneous Blood Gas Monitoring. Original Article Series - Birth Defects. The National Foundation March of Dimes. Huch A, Huch R, Lucey FJ (Eds). New York, Alan R Liss, 1979, pp 599-605

57. Fall O, Johnsson M, Nilsson BA, et al: A study of the correlation between the oxygen tension of the fetal scalp blood and the continuous, transcutaneous oxygen tension in human fetuses during labour. *In*: Continuous Transcutaneous Blood Gas Monitoring. Original Article Series - Birth Defects. The National Foundation March of Dimes. Huch A, Huch R, Lucey JF (Eds). New York, Alan R Liss, 1979, pp 223-233

58. Pace NL, Stanley TH, Adriano KP, et al: Transcutaneous Po_2 poorly estimates arterial Po_2 in adults during anesthesia. *International Journal of Clinical Monitoring and Computing* 1985; 1:227

59. Clyne CAC, Ryan J, Webster JHH, et al: Oxygen tension on the skin of ischemic legs. *Am J Surg* 1982; 143:315

60. Kram HB, Appel PL, White RA, et al: Assessment of peripheral vascular disease by postocclusive transcutaneous oxygen recovery time. *J Vasc Surg* 1984; 1:628

61. Lund N, Jorfeldt L, Lewis DH: Skeletal muscle oxygen pressure fields in healthy human volunteers. *Acta Anaesthesiol Scand* 1980; 24:272

62. Ehrly AM, Schroeder W: Oxygen pressure in ischemic muscle tissue of patients with chronic occlusive arterial diseases. *Angiology* 1977; 29:101

63. Ehrly AM: Measurements of oxygen tension in muscle. *In*: Pharmacological Approach to the Treatment of Limb Ischemia. Spittell JA Jr (Ed). Philadelphia, American College of Clinical Pharmacology, 1983, pp 65-72

64. Kunze K: Das Sauerstoffdruckfeld im normalen und pathologischveran- derten Muske. Schriftenreihe Neurologie. Berlin, Springer-Verlag, 1969

65. Creutzig A, Alexander K: Drug-induced alterations in muscle tissue oxygen pressure in patients with arterial occlusive disease. *Int J Microcirc Clin Exp* 1985; 4:173

66. Singagowitz E, Golsong M, Halbfass HJ: Local tissue Po_2 in kidney surgery and transplantation. *Adv Exp Med Biol* 1978; 94:721

67. Broelsch C, Hoper J, Kessler M: Oxygen supply to the cirrhotic liver follow- ing various portacaval shunt procedures. *Adv Exp Med Biol* 1978; 94:633

Chapter 17

Circulatory Assist Devices: A Review

Jack G. Copeland, III, MD, Marilyn R. Cleavinger, MSBME, and Richard G. Smith, MSEE, CCE

Outline

Educational Objectives

In this chapter the reader will learn:

1. to identify the different types and applications of circulatory assist devices.

2. to understand the criteria used in selecting and applying a circulatory assist device.

3. to describe the support, cost, and complications associated with the technology of each circulatory assist device.

Introduction

The use of circulatory assist devices (CAD) has expanded dramatically within the past few years. Since 50% of all deaths in the United States involve cardiovascular disease (1), there is a significant need for devices to assist an impaired myocardium, and many variations of mechanical circulatory support have been developed and tried during the past 30 yr. Ongoing improvements in biomaterials, surgical techniques, patient management, and engineering designs have produced this class of devices which today are being used with increasing success in applications requiring support of the failing heart.

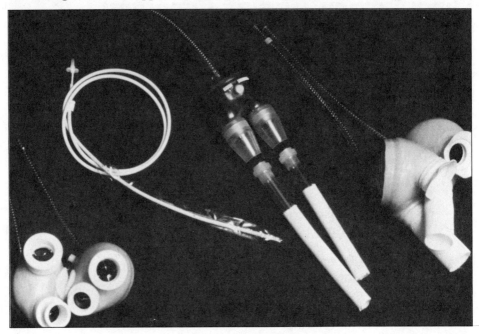

Fig. 1. An assortment of CADs. From left to right are: Jarvik 7-70 TAH, intraaortic balloon, Symbion pneumatic pulsatile VAD, Jarvik 7-100 TAH.

Mechanical assistance is currently indicated for two groups of patients: those in cardiac failure where the possibility of myocardial recovery exists (such as following a cardiotomy or an ischemic event) and those requiring support while awaiting cardiac transplantation (2). CADs available at this time are for temporary use only and include the intra-aortic balloon pump (IABP), ventricular assist device (VAD), and the total artificial heart (TAH), such as those shown in Figure 1. Work is also in progress at several centers under the guidance of the National Heart, Lung, and Blood Institute to develop totally implantable circulatory support systems which will perform faultlessly for a minimum of 2 yr. These permanent systems are targeted for use with irreversible cardiac damage where transplantation is not an option (3).

CADs reduce or totally replace the work effort required of the heart while providing circulatory support throughout the body. Studies have also shown that decreasing the workload of the heart while reperfusing the myocardium after an acute ischemic event may provide significantly better recovery of myocardial tissue (4, 5). CADs also provide an increase in myocardial perfusion which further aids in the recovery of tissue compromised by ischemia.

The prevalence of heart disease produces many people who need surgical intervention to improve their cardiac function, but whose existing myocardial impairment will put them at significant risk from surgery. A compromised myocardium may not contain the reserve necessary to withstand the trauma of surgery; approximately 2,000 patients per year are unweanable from cardiopulmonary bypass (6). CADs provide the surgeon with a tool to use in salvaging patients who exhibit a stunned myocardium postoperatively. In a recent series of cardiotomy cases, approximately 7% required IABP support with an additional 1% requiring further assistance in the form of a VAD (7, 8).

It has been recently estimated that 20% to 40% of transplant candidates will die before receiving a donor heart (9). The current wait for a heart transplant at our hospital is 36 days (10) and continues to increase due to the expanding discrepancy between the number of qualified recipients and the number of suitable organs available. Many successful bridges to transplant experiences have been reported following the employment of mechanical cardiac assistance to prevent or reverse the effects of cardiac decompensation occurring prior to transplantation (11-13). Registry data collected for 1986 indicates that mechanical bridges were used in over 4% of the total number of reported orthotopic cardiac transplantations for that year (14, 15).

Description of Devices

Intra-Aortic Balloon Pump

The intra-aortic balloon pump is the most commonly used mechanical assist device, with approximately 10,000 uses per year in the United States (9). Most hospitals with active cardiac catheterization laboratories or cardiovascular surgery facilities are already equipped with this technology. IABP is relatively inexpensive and easy to use. Although it requires the percutaneous femoral insertion of the balloon within the aorta, this is minimally invasive in comparison to the insertion of a VAD or TAH.

The first IABP was developed in 1962 by Moulopoulos, et al. (16) according to the principles of counterpulsation described by Clauss et al (17). A long, thin, flexible balloon is inserted via the femoral artery into the thoracic aorta to act as a blood displacement device. The balloon is filled with helium or CO_2 and pulsed, or alternately inflated and evacuated, in phase with events in the cardiac cycle. The principle of counterpulsation requires that the balloon be deflated during ejection of blood from the ventricles (systole) and inflated during ventricular filling (diastole). Proper timing with events in the cardiac cycle is crucial to the success of this therapy.

During systole, deflation of the balloon allows the left ventricle to eject blood into a lower aortic end-diastolic pressure, thereby decreasing the workload of the left heart. This concept, known as afterload reduction, has been demonstrated to decrease myocardial O_2 consumption by about 10%. Inflation of the balloon augments myocardial perfusion by increasing pressures in the coronary arteries during diastole. Counterpulsation also provides systemic circulatory support by increasing the mean arterial pressure. As a result, cardiac output is usually augmented by about 10%, or in the range of .5 to .8 L/min (18).

Since increases in cardiac output are limited by the ability of the left ventricle to eject blood, the IABP provides its best support to patients with normal or greater-than-normal cardiac output. Its use has been most successful in those patients with reversible cardiac damage related to myocardial ischemia and/or cardiac surgery (10). Low-output heart failure in patients with cardiomyopathy degenerating into cardiogenic shock is associated with a high mortality that is not significantly decreased by intra-aortic balloon pumping. IABP is also of limited benefit in patients with severe ventricular arrhythmias or right ventricular failure (19).

Table 1. A comparison of VAD characteristics for devices currently in use

Manufacturer	Pulsatile Flow?	Drive Mechanism	IDE Required?	VAD Placement?
Sarns / 3M Ann Arbor, MI	No	Centrifugal	No	Extracorporeal
Bio-Medicus Eden Prairie, MN	No	Centrifugal	No	Extracorporeal
Abiomed Danvers, MA	Yes	Pneumatic	Yes	Extracorporeal
Elecath Rahway, NJ	Yes	Hydraulic	Yes	Extracorporeal
Sarns / 3M Ann Arbor, MI	Yes	Pneumatic	Yes	Paracorporeal
Symbion Salt Lake City, UT	Yes	Pneumatic	Yes	Paracorporeal
Thoratec Berkeley, CA	Yes	Pneumatic	Yes	Paracorporeal
Novacor Oakland, CA	Yes	Electromechanical	Yes	Intracorporeal
Thermedics Woburn, MA	Yes	Electromechanical	Yes	Intracorporeal

The incidence of device-related complications has been reported at about 20% of all IABP insertions. Vascular complications include dissection of the aorta, dislodgement of atherosclerotic deposits, thrombosis, emboli, and limb ischemia which occasionally results in amputation of the affected extremity. Infection, bleeding, thrombocytopenia, and balloon rupture have also been reported (20). Inability to place the balloon occurs in about 12% of attempted insertions. Contraindications to IABP assistance include aortic valve insufficiency, vessel tortuosity, peripheral vascular atherosclerosis, and the presence of an aortic aneurysm.

Ventricular Assist Devices

There are many patients with various low cardiac output syndromes who require more than the 10% augmentation of systemic circulatory flow that the intra-aortic balloon pump provides. A higher level of circulatory support can be provided by the placement of a VAD. A VAD provides support for a single ventricle and may be used for left (LVAD) or right (RVAD) assistance. Two devices may be used together for biventricular (BVAD) support.

Several types of VADs have been developed and are in clinical use; Table 1 lists a comparison of characteristics for VADs currently in use. Devices range from simple, inexpensive, readily available devices to complex, costly, investigational devices whose use is restricted by the United States Food and Drug Administration (FDA). A representative description of each type of VAD is presented below.

Most VADs are designed to pump blood in parallel with an impaired ventricle. They can bypass all or part of the blood intended for the affected ventricle. This process greatly decreases the preload, or end-diastolic volume, in the ventricle. Cardiac output is maintained or improved while allowing the ventricle to rest and recover. Current estimates are that over 500 patients have been treated with short-term VADs with survival rates close to 50% (21).

On the average, reversible myocardial injury may require about 7 days of ventricular bypass assistance before recovery is adequate for VAD removal (22, 23). Likely recovery mechanisms are the return of ventricular wall tension, the reduction of myocardial edema over time with an associated decrease in myocardial compliance, and the rebuilding of high-energy phosphate stores necessary to restore adequate systolic function (24). VADs have been shown to decrease the myocardial O_2 consumption requirements by about 50% (25). Animal studies by Reimer et al. (26) show that a 15-min period of myocardial ischemia will deplete 50% of the total adenine nucleotide pool from the myocardium. Four days after the ischemic episode, these values were restored to 91% of control levels (26).

VAD insertion requires the attachment of two large-bore cannulae: one to carry blood to the VAD, and one to return it to the circulation. Cannulation sites can vary, but atrial placement is most often used for the VAD inflow, while an aortic (LVAD) or pulmonary artery anastomosis (RVAD) typically serve as the return site. Atrial cannulation does not unload the ventricle as completely as ventricular cannulation, but has the advantage of being easier to insert and remove, avoids additional damage to ventricular myocardium, and reduces the risk of intraoperative bleeding (24). Mobility of the ventricular apex is retained, allowing normal apical movement during systole and better access within the mediastinum during implantation.

For the purposes of illustration, the insertion of cannulae for a left atrial to aorta (LA-aorta) bypass will be described. The insertion and removal of a VAD typically requires a median sternotomy, which will already exist in the case of failure to wean from cardiopulmonary bypass. After checking for a patent foramen ovale, the atrial cannula is securely sutured within the left atrial appendage. Next, the Dacron conduit of the arterial cannula is anastomosed to the ascending aorta. Most VADs are placed extracorporeally; thus, both cannulae must be brought through the chest wall, usually just below the subcostal margin. The VAD and cannulae are then primed and connected together, the circuit is de-aired, and VAD pumping is started as weaning from bypass proceeds. A pulsatile pneumatic VAD in situ is shown in Figure 2.

The VAD is removed by reopening the sternotomy and clamping the cannulae as the device is turned off. Systemic heparinization at the time of removal reduces the risk of thrombus formation. Cardiopulmonary bypass is not usually necessary during the extraction of the VAD cannulae. The atrial incision is repaired by tightening the previously placed purse string sutures as the atrial cannula is withdrawn. The aorta is side-clamped, the Dacron graft is removed, and the aorta is oversewn to repair the arterial graft site.

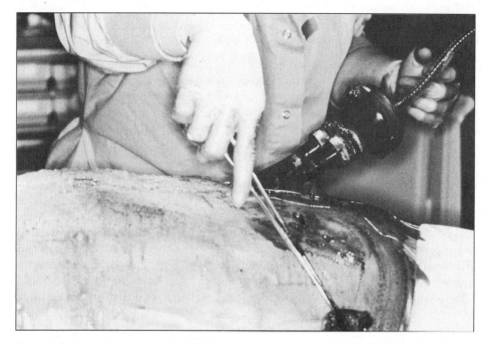

Fig. 2. The Symbion pneumatic VAD in situ, shown in preparation for the explant.

Nonpulsatile Pumps

The simplest and least expensive ventricular assist systems are the nonpulsatile pumps. The use of cannulas and tubing employed in cardiopulmonary bypass (CBP) facilitate the conversion from cardiopulmonary bypass to ventricular bypass (19). These pumps maintain continuous blood flow and therefore do not require artificial valves. Flows are controlled via compact, tabletop units which are relatively easy to set up. One disadvantage to nonpulsatile flow is that it may not be possible to maintain adequate end-organ perfusion over long periods of time. Flow rates are dependent upon cannula sizes (typically 26 to 34-Fr) and small cannulae may not be adequate for the level of circulatory support required (2). Pulsatile flows can be generated by putting an IABP in series with a nonpulsatile VAD.

Nonpulsatile pumps are the most widely available VADs. This type of device was in existence as a cardiopulmonary bypass (CPB) pump prior to the enactment of the Medical Device Amendments of 1976. As a result, these pumps have thus far been exempted from the stringent FDA regulatory process required for all types of pulsatile CADs. In addition to CPB and ventricular device applications, nonpulsatile pumps are also commonly employed in extracorporeal membrane oxygenation systems.

Roller Pumps

As one of the primary components of the CPB machine, roller pumps are employed in approximately 200,000 open heart surgical cases in the United States each year (26). CPB causes damage in the form of hemolysis, destruction of platelets, and complement activation (27); thus, CPB support is limited to a few hours before its deleterious effects outweigh its possible benefits. Roller pumps alone have been used outside the operating room as a VAD when separation from bypass has not been possible in any other manner (28).

Inflow and outflow cannulae are attached internally and brought through the chest wall as described above. Externally, the cannulae are connected by a length of tubing which is placed into a channel in the pump. Rollers on a rotating assembly occlude the tubing, advancing the volume of blood contained in the tubing as they revolve. Pump flow rates are calculated from tubing diameter and pump rotational speed.

Atrial pressures must be carefully regulated since poor atrial filling will not provide adequate flow to the pump, and it may generate sufficient vacuum to collapse and possibly damage the atrial walls. This is a vicious cycle, since atrial collapse will further obstruct flow to the pump. These pumps are capable of pulling enough suction to pull air out of solution; hence, the incorporation of a blood reservoir to allow for inflow variability may be desirable. Often, perfusionists remain continuously present at the bedside during roller pump assistance to manage these potential problems. Roller pump tubing wears over time and requires changing at 8 to 12-h intervals. Each time the circuit is broken for a tubing change, the risk of infectious contamination increases. For these reasons, the use of roller pumps as a VAD seems to be diminishing.

Continuous heparinization is required during roller pump support. Activated clotting times or partial thromboplastin times (PTT) are maintained at twice control levels. The presence of heparin will further complicate bleeding diathesis, which has in some cases proved to be fatal.

Centrifugal Pumps

Centrifugal pumps are nonocclusive and cause less trauma to the blood than do roller pumps. These pumps are relatively easy to use and the disposable pump head costs are reasonable. These features, in combination with the relatively easy access to these devices, make them the most common extracorporeal assist system in use today.

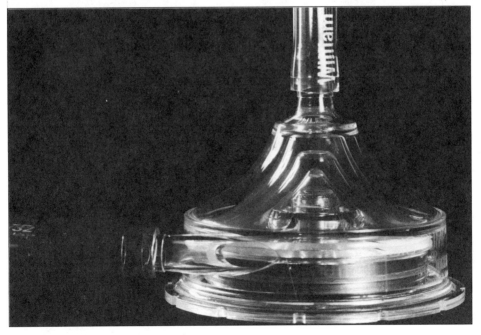

Fig. 3. The Biomedicus Bio-Pump, a centrifugal VAD.

A typical centrifugal system is represented by the Bio-Pump and Bio-Console (Bio-medicus, Eden Prairie, MN) system shown in Figures 3 and 4. The acrylic, conical pump head contains three concentric cones mounted on a circular magnetic plate. Inflow and outflow cannulae are attached internally, brought through the chest wall, and attached appropriately to the pump head. The head is fixed to the Bio-Console drive unit, which rotates the magnetic plate and therefore the cones. Rotation of the cones induces the blood within the pump to spin, and centrifugally forces it toward the outlet for return to the circulation. By design, centrifugal pumps reduce the possibility of air emboli by trapping air in the top of the cone (29).

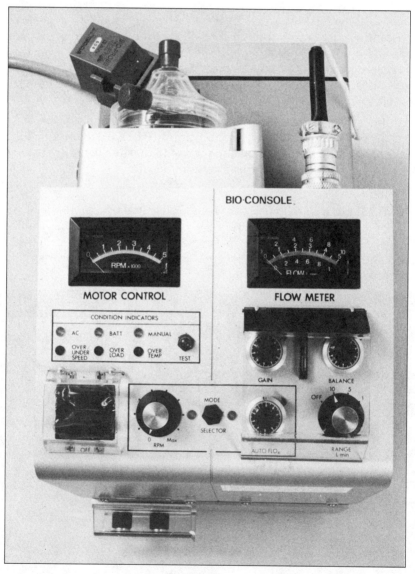

Fig. 4. The Bio-Com, the drive unit for the Bio-Pump.

Centrifugal pumps are known as nonpulsatile pumps because blood is continuously flowing through the pump. The operator chooses a rotational speed to achieve the desired flow rate. The drive motor then maintains the chosen pump speed, but changes in preload (pressure of the blood entering the pump) or afterload (resistance to outflow from the pump) may cause the flow rate to change dramatically. VAD flow rates are monitored by the placement of an electromagnetic flow probe on the VAD outflow cannula. Low flow rates (<2 L/min) can rapidly lead to the formation of thrombus within the device and should be avoided. As with roller pumps, continuous monitoring of the device is common. The pump head is replaced per the manufacturer's recommendations every 24 to 48 h to reduce the risk of thromboembolic complications. Heparinization is also used to decrease the incidence of thrombus formation.

Pulsatile Pumps

The merits of pulsatile vs. nonpulsatile circulatory assistance have been widely debated. Successful results have been reported using both types; thus, a pulsatile device is not an absolute requirement for maintenance of end-organ perfusion (2). Pulsatile flow is more physiologic and is likely to speed up the reversal of organ damage occurring prior to VAD intervention. Since length of time on a VAD correlates with the number of complications reported, a decrease in the length of time spent on a VAD is desirable. Pulsatile VADs require larger cannulae and can provide greater flows than nonpulsatile pumps (1). Pulsatile VADs are usually desirable for any long-term VAD support.

Pulsatile pumps are more expensive and complex to operate than their nonpulsatile counterparts. Large, complex control units may require special logistics for operation in the intensive care environment. In the United States, the use of pulsatile VADs is highly regulated by the FDA. Any physician wishing to use one of these devices must first be accepted into an investigational device study before the manufacturer can release the VAD. The device sponsor and the FDA determine the criteria for acceptance into these studies and the number of study sites is limited (30).

Pulsatile Pneumatic Pump

Pneumatic VADs use pressurized air to eject blood from the device. The pump has a rigid housing with two compartments which are physically separated by a flexible but fairly noncompliant diaphragm. One compartment contains the blood circulating through the pump and communicates with the inflow and outflow cannulae via unidirectional valves. The other compartment contains air and is attached to a pneumatic drive unit via a driveline.

Movement of the diaphragm increases the volume of one compartment while decreasing the size of the other chamber. Blood enters the device as pressurized air is vented from the ventricle, allowing displacement of the diaphragm to expand the size of the blood chamber. When ejection of the blood is desired, the air compartment is expanded by filling it with pressurized air, thereby "contracting" the blood compartment.

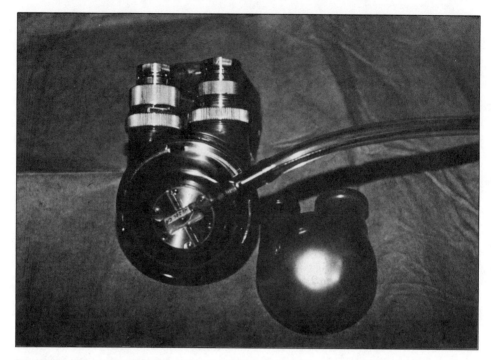

Fig. 5. The Pierce-Donachy pneumatic VAD and blood sac.

The most widely used pulsatile pneumatic VAD has been the Pierce-Donachy pump system shown in Figure 5. This investigational device is currently marketed by Thoratec (Berkeley, CA) and can be used to provide left, right, or biventricular assistance. Thirty-nine centers throughout the world are currently using this device.

The Pierce-Donachy pump employs a flexible, seamless blood sac made from Biomer (Ethicon™, Somerville, NJ) contained within a rigid polysulfone housing. A flexible diaphragm separates the blood sac from an air chamber. Ejection of blood from the pump takes place when the air chamber is sufficiently pressurized to overcome the afterload at the outflow cannula, open the outflow valve, and displace the diaphragm to collapse the blood sac. Bjork-Shiley (Shiley Laboratories, Irvine, CA) tilting disk valves regulate the direction of flow through the device. The pump lies paracorporeally on the anterior abdominal wall with the inflow and outflow cannulae exiting the chest below the costal margin (30). The pneumatic chamber of the pump is connected to its large drive unit by a 2-m vinyl air tube.

At the drive unit, ejection can be triggered by choosing one of three possible modes: by setting a constant heart rate (HR) (fixed rate mode); by filling to the maximum stroke volume (SV) of 65 ml (full-to-empty mode); or by timing in relation to electrical events in the cardiac cycle (synchronous mode). In theory, the synchronous mode has the advantages of diastolic augmentation of coronary flow and afterload reduction for any blood that the native ventricle is pumping. In practice, the full-to-empty mode provides a triggering mechanism which is more reliable and is usually the mode of choice. This mode provides maximal washout of the blood sac and decreases the possibility of thrombus formation within the device (31). Full-to-empty mode provides intermittent periods of counterpulsation as the ejection periods of the natural heart and of the VAD move in and out of phase with each other. VAD cardiac output is calculated from SV and HR information.

Drive pressures are adjusted at the console to allow for ejection against a wide variation of afterload conditions. The percent systole setting proportions the amount of time spent filling the pump relative to the total beat interval. Ejection can be triggered during diastole of the native heart by the use of the synchronous mode in conjunction with a delay interval. To increase the SV of the VAD, vacuum is applied to the air compartment during the filling interval.

Pulsatile Electromechanical Pump

In electromechanical assist devices, a rigid but movable plate replaces the function of the flexible diaphragm in pneumatic pumps. This obviates the need for pressurized air in the drive system. The flat pusher plates move in one direction to compress and eject the blood contained within the ventricle and in the opposite direction for filling of the pump.

The Novacor (Oakland, CA) pump, which is now in use at 11 locations throughout the world, is an electromechanical device designed for left ventricular assist only. This large, completely encapsulated pump, shown with its drive system in Figure 6, is implanted in a surgically fashioned pocket within the abdomen. Inflow and outflow cannulae are sutured to the left ventricular apex and ascending aorta, and then brought through the diaphragm for connection to the VAD. A vent tube containing power and control lines is tunneled subcutaneously before exiting the skin for connection to the drive unit.

Unlike the other VADs discussed, the Novacor pump does not pump blood in parallel with the native heart. Cannulation of the ventricular apex allows the entire volume of the left ventricle to be ejected during systole into the very low afterload of the empty VAD. The blood-contacting surface consists of a flattened, flexible sac made of segmented polyurethane. Two pusher plates are attached to opposing sides of the sac. Springs are electronically activated to push these plates toward one another, ejecting blood from the pump. Two modified Carpentier-Edwards (American Edwards Laboratories, Santa Ana, CA) pericardial valves provide unidirectional flow through the pump.

Ejection of the Novacor VAD can be triggered by three modes. Normally, the device is triggered by a decrease in the rate of blood flowing into the VAD as the natural ventricle empties during systole (fill-rate trigger). This allows the VAD to run at a rate identical to the natural HR without the reliance on ECG detection and its related problems. Alternatively, the VAD may be run at a fixed rate or with ECG trigger. Position sensors within the device measure its beat-to-beat fill volume. This volume is combined with the HR information to provide an accurate determination of the VAD cardiac output.

Total Artificial Heart

The TAH provides biventricular circulatory support, but following the complete excision of the natural ventricles. Since implantation is reversible only by transplantation, the TAH should only be considered for patients who are excellent candidates for cardiac replacement and used when clinical signs indicate impending death despite maximal inotropic support. Criteria for acceptance as a

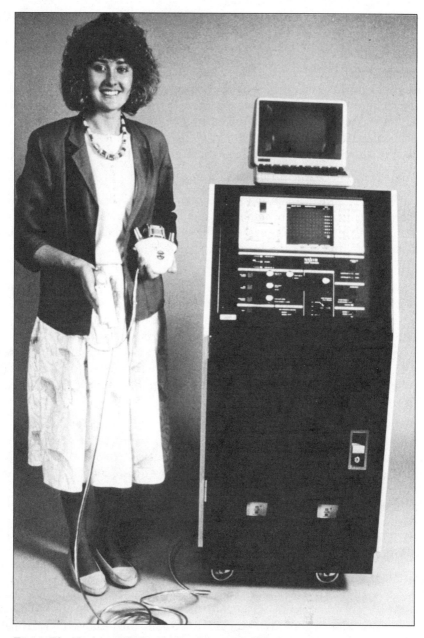

Fig. 6. The Novacor LVAD with its drive unit. The device pictured is a demonstration device and is not completely encapsulated as the clinical devices are.

cardiac transplantation candidate and a TAH implant candidates are listed in Tables 2 and 3. The most commonly used TAH, the Jarvik 7 (Symbion, Salt Lake City, UT), is produced in two sizes, one with a SV to 100 ml, and the other containing up to 70 ml. The 100-ml model is shown in Figure 7. TAH use is controlled by investigational device exemptions. The 26 centers which have this device available to them are shown in Figure 8.

Table 2. Criteria for transplant candidacy

End-stage cardiomyopathy

Less than 55 years of age

No pulmonary hypertension

No active infection

No malignancy or other life-limiting disease

No irreversible renal or hepatic disease

No severe cerebrovascular/peripheral vascular disease

No cytotoxic antibodies

No severe psychological handicaps

Table 3. Guidelines for using the TAH as a bridge to transplantation

Meets criteria for heart transplantation

Expected survival less than 48 hours

Donor heart not available

Chest large enough for device

Signed informed consent

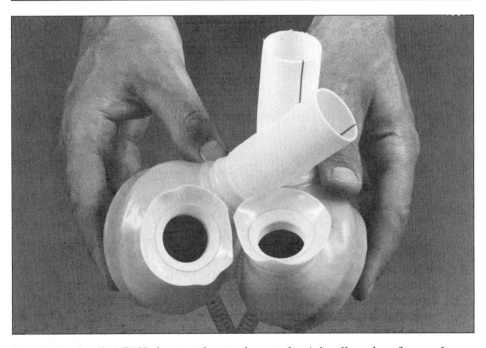

Fig. 7. The Jarvik 7 TAH showing the attachment of atrial cuffs and outflow grafts.

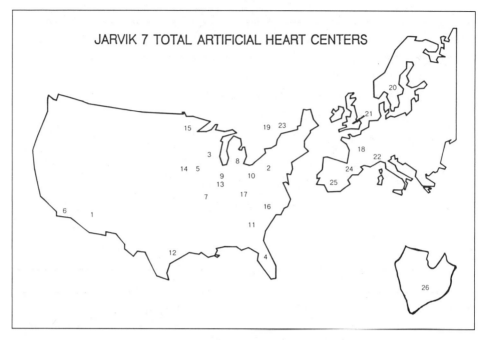

Fig. 8. Locations of the centers using the Jarvik 7 TAH:

1. University of Arizona Health
   Sciences Center
   Tucson, AZ

2. University of Pittsburgh
   Pittsburgh, PA

3. Midwest Heart Surgical Institute
   Milwaukee, WI

4. University of Florida
   Gainesville, FL

5. University of Iowa
   Iowa City, IA

6. Sharp Memorial Hospital
   San Diego, CA

7. Washington School of Medicine
   St. Louis, MO

8. University of Michigan
   Ann Arbor, MI

9. Loyola University
   Maywood, IL

10. University Hospitals
    Cleveland, OH

11. Emory University
    Atlanta, GA

12. Baylor College of Medicine,
    Texas Medical Center
    Houston, TX

13. St. Louis University Medical Center
    St. Louis, MO

14. Cardiac Surgical Associates,
    Mercy Medical Plaza
    Des Moines, IA

15. Minneapolis Thoracic Group
    Minneapolis, MN

16. Bowman Gray School of Medicine
    Winston-Salem, NC

17. Humana Hospital Audubon
    Louisville, KY

18. Groupe Hospital Pitie - Salpetriere
    Paris, France

19. University of Ottawa Heart Institute
    Ottawa, Canada

20. Karolinska Hospital
    Stockholm, Sweden

21. Papworth Everard Hospital
    Cambridge, England

22. Faculte de Medecine
    Creteil, France

23. Montreal Heart Institute,
    Institute of Cardiology
    Montreal, Canada

24. Hospital de la San Crue
    Barcelona, Spain

25. Jefe Del ep. DeCirugia de La Clinica
    Puerta De Hierro
    Madrid, Spain

26. Riyadh Al Kharj Hospital
    Riyadh, Kingdom of Saudi Arabia

Excision of the ventricles for TAH implantation is very similar to that required for the forthcoming cardiac transplantation. The native ventricles are removed at the level of the atrioventricular groove, just above the aortic and pulmonary valves. Aortic and pulmonary artery conduits and right and left atrial cuffs are sutured to the great vessels and atrial remnants, respectively. The left and then the right ventricles are snapped into place and the drivelines exit subcostally (32).

The spherical ventricles of the Jarvik 7 TAH are lined with Biomer, and contain two chambers separated by a multilayered flexible diaphragm. Like the pneumatic VAD, one chamber contains blood, the other air. Flow is channeled through each ventricle by two Medtronic-Hall (Medtronic Inc., Minneapolis, MN) clinical grade unidirectional valves. As blood enters the device, it displaces an equal volume of air from the air compartment. The drive unit used with the Jarvik 7 heart measures the amount of air exhausted to provide a SV estimate and uses this in conjunction with the HR setting to calculate cardiac output.

Cardiac output levels can be controlled by changing atrial filling pressures with intravascular fluid management or regulating device filling with vacuum-level adjustments or fill-interval timing. During ejection, the air compartment is pressurized sufficiently to eject the entire SV entering the ventricle. The driver has right and left drive pressure regulators which allow adjustment to ventricular afterload changes. The HR should be set so that the SV will be approximately 70% of the maximum SV of the ventricle. This provides a reserve filling capacity which allows the artificial heart to exhibit the Starling effect; thus, an increase in preload will produce an increase in cardiac output.

Clinical Experience

Reviews of recent VAD experience show that 40% to 50% of patients now receiving mechanical assistance can be successfully weaned or bridged to transplantation (2, 19). The success rate has continued to rise as surgical techniques, patient selection criteria, and management of the devices have improved. Attempts to predict survival have not been very successful (7, 19). The most important criteria to date has probably been the early use of a VAD to treat cardiac failure. Other factors affecting survival are: a) the condition of the patient at the time of insertion, since prior shock will predispose the patient to multi-organ failure; b) the length of time spent on bypass; c) the assessment and treatment of right ventricular failure; and d) the amount of ventricular necrosis in reversible injuries (33).

Clinicians using FDA-regulated investigational devices are required to provide detailed reports of all aspects of device use. These reports provide a useful mechanism for tracking device usage. However, IABP, centrifugal, and roller pump usage is not so controlled; consequently, information on their frequency of use is not readily available.

The registry of the International Society for Heart Transplantation reported 1,415 orthotopic heart transplantations in 1986 (14). During that same period of time, data collected by the Combined Registry for the clinical use of mechanical ventricular assist pumps and the TAH reported that 27 VAD and 32 TAH patients received mechanical assistance during bridge to transplantation. Of those 59 patients, 43 received transplants and 31 were still alive in mid-1987 (15). Outcomes were very similar between the VAD and TAH groups. Transplantation was performed in 19 (70%) VAD patients and 24 (75%) TAH patients with 15 (55%) and 16 (50%), respectively, surviving the early postoperative period.

The Thoratec pneumatic VAD was first used in 1982 for postcardiotomy support and in 1984 for bridge to transplantation. To date, 46 of 57 patients have

317

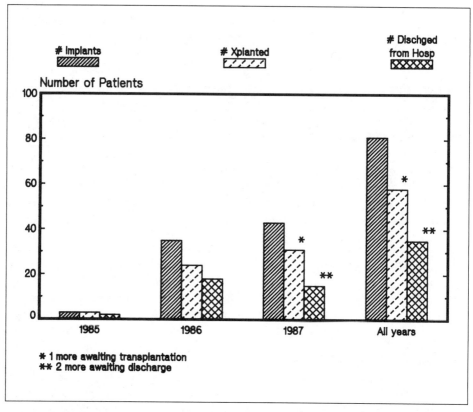

Fig. 9. Jarvik-7 bridge-to-transplant experience for the years 1985 to 1987.

received transplants with 38 surviving to hospital discharge. In postcardiotomy cases, 15 of 94 patients (16%) survived to discharge (Farrar DJ, personal communication, January, 1988).

The first clinical experience with the Novacor LVAD was for bridge to transplantation in 1984. Total bridge-to-transplant experience now numbers 17 patients, with eight receiving transplants, four surviving to discharge, and two still hospitalized (Strauss L, personal communication, January, 1988). There have been no survivors of the five Novacor implants for postcardiotomy support.

Since 1985, there have been 87 artificial hearts implanted as a bridge to transplantation. Eighty-one have employed Jarvik 7 devices. As seen in Figure 9, a summary of the Jarvik 7 experience shows that 58 patients were transplanted, with 31 surviving to date (Gaykowski R, personal communication, January, 1988). Figure 10 summarizes the clinical experience of all these devices to date.

Choosing a Device

In locations where there are multiple types of CADs available, selection of the most appropriate device becomes an issue. One must assess whether there is univentricular or biventricular dysfunction, whether the failure may be reversible, what level of assistance is likely to be required, and whether the patient would be a suitable candidate for transplantation. Figure 11 presents a synopsis of the criteria proposed for use in our institution for this decision-making process.

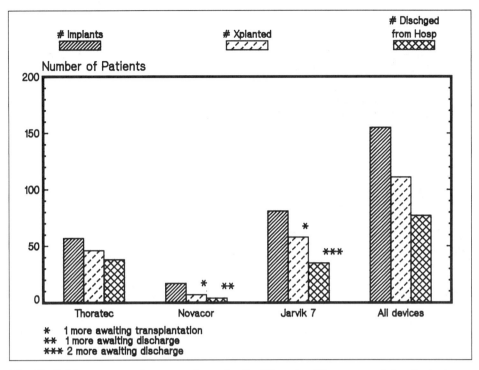

Fig. 10. Bridge-to-transplant experience for the Thoratec, Novacor, and Jarvik devices.

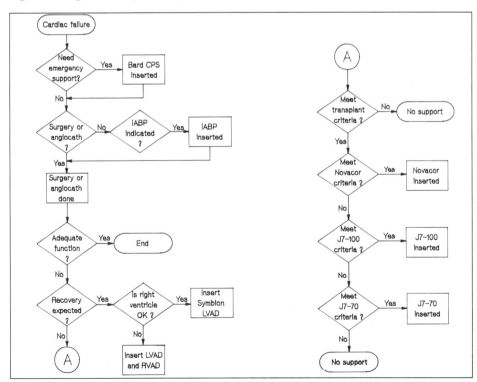

Fig. 11. Circulatory assist decision flowchart for devices used at University Medical Center, Tucson, Arizona.

We utilize the portable Bard (Billerica, MA) cardiopulmonary bypass system in emergency situations with patients who decompensate rapidly. This system allows the institution of bypass within 5 to 10 min and allows stabilization of the patient during the interval required for evaluation of the available options and institution of the selected therapy. Options might include coronary artery bypass grafting (CABG), the insertion of an intra-aortic balloon, LVAD, RVAD, or BVAD, implantation of a TAH, cardiac transplantation, or no support.

A Jarvik 7 TAH would be an option if the patient was a very good transplant candidate with definite biventricular failure and adequate chest size to accommodate the device. The replacement of both ventricles with the TAH should allow excellent regulation of cardiac output. This requires only two drivelines through the skin rather than the four exit sites that would be necessary for implantation of a BVAD. If the patient has only left ventricular failure, is a good candidate for cardiac transplantation, and is large enough to accommodate the Novacor pump, this device would probably be selected. Because this device requires coring through the apex of the left ventricle, we would prefer not to use this device in patients where there is possible recovery of the myocardium. Where recovery is possible or size limitations prevent utilization of the previously described devices, a pulsatile pneumatic VAD, centrifugal pump, or a combination of the two could be used for circulatory assistance.

Surgical Considerations

Once the need for a CAD has been established, implantation should proceed as quickly as possible. Delays may contribute to bleeding diatheses and/or end-organ damage which will complicate recovery. The surgeon must rapidly assess the situation and select a device based on criteria like those discussed in the previous section. An implant team must be ready to respond on short notice to prepare the device and driver. Informed consent must be obtained prior to the implantation.

All VADs and the TAH employ low-porosity, woven dacron grafts for attachment of the device outflow tract. These grafts must be preclotted prior to use. This can be done in advance if the implantation is elective but in the case of failure to wean from bypass, it will be necessary to reverse heparinization of about 100 ml of blood for this purpose. This can be done by adding 5 ml of protamine sulfate and 1 ampule of topical thrombin to the blood (34).

In terms of fit, the TAH is the most technically challenging device to implant. The current spherical shape of the ventricles does not maximize the use of the space remaining after the excision of the native ventricles. The limiting dimension is the anterior-posterior depth between the vertebrae and the sternum. Prior to surgery, estimation of chest size relative to the TAH can be accomplished by the use of x-ray masks as shown in Figure 12 (35). The ventricles are normally placed with the right ventricle anterior to the left ventricle as shown in Figure 13. If the anterior-posterior depth is inadequate, it may be possible to shift the left ventricle leftward, allowing the right ventricle to be moved a little deeper into the mediastinum. However, this may cause the device to compress surround-

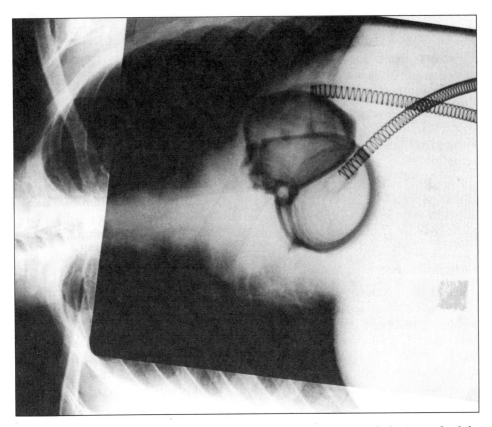

Fig. 12. Fit assessment for the Jarvik-7 TAH with overlay of a radiologic mask of the ventricles on a chest film.

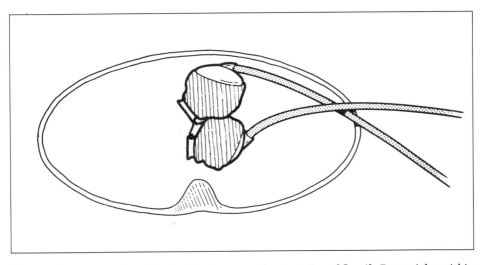

Fig. 13. A transverse view illustrating the normal orientation of Jarvik-7 ventricles within the chest.

ing tissues. All atrial cuffs and great vessel anastomoses must be inspected for kinking, which will lead to areas of poor flow and the development of thrombi. Flow obstruction due to compression of the vena cavae during closure of the sternum signals a significant complication to device function which must be remedied immediately.

If the excised ventricles were grossly dilated, it may be possible to fit the TAH within the pericardium. This is useful in preventing the development of adhesions around the device, and makes the explant procedure significantly less complicated.

Once VAD or TAH implantation is underway, it will be difficult to get exposure to tissues deep within the chest. This may complicate the maintenance of hemostasis by interfering with the visualization and access to bleeding sites. Placement of VAD cannulae must also avoid the compression of any coronary bypass grafts.

Complications

There are a number of complications associated with the use of mechanical circulatory assistance. The most common device-related complications are hemorrhage, neurologic events, infection, and hemolysis. The number of complications experienced generally correlates with the length of time spent on the support device. The level and duration of hemodynamic decompensation prior to the institution of mechanical assistance will affect the length of the postoperative recovery period; thus, once the need is established, mechanical assistance should be instituted at the earliest opportunity. Time spent on the device while waiting for the recovery of end-organ failure, such as kidney failure or pulmonary edema which resulted from delayed intervention, will expose the patient to greater risks.

Bleeding

There are a number of factors involved in CAD use that increase the incidence of bleeding complications. The attachment of grafts may be complicated by friable tissues due to atherosclerotic degeneration of the aorta or thinning of the pulmonary artery wall from chronic pulmonary hypertension (36). Platelet activity is dramatically reduced during cardiopulmonary bypass by dilution due to circuit priming, by mechanical trauma to the platelets from the pump and oxygenator, by consumption of platelets from the clotting of surgical incisions, and by deposition of fibrin and/or platelets on the artificial surfaces of the bypass circuit (27). Some data suggest that time on CPB is the single most important variable to predict severe postoperative bleeding and may be closely linked to the final outcome (37).

Anticoagulation in the postoperative period can cause bleeding complications. Septicemia may also exacerbate bleeding by causing thrombocytopenia. VAD or TAH patients are still at risk for tamponade and clinicians should be alert for its indications.

It is important to minimize transfusions for bridge-to-transplant patients. Exposure to antigens via blood transfusion can lead to the development of cytotoxic anti-human lymphocyte antibodies (HLA), which may prevent future cardiac transplantation by severely limiting the number of acceptable donors. Loss of blood due to laboratory draws becomes a problem. With CADs good cardiac output levels can usually be continuously maintained by controlling intra-vascular volumes and driver settings. This effect helps mitigate the problems of abnormally low Hct values. Whole blood transfusions are avoided and packed RBCs are cooled and filtered prior to transfusion to further decrease the risk of cytotoxic anti-HLA stimulation.

Thromboemboli

Thrombus formation is a common problem in CAD use. Thrombi can form as a result of blood exposure to foreign surfaces, episodes of low flow, hypercoagulable states, areas of poor flow within the device, or sepsis. Thromboemboli have been responsible for neurologic damage, and complications due to infarcts of kidney, liver, and other tissues have also been reported. Many of the neurologic events experienced have been transient ischemic episodes with spontaneous reversal.

All devices should meet certain criteria to reduce the likelihood of thrombus formation. Nonreactive, biocompatible materials with extremely smooth surfaces should be employed for all blood-contacting surfaces. Biomer is commonly used and has proven to be adequate in this respect. Device design should result in internal flow patterns with no areas of stasis (38). Connection sites between the cannulae and CAD should remain free of crevices or other imperfections where thrombus can be easily established (39). Figure 14 demonstrates the extent of thrombus formation in the crevices surrounding the valve during a Jarvik TAH implant of 9 days. The Jarvik 7 valve mounts are currently being redesigned in response to this problem.

Anticoagulation is often administered as an adjunct to mechanical circulatory assistance. Heparin is the most commonly chosen anticoagulant, but the use of

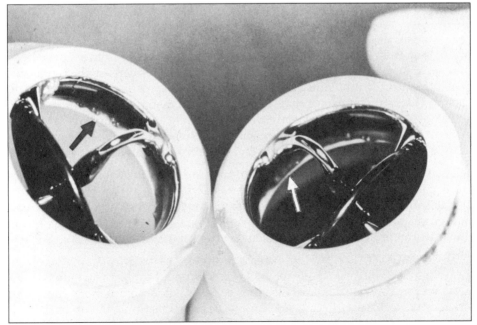

Fig. 14. Thrombus formation on the inflow valves of a Jarvik-7 TAH following implantation for 9 days.

Dextran 40, aspirin, and coumadin have also been reported (40). Heparin has the advantages of being easily reversed and rapidly titrated. A disadvantage is the need for intravenous administration. Dipyridamole is often added as an adjunct to anticoagulation as it reduces the ability of platelets to adhere to one another.

Anticoagulant management is complicated by the fact that many ongoing processes modify the effectiveness of a certain dose of the chosen agent. Therefore, the levels of anticoagulation required may change significantly during the postoperative course. Immediately postoperatively, the patient is usually thrombocytopenic and at greater risk for bleeding than for thrombus formation. An anticoagulation regimen should be started at a low level as postsurgical coagulopathies resolve. As liver, renal, and other organ systems begin to recover with time or as a result of augmented perfusion, levels will again require adjustment. Heparin levels are titrated based on frequent testing of clotting factors. Our protocol is to maintain the partial thromboplastin time at 1.5 to 2 times control levels.

The presence of infection further complicates therapy. If infected, these patients run the risk of developing septic emboli as well as hemorrhage, making the management of anticoagulation very difficult (41). Infectious complications may be one of the major reasons why strokes continue to occur despite carefully followed anticoagulation regimens.

DeVries (41) reported a correlation between rapid increases in platelet count, especially when there are many large, newly formed platelets, and stroke. Platelet counts are routinely tested on our CAD patients. Attention to the volume status is also important, since the development of thrombus is encouraged by hypercoagulability resulting from the contraction of the intravascular volume (39).

Infection

The incidence of infection has been a significant problem in the management of CAD patients. Interruptions in skin integrity due to the presence of drivelines or blood conduits and the placement of monitoring lines increase the number of possible sites for problems. Large amounts of clot resulting from bleeding around the artificial device may act as a culture medium for organisms. The irregular shapes of artificial ventricles or internal cannulae may make it more difficult for normal defense mechanisms to take place. Fit problems may lead to the compression of internal structures, and necrosis or atelectasis.

The prevention of infection is of paramount importance for the bridge-to-transplant patient. The presence of active infection is an absolute contraindication to transplantation. CAD-related infection may also appear following transplantation, when the immunosuppression required to prevent rejection of the allograft compromises the normal leukocyte-mediated defense mechanisms.

The use of a VAD or TAH requires a minimum of two mediastinal explorations: one for implant and one for explant. Additional exploration may become necessary to control excessive bleeding or relieve flow obstructions caused by suboptimal device positioning. Each entry to the mediastinum increases the risk of contamination with its attendant complications.

TAH implantation may result in lung compression, particularly if the depth of the chest cavity is not adequate for accommodation of the device. As mentioned above, one technique used to fit the device in a small chest is to position it to the left. As seen in Figure 15, this orientation may significantly compromise the lung, possibly leading to pulmonary collapse, impaired circulation, and the accumulation of fluids which will increase the risk of pneumonia.

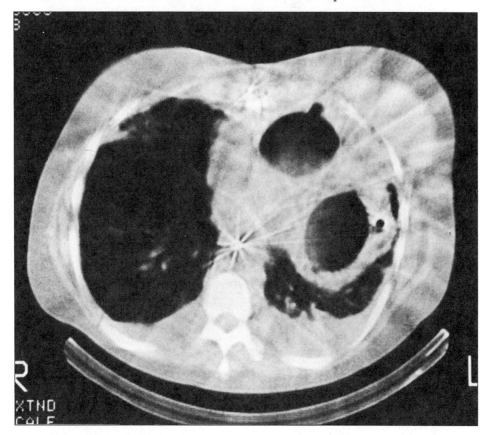

Fig. 15. CT scan showing left lung compression due to leftward positioning of the Jarvik-7 TAH.

Whenever mediastinal infection is likely, we have found it useful to prophylactically irrigate with an antimicrobial agent. The irrigation system consists of one or more small tubes placed in the mediastinum to infuse a dilute solution of an appropriate antibiotic or antifungal drug. This flush solution is drained by larger chest tubes under a small amount of continuous suction.

All CADs currently in use require penetration of the skin for the passage of pneumatic or electrical conduits. This is another likely site for infection to occur. Subcutaneous tunneling of these conduits decreases the likelihood that contamination from the exit sites will be carried to deeper tissues. Skin buttons, shown in Figure 16, help provide a barrier to infection by effecting a tight seal between the driveline and the skin button. The outer surface of the skin button has a textured coating to promote tissue ingrowth and impede vectoring of skin flora. Skin buttons also secure the drivelines in place, preventing them from sliding back and forth through the exit sites. Frequently, these areas must be carefully inspected and cultured if necessary, and aggressively cleaned and kept dressed at all other times.

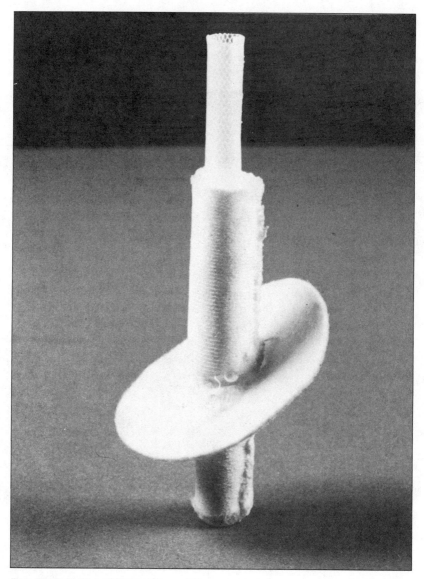

Fig. 16. Driveline skin button.

Cost

Many economic factors are considered with the introduction of CAD technology. The simplest devices require purchase of the hardware and disposables. The more complex systems could require further investment in backup equipment, training, building modifications, additional FTEs, annual fees, and future upgrades. These costs vary depending on the devices selected, the level of existing FTE support, the number of CAD systems at an institution, and the usage of these systems.

Balloon pump systems are widely used and cost $25,000 to $35,000. Existing staff (nurses and perfusionists) can usually provide the needed support. Non-pulsatile centrifugal blood pumps cost between $8,000 and $10,000, and demand more intense monitoring (usually necessitating a perfusionist), which could add to FTE costs.

Pulsatile VADs are under the FDA Investigational Device Exemption (IDE) restrictions which necessitate additional considerations. A device support team, usually consisting of surgeons, nurses, engineers, and perfusionists, must first receive training on animal implants. Consoles with built-in backup systems cost about $100,000, with $10,000 to $20,000 needed for each VAD (3 recommended). Further expenses are incurred if appropriate FTE support is not already present.

The TAH systems are also under FDA IDE restrictions. Training costs could exceed $100,000. Two consoles with complete backup systems are required, at a cost of $150,000 to $200,000. The TAHs are approximately $20,000 each. If both TAH sizes are required, a minimum of four hearts must be stocked. Additional expenditures may be required for building modifications for compressed air, future device upgrades, and FTE support.

CAD technology ranges from balloon pumps to complex TAH systems. The expense of supporting these technologies ranges from $20,000 to over $500,000 for each. If an institution invests in more than one technology, some of these costs can be shared. An example is the Utah Drive Console which can support both the Symbion TAH and VAD. Careful consideration of all direct and indirect expenses and the assessment of future directions is important for an institution, considering the investments required for the purchase of CAD technology.

Future Directions

The incidence of circulatory support device use will continue to expand as design improvements occur and more surgeons gain experience with them. No single device is likely to emerge as the ideal CAD, but instead a family of devices will expand to meet a number of needs. Statistics show that success is not entirely dependent on the device but on patient selection, team experience, and to some degree, luck. In general, early commitment to CAD support for patients with reasonable chances of recovery leads to successful outcomes. The longer a patient is supported on a CAD, the greater the chance of thromboembolic events and infection.

The current bridge-to-transplant devices are laying the foundation for totally implantable left ventricular assist pumps and artificial hearts. Estimates indicate that between 17,000 and 38,000 patients annually that could benefit from these devices which are powered electrically with energy transmitted across the skin (42). With the increasing shortage of donor hearts available for cardiac transplantation, implantable devices will provide an alternative therapeutic solution for patients with heart disease. Balancing the major issues of cost and ethics with technology and needs will decide the timetable and degree of availability of these devices.

References

1. Lederman DM, Singh PI: Cardiac assist: Many issues and some answers. *In:* New Developments in Cardiac Assist Devices. Attar S (Ed). New York, Praeger Publishers, 1985, pp 43-53

2. Pae WE: Temporary ventricular support. *Trans Am Soc Artif Intern Organs* 1987; 23:4

3. Altieri FD, Watson JT: Implantable ventricular assist systems. *Artif Organs* 1987; 11:237

4. Laschinger JC, Grossi EA, Cunningham JN, et al: Adjunctive left ventricular unloading during myocardial reperfusion plays a major role in minimizing infarct size. *J Thorac Cardiovasc Surg* 1985; 90:80

5. Cunningham JN Jr, Grossi E, Laschinger J, et al: Strategy for treatment of acute evolving myocardial infarction with a left heart assist device. Can this modality increase survival and enhance myocardial salvage? *In:* New Developments in Cardiac Assist Devices. Attar S (Ed). New York, Praeger Publishers, 1985, pp 79-91

6. DePaulis R, Riebman JB, Deleuze P, et al: The total artificial heart: Indications and preliminary results. *J Cardiac Surg* 1987; 2:275

7. Birnbaum PL, Henderson MJ, Weisel RD, et al: Extracorporeal circulatory assist devices. *Trans Am Soc Artif Intern Organs* 1987; 23:190

8. Pennock JL, Pierce WS, Wisman CB, et al: Survival and complications following assist pumping for cardiogenic shock. *Ann Surg* 1983; 198:469

9. Levinson MM, Copeland JG: The artificial heart and mechanical assistance prior to heart transplantation. *In:* Organ Transplantation and Replacement. Cerilli GJ (Ed). Philadelphia, JB Lippincott, 1987, pp 661-679

10. Copeland JG, Emery RW, Levinson MM, et al: The role of mechanical support and transplantation in treatment of patients with end-stage cardiomyopathy. *Circulation* 1985; 72:7

11. Copeland JG, Levinson MM, Smith R, et al: The total artificial heart as a bridge to transplantation. *JAMA* 1986; 256:2991

12. Hardy MA, Dobelle W, Bregman D, et al: Cardiac transplantation following mechanical circulatory support. *Trans Am Soc Artif Intern Organs* 1979; 25:182

13. Farrar DJ, Hill JD, Gray LA, et al: Heterotopic prosthetic ventricles as a bridge to cardiac transplantation. *N Engl J Med* 1988; 318:333

14. Kaye M: The registry of the international society for heart transplantation: Fourth official report - 1987. *J Heart Transplant* 1987; 6:63

15. Pae WE, Pierce WS: Combined registry for clinical use of mechanical ventricular pumps and the total artificial heart: First official report - 1986. *J Heart Transplant* 1987; 6:68

16. Moulopoulos SD, Topaz S, Kolff WJ: Diastolic balloon pumping (with carbon dioxide) in the aorta — A mechanical assistance to the failing circulation. *Am Heart J* 1962; 63:669

17. Clauss RH, Birtwell WC, Albertal G, et al: Assisted circulation. I. The arterial counterpulsator. *J Thorac Cardiovasc Surg* 1961; 41:447

18. Pennock JL, Wisman CB, Pierce WS: Mechanical support of the circulation prior to cardiac transplantation. *Heart Transpl* 1982; 1:299

19: Park SV, Lieblet GA, Burkholder JA, et al: Mechanical support of the failing heart. *Ann Thorac Surg* 1986; 42:627

20. Quall SJ: Comprehensive Intra-Aortic Balloon Pumping. St. Louis, CV Mosby Co, 1984

21. Ruzevich SA, Pennington DG, Kanter KR, et al: Long-term follow-up study of survivors of postcardiotomy circulatory support. *Trans Am Soc Artif Intern Organs* 1987; 23:177

22. Pierce WS, Rosenberg G, Donachy JH, et al: Postoperative cardiac support with a pulsatile assist pump: Techniques and results. *Artif Organs* 1987; 11:247

23. Braunwald E, Kloner RA: The stunned myocardium: Prolonged postischemic ventricular dysfunction. *Circulation* 1982; 66:1146

24. Pierce WS: Effective clinical application of ventricular bypass. *Ann Thorac Surg* 1985; 39:2

25. Pennock JL, Pierce WS, Prophet A, et al: Myocardial oxygen utilization during left heart bypass. *Arch Surg* 1974; 109:635

26. Reimer KA, Hill ML, Jennings RB: Prolonged depletion of ATP of the adenine nucleotide pool due to delayed resynthesis of adenine nucleotides following reversible myocardial ischemic injury. *J Mol Cell Cardiol* 1981; 13:229

27. Austin JW, Harner DL: The heart-lung machine and related technologies of open heart surgery. Phoenix, AZ, Phoenix Medical Communication, 1986

28. Litwak RS, Koffsky RM, Jurado RA, et al: A decade of experience with a left heart assist device in patients undergoing open intracardiac operation. *World J Surg* 1985; 9:8

29. Marchetta S, Stennis E: Ventricular assist devices: Applications for critical care. *J Cardiovasc Nurs* 1988; 2:39

30. Rahmoeller GA: FDA requirements for clinical approval of left ventricular assist devices. *In:* New Developments in Cardiac Assist Devices. Attar S (Ed). New York, Praeger Publishers, 1985, pp 36-38

31. Gaines WE, Pierce WS: Left and right ventricular assistance for postoperative cardiogenic shock. *In:* New Developments in Cardiac Assist Devices. Attar S (Ed). New York, Praeger Publishers, 1985, pp 191-200

32. DeVries WC, Joyce LD: The artificial heart. *CIBA Clinical Symposia* 1983; 38:1

33. Pae WE, Gaines WE, Pierce WS, et al: Mechanical circulatory assistance for postoperative cardiogenic shock. *Surgical Rounds* 1985; 8:49

34. Pierce WS, Pae WE, Myer JL: Clinical Application of Mechanical Circulatory Assistance — Operations Manual, 1983. Hershey, PA, Pennsylvania State University, 1983

35. Jarvik RK, DeVries WC, Semb BHK, et al: Surgical positioning of the Jarvik 7 artificial heart. *J Heart Transplant* 1986; 8:184

36. Levinson MM, Smith R, Cork R, et al: Clinical problems associated with the total artificial heart as a bridge to transplantation. *In:* Proceedings of the International Symposium on Artificial Organs, Biomedical Engineering and Transplantation in Honor of the 78th Birthday of Willem J. Kolff. Andrade JD, Brophy JJ, Detmer DE, et al (Eds). New York, VCH Publishers, 1986, pp 169-190

37. Al-Mondhiry H, Pierce WS, Richenbacher W, et al: Hemostatic abnormalities associated with prolonged ventricular assist pumping: Analysis of 24 patients. *Am J Cardiol* 1984; 53:1344

38. Murray KD, Olsen DB: Design and functional characteristics of blood pumps. *In:* New Developments in Cardiac Assist Devices. Attar S (Ed). New York, Praeger Publishers, 1985, pp 84-78

39. Levinson MM, Smith RS, Cork RC, et al: Thromboembolic complications of the Jarvik-7 total artificial heart. *Artif Organs* 1986; 10:236

40. Schoen FJ, Clagett GP, Hill DJ, et al: The biocompatibility of artificial organs. *Trans Am Soc Artif Intern Organs* 1987; 23:824

41. Flamenbaum W: Coagulation problems in artificial organs. *Trans Am Soc Artif Intern Organs* 1987; 23:689

42. NIH: Artificial heart and assist devices: Direction, needs, costs, societal and ethical issues. May 1988, *NIH Publication* #85-2723

Self-Assessment Questions

1. CADs:
   A. reduce or totally replace the work effort required of the heart
   B. increase myocardial perfusion
   C. maintain or improve cardiac output
   D. all of the above

2. The TAH:
   A. counterpulsates with the natural heart
   B. supports only the left heart function
   C. is used only as a bridge to transplantation
   D. requires minimal surgical skills to insert

3. The most widely used CAD is:
   A. the TAH
   B. the nonpulsatile centrifugal pump
   C. the pulsatile pneumatic pump
   D. the IABP

4. Anticoagulation therapy is used with CAD support to:
   A. prevent thromboemboli
   B. reduce bleeding complications
   C. minimize the risk of infection
   D. speed up the surgical insertion of the device

5. Pulsatile pumps:
   A. are the least expensive of all the VADs
   B. are not regulated by the FDA
   C. can be synchronized with the cardiac cycle
   D. operate on the principle of continuous flow

Self-Assessment Answers

1. D

2. C

3. D

4. A

5. C

Chapter 18

Determinants of Care

Joseph M. Civetta, MD

Outline

Educational Objectives

In this chapter the reader will learn:

1. four frames of reference for determining care.

2. to separate the ICU illness into stages for evaluation of care.

3. the relationship between societal values and goals of medicine as a foundation for the delivery of care.

4. specific physiologic elements useful in determining the goals and implementation of care in acute illness.

5. to compare and contrast elements useful in determining therapeutic goals at different stages of illness.

Introduction

At the dawn of critical care, nearly 25 to 30 years ago, the selection of patients for admission and the objectives of treatment seemed to cause no great problems because, during this evolutionary phase, the major determinants of care were decided by the medical profession. Today this is no longer true because of profound legal, ethical, moral, religious, and financial aspects to the delivery of care. Webster's Dictionary defines "determinant" as, "A fact, circumstance or situation which identifies . . . the nature . . . of an issue" (1). Our problems are compounded because there are only a few facts and a rather large number of circumstances and situations that must be considered important determinants. We shall consider determinants of care from four separate frames of reference which have important interactions: a) medical considerations with respect to selection of patients; b) the standpoint of the resources of the facility, that is, the ICU; c) the patient's course as it evolves during the ICU admission; and d) the societal aspects which now impact on these three primary frames of reference. The first three can be treated separately; however, I shall discuss the societal aspects where relevant.

I would like to start by examining the implicit contract between society and the medical profession in the past, and try to pinpoint why recent technological changes have resulted in the conflict between these frames of reference which previously, at least on the surface, seemed free of major confrontation or incompatibility.

The Edwin Smith Surgical Papyrus is, perhaps, the oldest existing medical document. It was scribe-copied about 1600 B.C.E. from a much older document, possibly dating as early as 3000 B.C.E., "judging from the character of the glosses which were introduced to explain archaic terms" (2). It is a collection of 48 case descriptions but, of greatest importance for our consideration, each case is classified by one of three different "verdicts," the term used to describe the diagnosis: a) "an ailment which I will treat;" b) "an ailment with which I will contend;" or c) "an ailment not to be treated." Thus, in the earliest medical documents physicians were cautioned to recognize those ailments which were beyond their curative powers. One of the problems in the ICU today is that we have lost the ability to distinguish and separate these ailments. The definitions of treatment and therapy both contain the expectation that cure is possible. If we could recognize an ailment that "ought not be treated," we would realize that the term "life support" is misapplied; our interventions are futile as true therapy and can only prolong the patient's dying. However, this distinction is not clear and certainly is not fully accepted by either the medical profession or society in general.

Jerry Avorn (3) noted that, "Until a century ago, medical therapy was, for the most part, both cheap and useless, thereby posing no great problems of distributive justice. Quite the opposite is now the case. The remarkable progress of biomedical technology since World War II has made it possible for physicians to keep sicker and sicker patients alive longer and longer at greater and greater costs." Apparently, this ability was construed as true medical "progress," but we have learned that terms such as "sicker" and "alive longer" carry implications unknown in prior eras. Patients in the ICU may be kept in a state of prolonged dying, a period lasting days, weeks, months, and even years, if we maintain careful attention to numerous details of bedside care. The transition from life to death can now be artificially lengthened so that the process seems suspended or frozen in time. We then find it difficult to judge the severity of illness: is a patient sick but with a chance of survival following ICU treatment or so sick that the natural progression of death is just delayed by our, perhaps, poorly termed "life-support" techniques?

Even the term "alive" is no longer simple. Society values both the sanctity of life and the quality of life. Before the technological/ICU era and its unprecedented dying state, there were few occasions in which the two societal values relating to life came in conflict. The period of dying was, for the most part, mercifully short and instances such as prolonged vegetative states were more curiosities because of their rarity than a matter of major medical or societal concern. This is no longer true and society — and all of the members of the society, i.e., patients, lawyers, judges, physicians, and nurses — are often perplexed, anguished, and confused. Edgar Allan Poe, the master of horror stories, wrote "The Strange Facts in the Case of M. Valdemar" in 1845 (4). In the story, a patient was hypnotized (termed 'mesmerized') at the moment of death. The patient remained suspended in this state for months. It makes especially chilling reading today, as analogously, we and society are mesmerized by the technology which has created the suspended state of dying in the ICU. It will take time for society to sort out these values and definitions. At a recent conference, Dr. Thomas Starzl maintained that societal confusion is understandable, given the jolt to the definitions of life and death, unquestioned and undisturbed throughout human history. Until 30 years ago, cessation of vital signs (cardiac activity and breathing) was a sign of death. Now this state is termed "cardiac arrest" and, indeed, it may not be death, for after prompt resuscitation, many patients again function as active members of society, i.e., they are alive. On the other hand, cardiac and respiratory activity no longer necessarily signify life. The concept of brain death, stimulated by successful human organ transplantation, has now evolved and achieved both medical and legal status.

The problem reached public attention with the Karen Ann Quinlan case (6), but, in fact, this was not the beginning of the problem but rather the beginning of public debate. According to Justice Christopher Armstrong (7), before the Quinlan case and the enormous publicity that resulted from it, the public generally assumed that physicians would *always do everything* in their power to sustain the lives of critically ill patients. This was not strictly true; there were situations in which available measures such as hospitalization and antibiotic therapy for severely debilitated patients with fever in nursing homes were withheld (8). However, these matters were not discussed openly, perhaps because physicians were afraid that, in destroying the public misconception, confidence in the profession might also be impaired. The ethical principles of beneficence and autonomy were not as clearly articulated nor seemingly in as much conflict in those simpler days. While a competent patient should have the right to make his or her own treatment decisions (the principle of autonomy) everyone seemed comfortable that the physicians were the appropriate ones to suggest what was in the patient's best interest (the principle of beneficence). Also, society and the medical profession passively agreed that knowledge of the fact of choice would trouble many families unnecessarily. In this era, too, we see the physician as a "wise family physician," treating the family for an extended period of time, knowing the concerns and troubles intimately. Where difficult decisions had to be made, he (rarely she, for remember, this is an earlier day) would not hesitate to spare the family and take the burden on himself. Justice Armstrong (6) continues, "Three factors conspired to destroy the myth. One was the gradual breakdown of the once intimate relationship between the doctor and the family . . .; the second factor was the growth of malpractice litigation . . .; (and) the third factor was the revolution of drugs and technology." We certainly participate in the super-specialization by our choice of intensive care, so that we are complete strangers to the patient and family at the time of ICU admission. Malpractice litigation, without the bond between doctor and family, creates an atmosphere conducive to worry about potential legal liability and the dangers of acting in the absence of documented informed consent. As we well know, medical care is no longer "cheap and useless" (3), but the real issue is that the advances in our knowledge have exponentially increased the range of treatment options, thus making it virtually impossible to "always use everything" in Justice Armstrong's words. The ultimate result was that choice could no longer be submerged; it had to come, in Fried's words, "out of the closet" (9) and enter the public domain. In the last 10 years, there have been more than 30 cases of precedential significance concerning lifesaving treatment which have been decided in appellate courts. While there is a growing consensus (6), only certain issues have been addressed and, even in these situations, there are differing decisions in different states. None of this can delay us from setting objectives for critical care today and understanding the determinants of the care to be rendered. We might view the overall task as encompassing appropriate goals of medicine, the limitations of present care, an alignment of the hospital's mission and resources and, finally, congruence with overall societal values. Clearly, the medical determinants of care are only a small part of the picture.

Selection of Patients: Medical Considerations

Life was simpler when we believed that the selection of patients could be reduced, as it were, to a single criterion, "choose the sickest patients." This fundamental objective can be considered the stimulus for the formation of ICUs in the first place. Prior to establishing special care areas and at a time when new and expensive equipment had been developed, distribution of both sick patients and scarce equipment throughout the hospital seemed inefficient in terms of both efficacy and cost. So, from one perspective, ICUs were created to concentrate three critical components: the sickest patients, the highly technical and expensive equipment, and the persons with the knowledge and experience to treat these patients and to use the equipment. Simplistic even then, the concept of choosing the sickest patients had to be expanded into at least three groups which have, unfortunately, from a clinician's point of view, never been mutually exclusive: patients just right for intensive care, as well as those who might be considered "too sick" and "too well." In this conception, the patient would be just right for intensive care if the illness was deemed too severe for care in a routine hospital area, i.e., without specialized care death would be the inevitable outcome, and *the illness was likely to respond to treatment in the ICU*. To this date, unfortunately, few disease states and even fewer patients meet these criteria such that there is unequivocal evidence of the efficacy of intensive care (10). We might, for the sake of discussion, examine the other two classes of patients: "too sick," those whose illness was so severe that death was likely even after treatment in the ICU; and "too well," those who were likely to survive even if they did not receive the "benefits" of intensive care. I submit that this classification system fails to recognize that these distinctions are not always possible and, more important, not necessarily desireable. We will consider this further in the section concerning the resources of the ICU as we try to derive appropriate objectives for care, given the interrelationship of the four determinants today.

We can examine the theoretical basis for current attempts to exclude patients who are "too sick" or "too well" for ICU care. While terminally ill patients would experience little benefit from the ICU, neither clinicians nor patients and their families usually want or even think of ICU admission, in contrast to hospital admission. Although it is true that 80% or more of patients in the United States presently die in hospitals, and many patients with terminal illnesses are readmitted to the hospital primarily to die, the motivating force is not one last ditch effort to avoid death but rather comfort for the patient and relief of stress on the family. On the other hand, patients with acute devastating illness who are admitted to the ICU, if they die, usually do so quickly. Resource utilization is not a problem and efficient, rapid, crisis-oriented care can and does produce the dramatic success idealized if not exactly typical of intensive care. Exclusion of the patient "too sick" would have little salutary effect in terms of treatment goals and essentially no impact on resources in my own ICU because these patients use less than 1% of the patient-days (11). In fact, in order to choose all the appropriate patients, we must, by design, broaden the admission criteria including some patients who might retrospectively be deemed "too sick" because of our inability to only select the appropriate patients. In like manner, we often extend our selection process to include patients who may be considered "too well" for intensive care. This, again, is not necessarily purely a medical decision though, most worrisome, some other nonmedical determinants designed to exclude patients are currently proposed and others are in effect. Some (12, 13) have proposed that patients be excluded if the risk of mortality or morbidity is low or if the need for treatment is low (14). Conceptually, this, too, might be considered reasonable but only from a very restricted viewpoint. Any changes in current policy, if undertaken because of financial constraints, should have a significant potential benefit to justify the attendant risks which are at least implicit in excluding currently admitted patients from the ICU. In one study, if the estimated probability of needing ICU-type treatment was 10% or less, the intensive care admission would be considered unnecessary (12). Given the present hypersensitive medicolegal scrutiny, particularly blurring the distinction between bad outcome and negligence, it seems hard to believe that the negligible financial savings of a single day's observation in the ICU is likely to be considered a justifiable defense in a malpractice action. While unnecessary admissions are clearly wasteful, an analysis of the risk of complications proposed by the Consensus Development Conference (10) weighed two distinct factors: the risk of complication and likelihood of successful treatment. They believed that patients who were at a markedly increased risk deserved the observation currently available only in ICUs. If equivalent results of treatment of a developed complication can be reasonably expected in both routine care areas and the ICU, no advantage to ICU admission can be postulated. However, when delay in diagnosis or treatment can be predicted from the staffing and equipment levels currently available in a given hospital's routine areas, and this would compromise treatment, ICU admission would seem warranted. After all, if ICUs were created by clustering expensive equipment and knowledgeable and experienced personnel, we must consider what we left behind: routine care areas without extra equipment, staffed by persons neither trained nor experienced in the management of problems now routinely confined to the ICU. In fact, this effect upon routine care areas was considered to be one of the detrimental effects of the development of ICUs (10).

By omitting terminal patients and those who would fare well enough in routine care areas, we should be able to select patients appropriate for intensive care based on these medical factors, recognizing the organizational components just discussed. Today, however, we must remember the financial, legal, ethical, moral, and religious ramifications to our medical selection process in the delivery of care, termination of life support, utilization of scarce resources, malpractice, and rising medical costs, all of which impact and, perhaps, have greater weight than "mere" patient-physician-disease interactions. Because society can only be expected to resolve these complex and interrelated issues over time, and while the situation for us today is serious and even baffling, it is not hopeless. As we attempt to refine admission criteria for the proper use of the ICU, we must depreciate the current foci upon money and medicolegal considerations, notwithstanding their considerable visibility and impact. Unfortunately, continually rising costs for medical care have been cited as the reason to institute major changes in health-care financing; these now impact on the delivery of care. There is also an ominous specter to this emphasis on risking costs; cost containment, if poorly conceived and implemented, will reduce the access to care as well as the quality of care, and yet will fail to achieve true savings. Opinions are quite divergent with respect to the directions which should be undertaken. Proponents of prospective payment systems, such as diagnosis related groups (DRG) now utilized by Medicare, believe it will solve many of the ills now attributed to cost based reimbursement. Richard Schweiker, the former Secretary of Health and Human Resources, told Congress that a DRG-based system will provide hospitals with an incentive to improve efficiency, establish Medicare as a prudent buyer of hospital services, and reduce the administrative burden on hospitals while assuring the beneficiary access to quality health care (15). We should note that the DRG system was not designed as a tool for reimbursement and that no outcome criteria have been developed to assess the effects of the system, especially with regard to intensive care.

Even after 4 years of concerted efforts, medical costs rose at a 7.5% annual rate in 1986, whereas the overall inflation rate has fallen to below 2%. Meanwhile, all eyes focus on the spectacular successes achieved in transplantation, even though costs for an individual patient exceed $100,000 for just the hospitalization. George Orwell's major error in "1984" (16) was not in predicting the *type* of future but in attributing the *cause* of the changes to direct governmental intervention. Many of the changes have occurred without obvious "Big Brother" control. Many Newspeak concepts, if not the words, are with us today. For instance, the term "doublethink" referred to the developed ability to hold two contradictory ideas in the mind at the same time and not notice that they were diametrically opposed. Thus, it does not seem contradictory today to expect to lower costs and to introduce better and more expensive forms of effective therapy simultaneously. We must await society's realization that this is a problem which will not go away. If medical science is to continue to discover, refine, and improve therapy, the conflict between a desire to lower costs and to improve care will actually become more acute. Although improved efficiency could have been considered an initial realistic method to decrease spending, true improvements in care which may be costly must be factored into the overall equations. Stern and Epstein (15) wrote that although DRGs have a moderate chance of decreasing total health care costs, they were also likely to have deleterious effects upon the quality of patient care and access to care.

The simple time in terms of choices or selection of patients for intensive care is gone; furthermore, the currently proposed simple solutions based on exclusion criteria will have little impact upon the cost of ICU care, but rather are likely to have deleterious effects upon both quality and access to care.

ICU Resources

A qualitative basis for categorizing general goals of intensive care, based upon the commitment of hospital resources to the ICU, is needed (17). These categories were developed to distinguish patients from routine postoperative surgical patients but, in general, applied to all "specialty" ICU patients as well. The three categories are: monitoring/observation, extensive nursing requirements, and constant physician care. I would consider physiologically stable patients as appropriate candidates for ICU admission in the category termed "monitoring/

observation" if these patients have a recognized risk of complications, and if the likelihood of recognition and successful treatment is higher in the intensive care setting. We must remember that the focus on cost containment has not been confined to the ICU. In fact, ICU staffing levels and equipment have generally been affected the least of any area of the hospital. Intensive monitoring and observation were never particularly easy or effective in routine care areas; after all, one of the earliest forms of intensive care in this country, the coronary care unit, was created to correct this deficiency. However, we must address the issue of monitoring and observation quantitatively as well as qualitatively. The patient/nurse ratio is 12:1 during the night shift in my hospital's regular care areas. After allowing time for necessary administrative and physiologic functions, the nurse has less than 30 minutes per shift available for any individual patient. This staffing pattern was designed *because* patients needing intensive observation and monitoring are now admitted to the ICU. Should these patients now be excluded from the ICU, the hospital will have to increase its staffing in the general care areas to provide the still necessary monitoring and observation. This may be accomplished by establishing intermediate care areas (18) or "overnight recovery rooms;" in practice, the same patients must be provided the same level of nursing surveillance wherever they are physically located. The particular "solution" is not the issue; increased staffing and more equipment will be necessary to create the monitoring/observation environment, no matter where it is located or what name is issued. ICU care by any other name, to paraphrase, will still cost as much. However, the advantages of concentration of persons and resources, underlying the initial conception of the ICU, will be lost; the ICU will still be necessary for its other patients and the overall net result will be increased total hospital costs rather than the savings projected from the too restricted viewpoint based on the likelihood of interventions. By the way, if these less costly monitoring/observation patients are removed, only the more costly will remain and the bottom line figure (the average cost per ICU patient) will also increase. Monitoring/observation patients belong in today's ICU.

The same considerations apply to patients who have extensive nursing requirements. Frequent position changes, complex dressings, intake and output measurements and laboratory testing, and a myriad of additional nursing tasks are beyond the capabilities of the small nursing contingent now assigned to large care areas. The measures designed to improve efficiency which have been enacted over the past years have already eliminated the personnel necessary to accomplish these tasks; this was reasonable since these capabilities were included in the ICU as a part of the overall design. These patients make up approximately 60% of our patient population (19) but, for more than mere numbers, they are a most important focus. These patients are generally physiologically stable; in fact, using most indices of severity, they are classified in the mid-range, neither very sick nor very well. They remain in intensive care for a long period of time for this very reason. Patients in the monitoring/observation class are usually discharged within a day or two. Patients requiring constant physician care can only stay in this category for a short period of time (thereafter, the acute abnormalities are either resolved successfully, in which case they enter the extensive care category or, if therapy has been unsuccessful, these patients die). Although the extensive nursing patients may be physiologically stable, careful monitoring and observation are always necessary. However, the motivating force for ICU admission is the complexity and frequency of nursing tasks which exceed the realistic expectations of time available in general nursing units. These patients may develop complications related to the primary admitting diagnosis or subsequent failure of initially functioning organ systems, all of which create demands on nursing resources. Patients needing extensive nursing care must also be admitted to the ICU.

The third group, characterized as the patients requiring constant physician care, are physiologically unstable; physicians and nurses must remain at the bedside, reacting to changes in the patient's status by implementing and refining therapy. They conform to the popular image of intensive care because of the elements of high technology, rapid but efficient activity, crises and, perhaps, dramatic successes. There is no problem in the selection of these patients for the ICU admission, although they make up only 10% to 20% (19) of our ICU population. Yet, even in these circumstances, once this acute stage passes, as it must, the reality includes other elements as well, such as the nearness of death and illnesses lasting months — because it is unlikely that the devastating illness resulting in their initial classification can resolve rapidly. It is this form of intensive care, prototypic in initial concept, that must now evolve beyond crisis orientation in both medical and nonmedical areas to develop consonance with evolving societal values.

We must direct our efforts to understand the relationship between society's values and the goals of medicine; this has been well described by Young (20). The goals of medicine, the preservation of life, and the alleviation of suffering, are respectively derived from societal values of both the sanctity and quality of life. Today these two societal values are often in conflict. Because the passage from dying to death may almost be suspended through the application of technology, resolution of the conflict is now necessary. Prior to life support, death rapidly followed the onset of dying and there was "no real problem." Of course, the conflict existed; however, it was so rare or shortlived that nothing needed to be done about it. However, resolution did *not* occur; the conflict simply *disappeared* with the death of the patient. Now, the prolongation of dying and suspension of death, at least for potentially long periods of time, force recognition and resolution. We must make a choice. There seems to be an increasing awareness that sanctity and quality of life may not be attainable at the same time; there is a conflict between the preservation of life and the alleviation of suffering. There is also a growing tendency to evaluate quality of life as a valid criterion in making such decisions both within the medical profession and society in general.

Furthermore, the right of a competent patient to determine treatment, autonomy, has become increasingly well recognized both ethically and legally, leading to an increased awareness of the elements necessary to have truly informed consent. The three vital elements (21) are: disclosure by the physician, *understanding* by the patient, and a free choice. All three elements often lack a comfortable degree of certainty in the ICU. When we speak of a distinction between critical illness (a reasonable prospect of recovery) and dying (a patient whose disease process is irreversible), we have no way to do so conclusively. Current scoring systems have insufficient precision to forecast outcome for an individual patient. Most often, we act on consensus among treating physicians, gained from observation over time, about the trajectory of the patient's clinical course. This lack of certainty may make it even more difficult to explain the situation to the patient or the family. It is important to remember that informed consent is a process which, in these difficult cases, should evolve over time. Thus, when we are faced with a patient who is admitted with a poor prognosis, perhaps a 5% expectation of survival (however determined), this means, in a manner of speaking, that 95 out of every 100 patients with a similar clinical condition will ultimately die. We should be able to identify markers or milestones along the projected courses which can help us realize whether the patient will ultimately become one of the five survivors or join the 95 who die. On a day-by-day basis, we can then compare the patient's actual course to that projected for a survivor or, conversely, for a patient who dies. If we continue this process of repeated observation and comparison, we can gradually reach a firm conclusion with respect to prognosis.

The second element is equally difficult. Note that disclosure alone is not enough but that we must assure ourselves that the information is understood by the patient or in the case of an incompetent patient, by the family. This, too, is problematic. If the illness is unexpected or unexpectedly acute, as may occur in trauma or a devastating complication suffered during the course of elective surgery, the patient, of course, may be incompetent *and* the family may be incapable of understanding even the most lucid and careful explanation. One of the most primitive but temporarily effective defense mechanisms is that of denial. Patients and their families often just cannot accept the sudden reality of life-threatening illness and it may well be that this precludes true understanding necessary for informed consent. While we recognize that in a crisis we may proceed without such understanding, the patients of greatest concern are those who remain suspended between living and dying. We cannot proceed as if it were a crisis and must do our best to help families and patients adjust to these terrifying prospects. We often deal with the family of the incompetent patient and must judge their understanding and ultimately accept their choice (unless there is obvious conflict among family members or between a medical care team and family). Oftentimes, we could have obtained information directly from the patient concerning his or her values so when a choice would become necessary, it could be based upon information directly supplied by the patient. In addition to living wills and durable powers of attorney, oral declarations are considered valid in some jurisdictions. It is of more importance to remember that many patients with chronic illness could be questioned about their thoughts and values regarding prolonged ICU care and the inevitability of death — when they are still competent, that is, prior to hospitalization, or even at the beginning of their ICU stay. For elective surgical patients, particularly those with diseases of poor prognosis, the elderly, or those who have associated severe medical conditions, such information could be obtained as a "value history" (21) at the time patients are admitted to the hospital. The element of choice, too, is problematic in the ICU, especially for incompetent patients, but we can obtain information from the patient or family concerning the patient's identified values and wishes concerning quality of life decisions.

Thus, we can align our goals of care with societal values for this patient both prior to and after our recognition that further medical care will be fruitless, that is to say, the patient's condition is irreversible. Up to this point of recognition of irreversibility, care is appropriately directed toward cure. Our therapeutic efforts can be successful and we should strive for the preservation of life in concert with the societal value of sanctity of life. When the disease process is considered irreversible, when our care cannot achieve cure, it is all too easy to sense failure and frustration, but we actually have new and important goals for our caring efforts (22). Armed with conclusive knowledge of the irreversibility of the patient's disease and specific information relating to this patient's perceived quality of life, our continued care aligns the alleviation of suffering with the societal value of the quality of life. Pain and anxiety should be relieved, of course, but we must extend the concept of the alleviation of suffering to include efforts to aid the patient and family in adjusting to the nearness of death. When cure cannot be achieved, dying itself should not be prolonged with technology. If life cannot be extended with dignity and purpose, meaningless prolongation of dying is the inevitable outcome (20). This costly and ineffective utilization of resources during a patient's dying is neither necessary nor desirable for medicine, the patient, or society. This approach provides a suitable framework to approach problems of limited resources and distributive justice. Exclusion criteria discussed before will neither result in a more equitable distribution of limited resources nor effect true savings. Limitations of that type will result in an imposition of restrictions concerning the availability and quality of care.

Critical care today requires a focus beyond the needs of a specific patient and must encompass the total number of patients who could be considered eligible for care, given the number of available beds. Since the beds are so expensive, clearly the hospital cannot afford to maintain an excess of beds staffed to accommodate all potential emergency admissions. However, emergencies are actually predictable in the sense that we know, on average, how many can be expected per year and, by calculation, per day. Should all the existing care have already been allocated, some decision will have to be made to distribute resources in an ethical manner.

At the outset, however, it is important to remember that although the *problem* seems to require a solution to resolve the incompatibility of a "full" unit and admission of a new patient, the *solution* may be effected step-by-step so that, in reality, no patient is deprived of necessary care. This process, however, usually requires creativity, cooperation, and a great deal of work to bring a successful conclusion. The physical process of discharge from the ICU to routine care areas can be accelerated if we know the usual problems and take steps to solve them. Often hours elapse before the "recipient" bed is "ready," because of waiting for a family member or medications, for the bed and room to be cleaned, for transport personnel, a delay because the personnel on the floor may wish to wait until after shift report, etc., etc., etc. Each of these, subject to discreet pressure, can be influenced or solved. Other possible solutions include special duty nurses provided outside the unit for patients who might require extra monitoring, another ICU may temporarily "loan" a vacant bed, overnight care may be provided in a recovery room in place of intensive care admission, extra nursing personnel may be enticed to work overtime or give up a day off, nursing personnel may be added to the unit's staff temporarily from another ICU, from the floor, supervisory personnel, or an agency, and even physicians have been "recruited" to provide independent and dependent nursing role functions (23). Using overtime or "day off" personnel, though sometimes necessary and possible, has been a factor which, ultimately, increases the stress of daily ICU life since these crises, that is to say, more patients than can be cared for by the available assigned nursing staff, occur regularly. Staffing cannot be based on the peak requirements. Asking nurses continuously to work double shifts or to work on days off places them in a dilemma — to work when they really want and need their time off or to "let everyone else down" by refusing to work. This is part of the "burn out" phenomenon or feeling compelled (from within) to resign from a position previously highly desired.

Unfortunately, no matter how creatively and diligently the participants work, new patients will arrive when all beds are full and all the temporizing measures have been exhausted. This serious problem has existed for the last 20 years despite the incredible expansion of the number of ICU beds during that era. In terms of the ethical principle of distributive justice, one method commonly and effectively employed is "first come, first served." Care is apportioned to appropriate candidates seeking admission; these patients may continue to receive care until their outcome is determined. This seemingly simple principle was confounded during the evolution of critical care through the creation of the unprecedented prolonged dying state. The difficulty in making such choices was examined by the National Institutes of Health Consensus Development Conference on Critical Care Medicine in 1983 (10):

"It is not medically appropriate to devote limited ICU resources to patients without reasonable prospect of significant recovery when patients who need those services and who have significant prospect of recovery from acutely life-threatening disease or injury are being turned away due to lack of capacity. It is inappropriate to maintain ICU management of a patient whose prognosis has resolved to one of persistent vegetative state, and it is similarly inappropriate to employ ICU resources where no purpose will be served but a prolongation of the natural process of death."

These statements, I believe, are of great help in focusing attention upon this difficult problem. However, some major difficulties remain; for instance, it is extremely difficult to define "without reasonable prospect of significant recovery" in most clinical situations. The actual number of patients who can be certified as brain dead is small and usually, because of the urgent need for rapidly harvesting organs, such determinations are made rapidly. Most of the prognostic indices lack the accuracy to make such a definitive diagnosis; indeed, if the data were present already, prolongation of dying would have been terminated so that the bed would have been available when the new patient presented. It is also most difficult to develop and promulgate the definition of "reasonable prospect." In our ICU, I poll the assembled residents, students, nurses, and other personnel during rounds concerning their desires to treat given certain mathematical probabilities of success. At a 1:10 chance of survival, usually there is complete agreement to treat. In contrast, at a 1:1,000,000 chance, I can usually find full agreement to stop treatment. Everyone also usually agrees not to treat if the probabilities of success are 1 in 100,000 or 1 in 10,000. There are some, nearly every rotation, who would wish to continue treatment if there was 1 chance in 1,000 of success. At the same time, there are always individuals who would be willing to stop treatment if the chance of success were 1:100. Of course, none of the existing predictors have this degree of precision, but the disagreement concerning how to proceed, given a *theoretically precise* estimate, is striking to me. Until more accurate predictors are available *and* until there is a consensus concerning "reasonable prospect," the problem will continue. Society seems to be wrestling with this problem today, having finally reached reasonable consensus concerning brain death (most, but not all states, now have statutes).

An even more difficult problem concerns the distribution of limited care when the differences in outcome are only of degree, that is to say, when a patient with a

70% expected rate of recovery compared to a patient with, perhaps, only *but a realistic* 5% chance of survival. At the present time, it would seem that the only acceptable solution is to find an alternative to depriving one patient of care. We should not be forced to make an "either/or" choice. Some temporizing measure may be possible, perhaps until another patient recovers sufficiently for discharge or dies. The alternatives listed before, by the way, do not reflect all possible solutions. This exposition is not intended to resolve or solve the problem of limited resources and excessive demand. Rather, temporizing measures, creative thinking, extra effort, and cooperation will be necessary. This one problem has occupied more of my own professional life as an ICU Director than any other. I see no reason to believe it will either be solved or even ameliorated in the immediate future. If this is simply a matter of cost per life, surely society will want to compare such costs with other "scales of monetary value," perhaps in the arena of entertainment and sports or the costs expended by the military-industrial complex to *take* a life.

Evolution of the Patient's Course

We examined the determinants of care from the medical perspective, the ICU resources available, societal values concerning the sanctity and quality of life and, finally, have tried to coordinate these with the patient's wishes and values as expressed through informed consent. However, that resolution depends upon the particular stage of the patient's illness. In this area, we can look to the predictive indices or severity scoring systems for assistance, not so much to determine prognosis or severity in an individual case but, rather, to assess what information is useful in describing the patient's illness throughout its course.

Many methods have been proposed to assess severity of illness and risk of death or other outcome variables such as sepsis or other complications. The groups studied include: trauma patients, all ICU admissions, elective surgical candidates, patients for cancer surgery, and patients given a preoperative nutritional assessment. Parameters were found to be effective in prediction for each specific group of patients although, as we shall see, the important parameters differ markedly among the different groups. Although it had been hoped that the vast mass of data, when subjected to proper statistical techniques in sufficient quantities, would quantify the degree of illness and predict the likelihood of recovery prospectively, these expectations have not been realized (24). While it was hoped that precise mathematical models could replace the uncertainties of clinical judgment, this prior clinical uncertainty recognized that outcome is often later determined by the unpredictable occurrence of catastrophic events, development of new illnesses or complications, iatrogenic events, and, especially, ultimate failure of organ systems functioning early in the patient's course. These same events must effect the reliability of all mathematical predictive systems.

I wish neither to sound critical of these instruments nor to evaluate their potential to address severity of illness. My goal, rather, is to examine the predictive indices or scoring systems in order to extract the important elements at each stage of the patient's course in the ICU. We can focus our attention on the relevant physiologic processes which have the greatest effect on survival at that state (Table 1). In this way, we can identify the determinants for care, given the existing circumstances for *this* patient at *this* point in the illness. We must also balance the probable effects of disease and the wishes and values of the patient.

Algorithms describing the disease and treatment apart from the patient are incomplete and lack the necessary context desirable in describing all the determinants of care.

TABLE 1. Stages of illness

Presentation for ICU Care

Short-Term ICU Outcome

Necessity for Continued ICU Care

Long-Term ICU Outcome

Discharge from the ICU

Presentation for ICU Care

We should consider patients admitted from emergency and elective sources separately. Emergency patients have a higher mortality rate and serve to draw our special attention because of their initial acuity; thus, important parameters are usually related to cardiorespiratory integrity. Furthermore, little may be known or there may be little time to amass other relevant information at the time these patients are considered for ICU admission. In contrast, elective (usually surgical) patients are in a stable state even if chronic illness is present; furthermore, their course will be based on the capacity to withstand the future stress induced by operation, that is, their physiologic reserve rather than the capacity to respond to existing stress which characterizes the emergency patients.

The greatest wealth of analyzed data exists for the multitrauma patient. Many scales have been developed primarily for the purpose of triage within trauma systems. They usually rely on simple measurements to be performed by paramedics or other nonphysicians. The scores include: the Triage Index (25); Trauma Score (26); Trauma Index (27); Illness-Injury Severity Index (IISI) (28); and Circulation, Respiration, Abdomen, Motor and Speech (CRAMS) (29). The number of variables, must, of necessity, be small and there is considerable overlap, as seen in Table 2. That the identified factors are important rests upon the dependence of the multicellular organism on integrated cardiorespiratory function to transport O_2 from the external environment to the individual cells.

With respect to other types of emergencies such as GI inflammation, obstruction, or perforation, no similar triaging instruments exist. This is because the selection of these patients and their distribution in the hospitals of a community has not been identified as a problem, the principal reason leading to the creation of trauma systems and, thus, to the development of triage instruments. However, similar types of abnormalities in cardiorespiratory integrity and end-organ function exist. For instance, the decision for urgent operation in patients with bowel obstruction and metabolic acidosis is made because of the derangement in cellular O_2 utilization suggestive of ischemic or infarcted bowel.

TABLE 2. Common elements in triage systems

ELEMENTS	INDEX
Respiratory System:	Trauma Index, Illness-Injury Severity Index CRAMS
Expansion	Triage Index, Trauma Score
Rate	Trauma Score
Cardiovascular	Trauma Index
BP	Trauma Score, Illness-Injury Severity Index
Pulse	Illness-Injury Severity Index
CNS	Trauma Index
Eye Opening	Triage Index, Trauma Score
Motor Response	Triage Index, Trauma Score, CRAMS
Verbal Response	Triage Index, Trauma Score, CRAMS
Level of Consciousness	Illness-Injury Severity Index
Perfusion	
Capillary Refill	Triage Index, Trauma Score, CRAMS
Skin Color	Illness-Injury Severity Index
Other*:	
Age	Illness-Injury Severity Index
Mechanism of Injury	Illness-Injury Severity Index
Region of Injury	Illness-Injury Severity Index, CRAMS

*Age, mechanism and perhaps other factors of injury used in combination with Trauma Score and others for purposes of triage.

While elective patients usually have stable cardiorespiratory function and O_2 transport prior to surgery, descriptors of organ system function and physiologic reserve are important determinants of care. Using similar statistical methodology to the evolution of trauma triage instruments, various measures of nutritional status as predictors of both septic implications and mortality have been developed. Some of the components also reflect hepatic function. Since multiple organ system failure and sepsis are common clinical syndromes in patients who die after elective surgery, it is not surprising that these indices tend to be relatively similar and reasonably simple in construction. Three representative instruments are the Prognostic Nutritional Index (30), Hospital Prognostic Index (31), and Sepsis-Related Mortality (32). The components utilized are listed in Table 3. It is interesting that of all the complex measurements of immune response and hepatic function possible, serum albumin levels and the delayed-type hypersensitivity skin test response were found to be important predictors in all three instruments, the less reactivity and the lower the albumin, the higher the risk of complications, sepsis, and mortality.

TABLE 3. Elements used in nutrition-immune function prognostic indices

ELEMENTS	INSTRUMENT
Triceps Skin Fold	PNI
Albumin	PNI, HPI, SRM
Transferrin	PNI
Delayed Hypersensitivity	PNI, HPI, SRM
Sepsis/Cancer	HPI, PNI
Age/Sex	SRM

Definitions of Delayed Hypersensitivity and values assigned to diagnoses are different, although the categories are similar.
PNI = Prognostic Nutritional Index (30).
HPI = Hospital Prognostic Index (31).
SRM = Sepsis-Related Mortality (32).

Patients who are to undergo elective surgery and who are considered to have compromised hemodynamic function are often admitted to the ICU preoperatively for invasive hemodynamic monitoring and assessment of the physiologic reserve of the cardiovascular system. Creation of the physiologic profile also incorporates measurements of BP and pulse rate in addition to other parameters of cardiorespiratory function which require invasive monitoring (Table 4). These are also used to calculate O_2 transport and utilization parameters (33). If there is evidence of inadequate baseline function, such as decreased cardiac output or left ventricular stroke work, increased O_2 extraction or inadequate O_2 delivery, augmentation of ventricular function using preload, manipulation of afterload by vasodilators, and augmentation of contractility may be attempted. If none of the above measures can improve function and O_2 delivery remains diminished, the risk for developing cardiac complications and potential mortality is considered to be extremely high (33, 34). However, 95% of patients can be rendered suitable candidates for the intended surgery using this approach (33, 34).

TABLE 4. Measured physiologic parameters

Cardiovascular	Respiratory
Cardiac output	Hemoglobin
Systemic arterial pressure	Inspired O_2 tension
Heart rate	Arterial O_2 tension
Pulmonary arterial pressure	Arterial CO_2 tension
Left ventricular filling pressure	Arterial O_2 saturation
Right ventricular filling pressure	Venous O_2 tension
Height and weight	Venous O_2 saturation

Deterioration in clinical status may occur in the hospitalized patient. The parameters of sudden clinical deterioration necessitating emergency intensive care admission usually are related to cardiorespiratory and O_2 transport values similar to other emergency patients.

In summary, at the time of presentation for the ICU admission, in emergency cases, we can expect that the determinants of care will be predicated upon derangements in O_2 transport and cardiorespiratory variables. On the other hand, preoperative elective surgical patients, not surprisingly, must be considered in terms of immune and nutritional status and physiologic reserve of the cardiovascular system.

The Short-Term ICU Outcome

The relationships among mortality rate, duration of intensive care stay, and severity of illness are complex. In surgical ICUs, a significant number of patients are admitted for monitoring-observation and have short ICU stays. A small number of patients in all types of ICUs are so critically ill that they die within the same short time frame despite all efforts. The mortality *rate* for short-term ICU admissions is low since it is the ratio of the relatively few patients who die divided by the sum of these patients and the large number of the monitoring/observation patients who live. Clinical decision-making is relatively easy for both groups: little needs to be done for the monitoring-observation group and, although all considered therapy is attempted for the most critical group, it is only possible to intervene for a short time (35). The mortality rate for patients who have long ICU admissions is much higher, commonly approaching 50% (17). One might mistakenly conclude that, because the mortality rate is higher, these patients have a greater severity of illness. This is not true because the short-term ICU admission group actually contains the patients with the most severe illnesses. The long-term group is the most *problematic,* especially to differentiate between those who may survive or die, because we wish to intervene to achieve therapeutic success for the former, while, in the latter, our primary goal becomes the alleviation of suffering. In this latter group, our sense of urgency to effect a salutary outcome may not be satisfied but our actions will be appropriate.

We must distinguish between the aphorism of our training, focusing on crisis orientation, "Don't just stand there, do something," and, when we realize that the disease is irreversible, we must substitute, "Don't just do something, stand there." We must not continue futile activity but must restrain ourselves, recognizing our limitations and in awe of powers greater than ours which have decided the outcome. Collection of information from both medical and patient-related sources must continue to allow reassessment and reappraisal of both risks and benefits. The longer the illness and the graver the prognosis, the less medicine has to offer and the greater the weight which should be given to the patient's choice based upon personal values (21).

Most patients admitted for monitoring/observation do not and should not develop complications; therefore, the following day they are safely discharged to routine care areas. This decision is usually easy. In a certain number of cases, however, problems will develop; these patients may then require an increased level of nursing and physician care as well as an increased duration which also correlates with higher costs (35). Patients with the highest degrees of abnormal cardiac, respiratory, and O_2 transport function will have not only a high mortality rate but a short duration of intensive care before death occurs. These patients, clinically, are clearly the most severely ill and not surprisingly are so judged by predictive instruments. We must, therefore, determine the basis of the indices which can distinguish short-term survivors from early deaths. We can then focus upon the identified components to direct our decision-making.

The Acute Physiology Score and Chronic Health Evaluation (APACHE) was introduced in 1981 (36). Initially, 34 physiologic measurements were obtained from the patient's clinical record and weighted according to an assigned scale. Additionally, a four-category designation of pre-admission health status was made. More recently, APACHE II (37) reduced the physiologic measurements to 12 values routinely collected, plus age and previous health status. The Therapeutic Intervention Scoring System (TISS) assigned point values in a similar fashion to APACHE but to interventions rather than physiologic abnormalities (38). Patterns of evolving cardiorespiratory function in surviving and nonsurviving patients were the basis of a third instrument (39). While APACHE II and TISS had subjective weights assigned to the values of the variables, actual measurements form the basis of the frequency/distribution predictive system. Finally, simple variables available at the time of admission were analyzed mathematically (40) to form the basis of the fourth instrument, specifically designed to predict survival and mortality. Except for the complete listing of therapeutic interventions in TISS, the other three instruments contain approximately 12 individual components; seven of them appear in at least two, and four of them appear in all three instruments (Table 5). This similarity again underscores the fundamental biologic necessity for transport and cellular utilization of O_2. The fact that these parameters are few and have important statistical validation sup-

---

TABLE 5. Common elements in severity and prognostic indices*

ELEMENT	INDICES
Cardiovascular	
BP	APACHE II, TISS, CRV, MLR
Heart Rate	APACHE II, TISS, CRV, MLR
Cardiac Output	TISS, CRV
Respiratory	
Arterial Oxygenation	APACHE II, TISS, CRV, MLR
Neurologic Function	APACHE II, TISS, MLR
O_2 Transport	
Hemoglobin	APACHE II, CRV
Bicarbonate/pH	APACHE II, TISS, CRV, MLR
Renal Function	APACHE II, TISS, MLR

*Note that TISS reflects therapeutic interventions chosen to affect listed variables.
APACHE II = Acute Physiology Score and Chronic Health Evaluation (37).
TISS = Therapeutic Intervention Scoring System (38).
CRV = Cardiorespiratory Variables (39).
MLR = Multiple Logistic Regression (40).

ports the need for early and intense monitoring of cardiorespiratory function as well as O_2 transport in critically ill patients. These parameters, then, become determinants of care in terms of monitoring and the basis for the selection of interventions.

Necessity For Continued ICU Care

Since outcome has already been decided for patients with the least and most degrees of severity, the ICU now contains patients midway along the severity spectrum (11) who have expected mortality rates of 50% (21). The mortality rate should be 50% because the severity spectrum starts with patients with the least degree of illness (the mortality rate approaches zero) and as a continuum extends to the most severe, those with lethal illness (with a mortality rate of 100%). Thus, the initial period of easily separating patients is over — because the least severe have been transferred to routine care areas and the most severe have already died.

The remaining patients may also be considered "critical." The distinction between those patients who will live and those who will ultimately die is impossible to achieve on admission; time and intervention will both be necessary in order to achieve resolution or separate these groups. Decision-making is both more difficult and more necessary. "Critical" in this context should be used to underscore the need for effective intervention and the realization that such intervention does not produce immediate results; rather, a successful outcome can only be determined after a considerable investment of time. In a study of long-term patients (11), the average duration of stay was approximately 3 weeks in both patients who ultimately lived and died. If resolution took this length of time, it is clear that the initial physiologic state must have been similar in both groups. When the "early" indices (APACHE and TISS) were calculated on admission and then repeated over the next 2 weeks, statistical separation of those who ultimately survived from those who died was not possible until after 2 weeks of applied interventions. It is not surprising that these indices were not helpful. They were designed to assess patients early in their course and are heavily weighted to cardiorespiratory and O_2 transport parameters. These variables do not ultimately determine outcome in this small subgroup (7% of total) of patients. On the other hand, these patients use 35% of the total patient-days of care. Decision-making is a long and arduous problem, balancing benefits and resource utilization, and developing a medical judgment. An index, based on data available at the time it is calculated, can predict with an accuracy determined by the impact of these data upon outcome. If other events actually determine outcome, such as evolution of the illness, unforeseen illnesses or complications and, especially, failure of organs functioning earlier, the index lacking these elements cannot be predictive. The ICU patient is not like a train with both destination and direction fixed by the tracks. Rather, the patient's course must be "driven" by clinical judgment, much as a car is guided through traffic and around obstacles.

Long-Term ICU Outcome

We must focus our attention upon what *not* to do as well as what we should do; this is not simply a matter of resource utilization but a matter of remembering what our "therapy" can accomplish. These long-term patients, midway along the severity spectrum, have survival rates of approximately 50%. We must continue to treat these patients because half will survive. Their degree of physiologic abnormality, utilizing our best quantitative methods, is not particularly high, nor is there any accurate way of predicting outcome. Since O_2 transport and cardiorespiratory parameters are not grossly deranged, it should be clear that our familiar "crisis interventions," such as cardiovascular monitoring/interventions and ventilatory support, have little chance to reverse the current problems faced by these patients. We must remember that we have little true treatment to offer when renal, hepatic, and immune function deteriorate despite maintaining cardiorespiratory function and nutritional support.

We must temper the "technological imperative," that is to say, to use everything in the therapeutic armamentarium continually until the moment of death. We must also recognize the impact of the uncertainty of outcome upon the patient and family as well as the ICU staff. Our desire to restore health to all of our patients must face the reality that nearly 50% of these patients ultimately die.

Based upon this realization that death is a likely possibility in the long-term patients and recognizing the limitation of early physiologic assessors for differentiating between patients who ultimately live or die, we must look to other processes, such as methods of quantitating protein metabolism and immune function. These are often the factors which differentiate success from failure in prolonged and critical illness. The multiple organ failure syndrome is believed to have a metabolic basis in substrate:energy failure (41). Many, if not most, of these long-term patients have primarily or secondarily developed the sepsis syndrome. Analysis of long-term patients who survived and died showed significant differences (42) such that patients who later succumbed could be identified more than a week before death with a high degree of certainty (Table 6). Note that many of these variables are based upon the failure of substrate metabolism including increased urea, lactate, and glucose. These represent alterations in metabolic pathways that are beyond our capacity to influence. The majority of the parameters which have been found to be discriminatory in these patients are not related to acute cardiorespiratory dysfunction nor to the types of bedside assessments which were so prevalent in the early predictors and are deemed so responsive to active early ICU treatment.

Our role now has a different tone, direction and even destination, at times. Although informed consent contains three elements, it is most important to remember that it is not a one-time thing, a form to be signed, but a process, one that must undergo continual evolution, particularly if we are to promote understanding by the patient and family to arrive at a valid choice. At times, we tend to see the ethical principles of beneficence and autonomy at opposite ends of a spectrum. This should not be the case. Beneficence, as a principle, means the protection and promotion of the best interests of the patient. In recognizing autonomy, we should acknowledge and implement the decisions of others, even if they differ from our own conception. To the physician who values cure, beneficence may seem in conflict with autonomy; the patient refuses care, yet the dedication of the physician is expressed by willingness to continue treatment. The patient may be considered illogical or stubborn in his or her refusal, rather than making an informed choice under the principle of autonomy. Conversely, to the patient who makes a choice based on intensely personal values, the physician's insistence that he or she "knows what is right" for the patient may be seen as

TABLE 6. Differences between surviving and dying septic patients

Differences	No Differences
Urea	pH
Lactate	Arterial P_{O_2}
Z* nonessential amino acids	Systemic BP
Alpha-aminobutyrate	Heart rate
Glucagon	Respiratory rate
Z* valine	
Z* aspartate	
Z* glutamine	
Glucose	

Adapted from Moyer (43).

Z* = fractional concentration total group of amino acids rather than absolute amount of particular listed component. Note that common components used in early predictors were of no value in these patients.

paternalistic or dictatorial. In fact, such an attitude on the part of a physician would not truly be promoting the best interests of the patient but, rather, promoting what the doctor views as the patient's best interest. The conflict is not between beneficence and autonomy but, rather, a conflict of individually assessed values. The process of informed consent should blend beneficence and autonomy. In fact, the interaction has many stages: the patient must decide to seek treatment in order to contact the medical system; the physician, then, performs an evaluation based upon information provided by the patient; when the physician arrives at a diagnosis, it is communicated to the patient; the impact of the diagnosis affects the patient and the impact is perceived by the physician; the prognosis can then be discussed, following which the patient's values should be explored; alternative forms of treatment can then be discussed; the patient can make a choice and, because of this process, the physician should be able to support the patient in this choice. Furthermore, the process of informed consent in the ICU must be considered from the standpoint of expected outcome. As the likelihood of survival diminishes, the importance of autonomy increases. In other words, if our treatment plan holds less and less chance of success as the illness progresses, then our very intention to promote the best interests of the patient with respect to cure becomes less and less possible and, therefore, we should give an increasing weight to the patient's wishes. The alignment of the objectives of medical care can now be considered to be consonant with both societal values and the patient's wishes. As our chances for cure diminish, we recognize that preservation of life is less likely and emphasize the alleviation of suffering. We focus upon the quality of life and, rightly, seek the patient as the appropriate source of this information.

We must redirect our efforts from the common technological ICU procedures to measures by which to alleviate the patient's suffering as we support the patient and await resolution based on the patient's ability to restore normal metabolic processes or, if this is impossible, to succumb. We must maintain efforts and continue our support. Once patients are admitted and as long as a reasonable, however defined, hope remains, we must remain committed to care. Cost containment is not to be concerned with stopping care after a specified time or dollar limit. However, we also have an equal imperative to avoid unnecessary manipulations which cannot influence the outcome and can only prolong dying, increase stress to patients and families, and drain already limited ICU resources. This is the proper place for an emphasis on cost containment.

Discharge from Intensive Care

One might believe that, if discharge from the ICU were delayed until all major physiologic abnormalities had been resolved, patients would continue their recuperation in a routine hospital area and be discharged. However, 20% of the total deaths in patients admitted to our ICU occurred after ICU discharge but before discharge from the hospital. Because we rarely discharge dying patients to the floor, these deaths occurred in patients discharged with the expectation of survival, yet they died during their subsequent hospitalization. The decision for discharge is not an easy one, even if the acute physiologic abnormalities prompting admission had resolved. Certain problems, such as a late dysrhythmia or pulmonary embolism, to be sure, account for some unexpected deaths. However, if a patient treated for respiratory failure suffers a respiratory arrest soon after discharge, we must examine our decision retrospectively to learn for the future. During the final days of ICU care, high technology and repeated measurements related to cardiorespiratory function, which are so important as immediate determinants of outcome, must be restrained. Our role in caring is educating the patient and family with respect to prognosis and the adjustments to lifestyle which may now be necessary. It is important to provide the necessary information in a sympathetic and understanding way so that the patient or, in the case of incompetent patients, the family, can properly exercise autonomy to choose the course most consistent with the patient's values. In this manner, when patients reach the point of consideration of discontinuation of interventions so as to shorten the dying process, consensus will already be present among the patient, family, and physicians. The burden of decision will not be placed upon distressed family members, quasi-incompetent patients, nor well meaning but, perhaps, poorly informed physicians.

Conclusion

When faced with the wide spectrum of current determinants of care, we recognize that we are back in the realm of clinical judgment, long described as part of the art of medicine. In our highly technological society and the environment in today's ICU, we hoped, perhaps, that the uncertainty of clinical judgment could have been dispelled by accumulating and analyzing a massive data base. All numerical indices have approximately a 15% misclassification rate for survival or death (24). Interestingly, this is essentially the same rate as reported for prospective analyses of clinical judgment (43, 44). Thus, quantitative instruments have not supplanted clinical judgment nor do they improve it. Clinical judgment should not be dismissed with its categorization as part of the art of medicine, but we should recognize that the expression of the art is as dependent upon education and experience as music, theater, and painting. If we wish to be artists, we must emulate the artistic method and concentrate upon learning the fundamentals of technique. The important elements at each stage of the illness were few in number and remarkably consistent among different scoring instruments. We can, therefore, learn to focus upon these elements. When the possibility of death increases, however, we must learn to restrict useless interventions and focus on caring for the patient and his family. Our time should be spent in communication, explanation, and clarification rather than ordering new drugs, tests, or procedures. Patients seek medical *care,* without necessarily expecting *cure.* Technology, including intensive care, can then be seen as a method to enhance our clinical judgment when appropriate, but we should not look to technological solutions for social and societal issues which are especially important in prolonged ICU care.

It is a common axiom that to learn about the future we must often return to a study of the past. We must re-emphasize the marvelous therapeutic quality of the physician/patient relationship, the principal tool possessed by our predecessors. We must also remember the lesson taught in the first medical text — to recognize when we should not treat. Medical "success" needs human dimensions to achieve fulfillment and be sustaining for both patient and staff. For the patients who survive, we can make the experience less fearful. We need to remember how helpless the patients must feel. A sympathetic approach will help, but we should strive to diminish their dependency when possible by giving them some control. For the dying patient, we will supply the only needs which matter and can be met, an easing of the lonely, frightening, and often painful transition to death. For society, we will preserve the scarce resources. For ourselves, as professionals, we must learn the fundamentals of the art of medicine. For ourselves, as just those members of the human race who happen to have chosen medicine as a profession, we can more confidently approach the future, secure in the knowledge that our human qualities are society's greatest medical resource. Effective decisions for clinical care, at this point in time, still depend primarily on the processor, a knowledgeable and caring physician.

References

1. Webster's Third New International Dictionary. Gove PB (Ed). Springfield, MA, G & C Merriam Co, 1976, pp 616

2. Hook D: The Edwin Smith surgical papyrus. *In:* Bulletin of the Cleveland Medical Library Association. Partington MM (Ed). Cleveland, 1973, p 22

3. Avorn J: Benefit and cost analysis in geriatric care: Turning age discrimination into health policy. *N Engl J Med* 1984; 310:1294

4. Poe EA: The Facts in the Case of M. Valemar. *In:* The Book of Poe. Hubbard A (Ed). New York, Doubleday, Doran & Co, 1934

5. Fein R: On measuring economic benefits of health programmes. *In:* Medical History and Medical Care: A Symposium of Perspectives. McLachlan G, McKeown T (Eds). London, Oxford University Press, 1971

6. *Matter of Quinlan,* 70 N.J. 10 (1976)

7. Armstrong CJ: Judicial involvement in treatment decisions: The emerging consensus: *In:* Critical Care. Civetta JM, Taylor R, Kirby RR (Eds). Philadelphia, JB Lippincott Co, In Press

8. Brown NK, Thompson DJ: Non-treatment of fever in extended-care facilities. *N Engl J Med* 1979; 300:1246

9. Fried C: Terminating life support: Out of the closet! *N Engl J Med* 1976; 295:390

10. Critical Care Medicine, Consensus Development Conference Summary, National Institutes of Health 1983; 4(6)

11. Civetta JM, Hudson-Civetta JA: Cost effective use of the ICU. *In:* Cost Effectiveness in Surgery. Eiseman B (Ed). Philadelphia, WB Saunders Co, 1987, p 13

12. Fogel R: United States General Accounting Office. Medicare: Past overuse of intensive care services inflates hospital payment. *In:* Report to the Secretary of Health and Human Services. GAO/HRD-86-25, March, 1986

13. Knaus WA: When is intensive care inappropriate? New "prognostic" measures provide answers. *Hospital Management Quarterly* 1986; 1:14

14. Henning RJ, McClish D, Daly B, et al: Clinical characteristics and resource utilization of ICU patients: Implications for organization of intensive care. *Crit Care Med* 1987; 15:264

15. Stern RS, Epstein AM: Institutional responses to prospective payment based on diagnosis related groups: Implications for cost, quality, and access. *N Engl J Med* 1985; 312:621

16. Orwell G: 1984. New York, Harcourt Brace Jovanovich, 1949

17. Civetta JM: The inverse relationship between cost and survival. *J Surg Res* 1973; 14:265

18. Teres D, Steingrub J: Can intermediate care substitute for intensive care? *Crit Care Med* 1987; 15:280

19. Civetta JM, Hudson-Civetta JA: Maintaining quality of care while reducing charges in the ICU: 10 ways. *Ann Surg* 1985; 202:524

20. Young EWD: Life and death in the intensive care unit: Ethical considerations. *In:* Critical Care. Civetta JM, Taylor R, Kirby RR (Eds). Philadelphia, JB Lippincott Co, In Press

21. McCollough LB: Informed consent: Conceptualization and application. *In:* Critical Care. Civetta JM, Taylor R, Kirby RR (Eds). Philadelphia, JB Lippincott Co, In Press

22. Civetta JM: Beyond technology: Intensive care in the 1980s. *Crit Care Med* 1981; 9:763

23. Gallagher TJ: Personal communication. 1975

24. Kirby RR, Civetta JM: Critical care outcome. *In:* Risk and Outcome in Anesthesia. Brown DL (Ed). Philadelphia, JB Lippincott Co, In Press

25. Champion HR, Sacco WJ, Hannon DS, et al: Assessment of injury severity: The triage index. *Crit Care Med* 1980; 8:201

26. Champion HR, Sacco WJ, Carnazzo AJ, et al: The trauma score. *Crit Care Med* 1981; 9:672

27. Ogawa M, Sugimoto T: Rating severity of the injured by ambulance attendants: Field research of trauma index. *J Trauma* 1974; 14:934

28. Bever DL, Veenker CH: An illness-injury severity index for non-physician emergency medical personnel. *Emergency Medical Technician Journal* 1979; 3:45

29. Gormican SP: CRAMS scale: Field triage of trauma victims. *Ann Emerg Med* 1982; 11:132

30. Buzby GP, Mullen JL, Matthews DC, et al: Prognostic nutritional index in gastrointestinal surgery. *Am J Surg* 1980; 139:160

31. Harvey KB, Moldawer LL, Bistrian BR, et al: Biological measures for the formulation of a hospital prognostic index. *Am J Clin Nutr* 1981; 34:2013

32. Christou NV: Predicting septic related mortality of the individual surgical patient based on admission host defense measurements. *Can J Surg* 1986; 29:424

33. Orlando R, Nelson LD, Civetta JM: Invasive preoperative evaluation of high-risk patients. *Crit Care Med* 1985; 13:263

34. Shibutani K, Del Guercio LRM: Preoperative hemodynamic assessment of the high-risk patient. *Seminars in Anesthesia* 1983; 1:231

35. Civetta JM, Hudson-Civetta J: Costly care: Data, problems and proposing remedies. *Crit Care Med* 1986; 14:357

36. Knaus WA, Zimmerman JE, Wagner DP, et al: APACHE—Acute physiology and chronic health evaluation: A physiologically based classification system. *Crit Care Med* 1985; 13:263

37. Knaus WA, Draper EA, Wagner DP, et al: APACHE II: A severity of disease classification system. *Crit Care Med* 1985; 13:818

38. Cullen DJ, Civetta JM, Briggs BA, et al: Therapeutic intervention scoring system: A method for quantitative comparison of patient care. *Crit Care Med* 1974; 2:57

39. Shoemaker WC, Pierchala BS, Chang P, et al: Prediction of outcome and severity of illness by analysis of the frequency distribution of cardiorespiratory variables. *Crit Care Med* 1977; 5:82

40. Lemeshow S, Teres D, Pastides H, et al: A method for predicting survival and mortality of ICU patients using objectively derived weights. *Crit Care Med* 1985; 13:519

41. Siegel JH: Cardiorespiratory manifestations of metabolic failure in sepsis and the multiple organ failure syndrome. *Surg Clin North Am* 1983; 63:379

42. Moyer E, Cerra F, Chenier R, et al: Multiple systems organ failure: VI. Death predictors in the trauma-septic state — The most critical determinants. *J Trauma* 1981; 21:862

43. Rodman GH, Etling T, Civetta JM, et al: How accurate is clinical judgment? *Crit Care Med* 1978; 6:127

44. Civetta JM, Caruthers-Banner TE: Does clinical judgment correctly allocate surgical intensive care? *Crit Care Med* 1983; 11:236